T0215305

General Practice Under the NHS

This accessible text covers the entirety of General Practice and the General Practitioner, from student to retirement and from the beginning of the NHS to the present day. It provides a comprehensive historical overview representing both academic and front-line perspectives, describing what has changed, beneficial or otherwise, as the specialty has evolved. The details within each chapter represent the views of the average working British GP and illustrate how the changes over the decades have impacted patient care and its delivery. The perspective often differs from that which prevails in many academic tomes on the subject.

The topics covered, from the primary care team, changes to out-of-hours provision, the impact of IT, training, and regulation, to the future of General Practice, will be essential reading for all doctors considering a career in the specialty and will also be of interest to GP vocational training scheme course organisers and trainers, overseas medical educators and healthcare policy makers, social and medical historians, and the general public.

General Practice Under the NHS

Past, Present and Future

James Sherifi

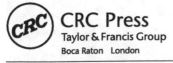

CRC Press
Taylor & Francis Group
Boca Raton   London

CRC Press is an imprint of the
Taylor & Francis Group, an **informa** business

First edition published 2023
by CRC Press
6000 Broken Sound Parkway NW, Suite 300, Boca Raton, FL 33487–2742

and by CRC Press
4 Park Square, Milton Park, Abingdon, Oxon, OX14 4RN

CRC Press is an imprint of Taylor & Francis Group, LLC

© 2023 James Sherifi

ISBN: 978-1-032-18831-7 (hbk)
ISBN: 978-1-032-18829-4 (pbk)
ISBN: 978-1-003-25646-5 (ebk)

DOI: 10.1201/9781003256465

Typeset in Minion
by Apex CoVantage, LLC

Contents

Preface

The history of the NHS has been sorely neglected in published literature and that is particularly so for the key part played by General Practice in ensuring that the founding principles, universality, free at the point of delivery, based on clinical need, were enacted and sustained.

Whilst there have been a number of texts that have dealt with various aspects of primary care, none have included a comprehensive history and current guide to the work of a GP, under one cover. This book seeks to address that omission.

It is written from and represents the perspective of the average front-line GP, and covers every aspect of a GP's life, from medical school to retirement. For the sake of brevity, the book is liberally referenced and focuses on England as the largest of the four nations.

This book is both a tribute to and a guide for the generations of doctors who have conscientiously, selflessly and professionally worked, under-resourced and in often trying circumstances, to successfully deliver on the NHS promise of universal, free healthcare. GPs were and are the foundation on which that promise has been sustained for over seven decades.

I am privileged to have led a life with no regrets. Most of that life has been spent doing a job that was emotionally challenging, intellectually stimulating, varied, all-consuming, fun and rewarding. Most of all, I was allowed to be a part of my patients' lives and to listen to their wonderful stories. Quite honestly, what could be better than that?

Jim Sherifi

About the Author

James Sherifi, the author, having succumbed to polio as an infant, subsequently developed a lifelong vocation to be a doctor, a dream realised when he graduated from Dundee University Medical School in 1975. He spent the following five years rotating through various hospital posts before finally settling down to a career as a GP principal in a practice in Colchester UK. Over the following 20 years, he added roles as GP vocational training scheme course organiser, GP with special interest in neurology, occupational health physician and occasional contributor of opinion pieces to GP journals.

The advent of a new millennium led him to seek new challenges. He left general practice and became a consultant at an international executive search agency specialising in the pharmaceutical and healthcare industry. However, his heart remained in clinical medicine and after four years he returned once more to the front line as a salaried GP in a semi-rural practice in Suffolk. The following 13 years saw him add to his portfolio of experiences in roles including GP appraiser, medical undergraduate tutor and examiner, CQC inspector, medical member of benefits tribunal for HM Courts and Tribunals and contributor of opinion pieces and learning modules to a variety of journals.

His enduring love of the subject impelled him to write this book.

Abbreviations

AKT	Applied Knowledge Test
BMA	British Medical Association
BMJ	*British Medical Journal*
BNF	British National Formulary
BPA	Basic Practice Allowance
CCPME	Committee on Postgraduate Medical Education or Central Council for Postgraduate Medical Education
CCT	Certificate of Completion of Training and Certificate of Competence of Training
CFA	Counter Fraud Agency
CFH	Connecting for Health
CHI	Commission for Healthcare Improvement
CHP	Community Health Partnerships
CPD	Continuing Professional Development
CPME	Council for Postgraduate Medical Education
CQC	Care Quality Commission
CSA	Clinical Skills Assessment
DES	Directed Enhanced Services
DH	Department of Health
DHSC	Department of Health and Social Care
ES	Enhanced Services
GMS	General Medical Services
GPF	GP Federation
GPC	General Practitioners Committee of the BMA
GPFC	General Practice Finance Corporation
GPSoC	GP Systems of Choice
GPVTS	GP Vocational Training Scheme
GS	Global Sum
HA	Health Authority
HEE	Health Education England
HMRC	Her Majesty's Revenue and Customs
IT	Information Technology

JCPTGP	Joint Committee for Postgraduate Training in General Practice
LHCRE	Local Health and Care Record Exemplars
LEC	Local Executive Council
LES	Local Enhanced Services
LETB	Local Education and Training Boards
LIFT	Local Improvement Finance Trust
LMC	Local Medical Committee
MAAG	Medical Audit Advisory Group
MADEL	Medical and Dental Education Levy
MHRA	Medicines and Healthcare Products Regulatory Agency
MIMS	Monthly Index of Medical Specialties
MMC	Modernising Medical Careers
MPIG	Minimum Practice Income Guarantee
MRCGP	Membership of the Royal College of General Practitioners (exam and membership)
MRCP	Membership of the Royal College of Physicians (exam and membership)
NASGP	National Association of Sessional GP
NES	National Enhanced Services
NPfIT	National Programme for Information Technology
NHSBSA	NHS Business Services Authority
NHSPS	NHS Prescription Services
NHSPS	NHS Pension Scheme
OOH	Out-of-Hours
PCN	Primary Care Network
PGMEC	Postgraduate Medical Education Committee
PMETB	Postgraduate Medical Education and Training Board
PMS	Personal Medical Services
PPG	Patient Participation Group
PPP	Public-Private Partnership
PUNs/DENs	Patient's Unmet Needs/Doctor's Educational Needs
QALY	Quality Adjusted Life Years
QOF	Quality and Outcomes Framework
RCOG	Royal College of Obstetricians and Gynaecologists
RCS	Royal College of Surgeons
SCoPME	Standing Committee on Postgraduate Medical Education
SCR	Summary Care Record
SFA	Statement of Fees and Allowances, Red Book
SFE	Statement of Financial Entitlements
SIFT	Service Increment for Teaching

1

Patients and Their Doctors

Self-employed with 2000 bosses

1.1 INTRODUCTION

If people did not become ill, there would be no need for doctors. Everyone becomes ill, and interacts with a doctor, at some time in their life. The dictionary definition of the noun 'patient' is 'a person receiving medical treatment.' Persons seeking medical treatment are not clients, customers, or service users. They do not choose to be ill.

The prime purpose of a general practitioner is to help people; to effect a beneficial outcome for those with healthcare needs, vulnerable people, 'patients.' The place in which they do this, and most patient-doctor interactions take place, is the consulting room. The consultation lies at the heart of the relationship between the patient and his or her doctor. This chapter will initially look at how the British population adapted to the changes in primary care over the past 70 years, before exploring the doctor-patient relationship and intricacies of the consultation in greater depth.

1.2 1948

The NHS was set up in 1948 with the altruistic aim of providing universal and free (at least at the point of delivery) access to healthcare for every man, woman, and child in the UK, from cradle to grave.

The founding core principles of the NHS were that it should:

- Meet the needs of everyone
- Be free at the point of delivery
- Be based on clinical need, not the ability to pay

As a historic declaration, this was on a par with the Magna Carta. The NHS was created to slay one of the five giants (Want, Disease, Ignorance, Squalor, and Idleness) set out in the farsighted Beveridge Report[1] of 1942. A utopian vision of

---

[1] Social Insurance and Allied Services. Report by Sir William Beveridge. HMSO. 1942
Pombo.free.fr/beveridge42.pdf

DOI: 10.1201/9781003256465-1

a society healthy in body and mind beckoned. The citizens of the UK were truly blessed.

With ease of access, patients' medical needs would be promptly addressed, thus reducing the burden of disease on society. The GP would facilitate that access, an individual with the medical knowledge, skills and experience to eliminate all illness; or, if not, then to act as the gateway to a professional who could. Sadly, all collaborators in this seductive hypothesis would soon be disillusioned.

Patients flocked to see their GP as soon as the ink dried on the enabling act for the NHS. Initially, they came with serious complaints that they had neglected, due to the financial constraints of the pre-existing, fee-driven medical system. Dickensian scenes of an undernourished infant, coughing pitifully on a threadbare sheet in some dark and dank garret whilst fretful mothers bathed their feverish brows and prayed to the Almighty to spare their dearest, were still common in the mid-20th century. The creation of the NHS put an end to such misery. However, once that tsunami of medical neglect had abated, patients began arriving in increasing numbers with minor self-limiting conditions that they had previously allowed to run their natural course. Those numbers continued to grow, with familiarity leading to patients developing an intimate, albeit professional, relationship with 'their' family doctor. They were beholden to the NHS for providing them with this bounty and to their GP for embodying the NHS. This relationship between patient and doctor prevailed thereafter and persists to this day, the seventh decade of this social experiment.

1.3 1948–1966

Between 1948 and 1966, most patients attended single-handed or small practices. Theoretically, they could see the same familiar face any time of the day or week. In practice, that was not always so. Patients were placed on a doctor's list that could number into the thousands. Doctors ran open-ended surgeries without appointments. Premises were old and cramped; queues, usually outside regardless of inclement weather, were common. This was particularly so in inner-city practices, but conditions in rural practices were hardly better. A general practice was overwhelmed from the outset, and there is no reason to believe that in those days, receptionists, often the doctor's spouse, were any less protective of their charges than they are now.

The image of the fatherly physician undertaking a consultation over a cup of tea, commonplace in the literature of that era, was never likely to have existed in the real world. GPs were always struggling with time, and a short and brusque consultation would have been the rule rather than the exception. Many practitioners had graduated through the army following the World War II. The majority came from a higher socioeconomic group or 'class' than their patients, inclined to view patients in a paternalistic manner at best and, at worst, a dismissive one. Yet, seemingly with no regard for such imperfections, patients remained forgiving of their doctor and continued to attend the practice in large numbers.

Between 1939 and 1957, particularly following the 1944 Goodenough Committee's report[2] on medical training, medical school output expanded to meet the projected demand for healthcare. However, by 1955, those in authority felt that the output of doctors would soon outstrip demand, resulting in a further review, the Willink Report,[3] recommending the reduction of student numbers by 10%, with that figure to be maintained until a further review 20 years later! Willink was the first, but certainly not last to underestimate the numbers required to meet the population's infinite demand for healthcare. Seventy years on, the number of UK medical graduates remained half of those needed.

1.3.1 Commonwealth Doctors

The shortfall in home-grown doctors was met by recruiting overseas. The Willink Report was so short-sighted that three years after its publication, 40% of all junior doctors in the NHS were recruits from the Indian subcontinent.

In 1961, Lord Cohen of Birkenhead told the House of Lords:

> The Health Service would have collapsed if it had not been for the enormous influx of junior doctors from such countries as India and Pakistan[4].

The logical source for the recruitment of doctors from overseas lay in the old British Empire, especially the Indian subcontinent.[5] As a serendipitous result of colonial rule, medical training and administration in India, Pakistan, and Sri Lanka followed the same structure and curriculum as the UK and met the General Medical Council (GMC) standards. Doctors from those countries were encouraged to come to the UK, to gain further training and experience that would benefit the healthcare system of their country of origin. On arrival in the UK, many received encouragement to stay. Meanwhile, UK-trained doctors emigrated in large numbers to the United States and Canada, driven by the comparatively poor NHS pay and working conditions. By the late 1960s, 400 doctors were emigrating each year, the equivalent of three medical schools' annual output.

In 1963, the Conservative Health Minister, Enoch Powell (1912–1998), who, ironically, would later call for stricter controls on immigration, launched a campaign to recruit trained doctors from overseas to fill the manpower shortages endemic to the NHS. Some 18,000 were recruited from the Indian subcontinent, with Powell stating on record that they

---

[2] Goodenouigh W. The Training of Doctors. https://www.ncbi.nlm.nih.gov/pmc/articles/PMC2285893/pdf/brmedj03895-0021.pdf

[3] Committee to consider the future numbers of medical practitioners and the appropriate intake of medical students. Report. London: HMSO, 1957. (Willink Report.)

[4] https://api.parliament.uk/historic-hansard/lords/1961/nov/29/the-shortage-of-doctors

[5] Esmail A. Asian doctors in the NHS: service and betrayal. Br J Gen Pract. 2007 Oct;57(543):827–34. PMID: 17925142; PMCID: PMC2151817.

provide a useful and substantial reinforcement of the staffing of our hospitals and who are an advertisement to the world of British medicine and British hospitals.[6]

In 1968, the Todd Committee's[7] predictions of further medical manpower shortages promoted additional overseas recruitment of doctors, before finally recommending the expansion of undergraduate numbers to meet the shortfall.

The outcome of the rollercoaster of conflicting reports on medical manpower was that by 1971, a third of all doctors had qualified overseas, with most filling vacancies in locations and specialties that were unpopular with UK-trained doctors. The proportion increased: in 1997, 44% of the 7,229 newly registered doctors had received their primary medical education overseas.

The prescient creators of the NHS had recognised that British doctors, the majority of whom came from middle-class backgrounds, would be reluctant to work in the socially and economically deprived regions that needed them most. The Medical Practices Committee (MPC)[8] (1948–2001) was created to ensure an equal distribution of doctors across the country. The committee had the power to classify areas as 'over-doctored,' restricting an influx of any additional practitioners, or 'designated,' allowing freedom of movement. Nevertheless, designated areas remained profoundly 'under-doctored.' Its impact was variable.

Overseas doctors continued to take up general practice positions in the most deprived regions of the UK. They were brave to do so. They went to inner cities where the population had limited experience with those from outside their own communities, let alone abroad. Local dialects and customs were difficult to understand. Attitudes of the time differed from those of today, and thinking that doctors from India, Pakistan, or Sri Lanka were immediately welcomed and instantly integrated into the community would be naïve. Britain in the 1950s was a country of casual racism. Infamously, signs in boarding-house windows declaring 'No blacks. No dogs. No Irish' were commonplace. An exclusively white population was suspicious at best and, at worst, horrified at having to see a foreign doctor. Yet, despite the initial antipathy, and to their credit, the community gradually assimilated these doctors, aided by their respective needs to live and to make a living. Overseas doctors became stalwart members of communities where they worked and, decades later, retired. One of the earliest victims of the COVID pandemic in 2020 was a GP of Pakistani origin, who had run a single-handed practice in a deprived coastal town of Essex for over 40 years. At his death, he was still practising at the age of 84. Despite the lockdown, his patients lined the

6 https://api.parliament.uk/historic-hansard/commons/1963/may/08/national-health-service

7 Report of the Royal Commission on Medical Education 1968 (Todd Report) The National Archives Ref: UGC7/1135. https://discovery.nationalarchives.gov.uk/details/r/C179709

8 Whowell WB. Medical practices committee. Br Med J (Clin Res Ed). 1981 Nov 28;283(6304):1485–6. doi: 10.1136/bmj.283.6304.1485. PMID: 6797586; PMCID: PMC1507654.

streets in tribute as the hearse carrying his coffin made its slow journey to the cemetery. Although tragic, the story serves as an example of the strong bond that existed between patients and their caring, devoted, and conscientious family doctor, testimony to the invaluable service the overseas doctors provided to the NHS.

1.3.2 Patients' Expectations

1.3.2.1 1948–1965

At the NHS's outset, the publicity guided patients' expectations towards being able to see a doctor at a time and place of their choosing. However, as much as the lack of doctors stymied those expectations, so did infrastructure. Few homes had access to telephones. Patients could only contact their GPs in person or through family or friends. Naturally, telephone consultations did not exist. Other parts of the NHS, secondary care or Accident & Emergency (A&E) were only accessible in an absolute emergency or with a GP referral.

As a child of ten, I broke my tibia playing football in our back garden. No one considered calling an ambulance. The family doctor was summoned by phone, arrived immediately, gave me a painkilling injection, carried me to his car, and drove me to the hospital. Fifty years later, I happened on an accident at our local supermarket where an employee had crushed his fingernail in a door. I offered to examine him, but the manager declined my offer since an ambulance was already on its way. The intervening years had moved the spectrum of concern from stoic to risk-averse. Changing times!

The elderly, immobile, and chronically ill all expected regular and frequent doctors' visits. GPs had rounds, much as milkmen did, delivering medicines and providing social support for the patient and family. Anecdotal tales spoke of householders requesting a visit by tying a coloured ribbon to their front gate or getting a neighbour to post a note in the GP's letterbox. Patients expected to be seen in their own home, and doctors expected to be called out.

Patients trusted their doctor and never doubted that he would always act in their best interests. Patients were also sympathetic to their GP's heavy workload and long hours. They tried not to 'bother' the doctor. They were grateful for the service offered and expressed their thanks at Christmas, when a GP might expect a card and a gift, a box of chocolates or a bottle of spirits. Others undertook a barter system reminiscent of pre-NHS days: a free car service from a garage owner admitted in a timely manner for appendicitis, or a joint of meat from the butcher for minor surgery on an ingrown toenail. Patients may have had high expectations of their local practice, but they never took their GP for granted. Sadly, in the course of time, the novelty of the NHS began to wear off as did the sentiment in that last sentence.

Doctors were embedded in their locality. Partners were expected to be always available to their patients, and any emergency demanded that they should be on-site quickly, before rigor mortis set in. The doctor, a patrician figure akin to a judge or senior civil servant, would be asked to open the village fete. The doctor's wife was seen shopping. Their children attended the local school.

The doctor's household was viewed as a kind of common enterprise in which everyone took an interest. People gossiped, apportioning comments (good or bad) based on the latest interaction they had had at the surgery. Yet, no matter how grim the doctor's reputation, they always flocked to the surgery on a Monday morning.

Patients interacted professionally with their GP in the setting of the surgery. They attended when they felt ill, saw the doctor, received a prescription, and felt better. The model's simplicity allowed for few mishaps and misunderstandings. Consultations were limited to five minutes, considered adequate for most presenting problems. Time was saved by keeping the clinical notes to a bare minimum with scribbled abbreviations or acronyms. The benefits of the process were accessibility and familiarity. The drawbacks were long waits; inhospitable, cold, damp, dark waiting rooms; lack of female doctors; rushed consultations; unhelpful receptionists. The system generally worked well, provided the medical presentation was simple and straightforward. However, it quickly unraveled if the consultation highlighted a more complex matter requiring investigation or referral to a specialist.

As they do today, the hospital pathology department did blood and urine tests, but those departments also had to take the samples since GP surgeries had no phlebotomy services. GP access to radiological investigations was the stuff of dreams. Hospital outpatient waiting times often ran to years.

This less-than-idyllic situation began to change following the 1966 GP Charter that arose in response to the dire conditions and poor facilities and pay under which GPs had laboured for the previous two decades. The posited solution was to bring GPs together under one roof, group practice. Patients could continue to see 'their' doctor, but they could now also choose, or more likely be directed, to see another, particularly on nights or weekends. Nevertheless, a conservative population tended to remain loyal to one individual, regardless of any misgivings they might have had regarding his or her performance.

Patients welcomed and were impressed by the modern, professional medical centres that began to spring up following the move to group practice. The dingy garrets of the past were reminders of post-war austerity. The new buildings heralded better times. Expectations began to rise of what they could expect from a healthcare service.

1.3.2.2 1966–1999

Little research exists on patients' expectations of the NHS, but in its first half-century, the citizens of the UK were generally blissfully ignorant of medical matters and happy to rely on the judgement of their GP or hospital doctor for any medical opinion. They attended the surgery with symptoms and expected them to be alleviated in short shrift. The increasing complexity of patient presentations, effective medical interventions, and demands on the service forced many GPs to extend their consulting times by 50%. By the late 1970s, the seven-minute appointment was accepted as the minimum time required to deal with a patient's problems, and surgery hours were increased to maintain the same number of daily appointments. Whether patients noted or felt the benefits of these changes was hard to gauge since they were never asked!

In the 1980s, a wait of two years or longer for a hip-joint replacement was the norm. Patients recognised that these areas were out of their GP's control. Health budgets were set by the central government and administered by faceless bureaucrats at the Family Health Service Authority (FHSA). GPs had little influence in bringing forward hospital appointments, allowing both doctor and patient to indulge in that most British of pastimes, 'blame the manager.'

The 1990 GP contract introduced changes that had an immediate but subtle impact on the way patients perceived their doctor. At the heart of these changes was a shift towards a preventive model of healthcare delivery, allied with improved productivity attracting payments for results. Of course, as always, the hope remained that these innovations would ultimately lead to budgetary savings. Patients began to notice that a consultation for a minor acute condition now included an interrogation on seemingly unconnected matters, such as smoking, weight, and exercise. A typical lament of the time was 'I only went in with a sore throat but all he was interested in was when I had last had a smear test' Questioning why that was so, patients drew the conclusion, unfairly, that their doctor now viewed them as a human cash dispenser. They were also nonplussed by the introduction of chronic disease management clinics, run by nurses, but only at certain times of the week. Before, they had been used to seeing their doctor at a time of their choosing for their asthma or diabetes. That flexibility was removed and replaced by a nurse who could seemingly do a doctor's job, eroding the dependency on the doctor as the sole repository of medical knowledge.

Despite the introduction of prescription charges at its inception, the 'free at the point of delivery' NHS had initially engendered a subliminal sentiment in the population that GPs were an altruistic body of men who put charity above income. The move towards a more cost-effective service caused them to reassess that view. The national press now publicised every change in the NHS, and its readership closely scrutinised and invariably willfully misinterpreted what they read. Thus, a harmless policy, such as the introduction of the 'blacklist' of useless medications that would no longer be provided on prescription, would be interpreted as a money-saving measure to substitute ersatz, cheap, less effective ones for truly effective medications. Patients felt they were being short-changed, and that the doctor as the messenger was complicit in this fraud. An increasing minority held these views, but the vast majority of the population remained both loyal to and forgiving of their doctor.

The schism in general practice that became Personal Medical Services (PMS) and General Medical Services (GMS) practices in 1997 also dented one of the founding principles of the NHS, the 'universality of healthcare' provision. Patients in PMS practices discovered that their wait for an orthopaedic procedure was much shorter than their neighbour's in a GMS practice. The latter began asking their surgery why this was so. Some changed practice when alleviation of chronic pain trumped loyalty.

1.3.2.3 2000–DATE

The computer had become a ubiquitous feature on the doctor's desk by the mid-1990s. Google became the Internet search engine of choice in 2000. Arguably, both led to a step change in the relationship between patient and doctor.

Whilst computerisation provided undoubted benefits to clinical management, patients resented competing with a computer monitor for their doctor's attention, especially when the monitor seemed both more seductive and demanding than they were. Talking to a doctor gazing fixedly at a TV screen led patients to think that the doctor's focus was not entirely on the conversation. They were probably right to think so. The old lament of 'my GP began writing a prescription as soon as I sat down' gave way to 'my GP never stopped looking at that bl***y screen the whole time I was in there.'

Whilst some elements of the patient experience may have seemed worse, others were improving. The profession was becoming more diverse. The number of women entering general practice had dramatically increased. Doctors' list sizes were falling, premises were improving, and ancillary staff, including nurses and phlebotomists, were providing convenient services that were previously only available at the hospital. Repeat prescriptions were issued faster and less prone to errors. The NHS annual influenza vaccination programme for the elderly and medically compromised, introduced in 2000, dramatically reduced anxiety, morbidity, and mortality in those groups.

Collaborations between practices covered out-of-hours (OOH) care, which cooperatives or deputising services would soon replace, and a local GP could still see a patient at home if deemed medically necessary. Hospital services were also improving, benefitting from the sharp increase in funding that the Labour government provided at the turn of the millennium. Altogether, the service they were receiving increasingly satisfied patients, a situation reflected by the low level of complaints the GMC received against medical practitioners.

However, the improvement in the population's healthcare was only possible because of the vast injection of money into the NHS during this period. Stubbornly, the increased investment in the NHS had not resulted in an equivalent increase in productivity, and the money was about to run out.

The new GMS contract of 2004 led to further erosion of the way patients had viewed their doctors. The tabloid press universally demonised GPs as (to paraphrase) 'avaricious lazy gold-diggers.' Replacing the GP 'out-of-hours' provision in a panic with a woefully inadequate service funded by Primary Care Trusts (PCT), an apparently shorter working week, and a widely publicised big increase in GP income, thanks to the Quality Outcomes Framework (QOF), all gave the impression that general practice had become a morally bankrupt and self-enriching profession that had lost touch with its vocational roots.

Although the introduction of the QOF had the altruistic aim of improving clinical care and best practice across the UK, the fact that a sizeable chunk of a GP's remuneration was based on achieving as many points as possible led to an unexpected skewing of the consultation's emphasis. A third party, the computer, was constantly interrupting the interaction between patient and doctor. Whilst average consultation times had increased to ten minutes, less time went to the patient's complaint and more to inputting data. Other provisions within the contract, such as enhanced pensions, made early retirement both realistic and attractive, further diminishing the number of GP principals in practice and replacing them with salaried doctors with less stake in improving the overall performance of the practice. Although early retirement on a full pension remained an option, many more GP principals chose to stay on well into their 60s and even 70s, out of support for their colleagues, loyalty to their patients, and simply a reluctance to let go. Yet, fewer doctors were seeing more patients, and their stress levels were rising. Average list sizes, having dropped to 1,700 patients per doctor in 2004, rose to 2,000 a decade later. Access to primary care services became progressively more restricted despite directives from the Department of Health (DH), demanding that all urgent requests be seen within 24 hours. Frustrated patients began complaining, engendering an increased fear of litigation, parried by overly detailed, verbose records, in the hope of keeping the 'no win, no fee' lawyers at bay. By and large, personal lists had disappeared, leaving patients to complain that they could no longer see 'their' doctor. The bond between patients and their family doctor had been broken.

The variety of healthcare professionals available to patients had become far more complicated than the simple offer of 'a GP' in previous decades. By 2012, female doctors had achieved parity in number with their male counterparts, although many worked part-time. The GP workforce was diversifying with a significant number of medical students coming from first- and second-generation Asian and Afro-Caribbean backgrounds, as well as from the European Union. Patients, especially the elderly, whom one might have expected to complain, gratefully accepted GPs with differing dialects and cultures, so long as they could at least be seen when they wanted to be.

The patient's lament in the queue at the supermarket checkout became 'you can never get through on the phone to make an appointment, and when you do, they haven't got any.'

The Labour Party entered government in 1997 recognising the need to expand services. They responded by augmenting NHS GP provisions by allowing commercial enterprises to tender mainly non-core NHS services, under Alternative Provider Medical Service (APMS) contracts.

Prior to APMS, doctors had always had the choice of opting-out of the NHS and working in private practice, but few tended to do so because of the capital outlay, uncertain income, and ethical concerns. Some doctors worked independently, usually in affluent areas, but most found working for a commercial provider on a fixed income, with some adding the incentive of a share of the profits, attractive. Such clinics invariably opened in cities, near offices or transport hubs. They generally catered to a professional clientele who wished to be seen at a time of their choosing without impacting on their work. Consultation times were longer and took place in a well-appointed setting with a tranquil ambience. Patients became clients, willing to pay for the convenience, with the patina of a superficially more qualified doctor in a bespoke suit. Nevertheless, clients remained registered with the GP surgery near their place of residence and, thus, were free to continue seeing their local GP. This was especially so for out-of-hours requests since few private providers offered such a service.

APMS contracts increased in the decade following 2010. Some, such as Virgin Care, provided NHS primary care in areas that were significantly under-doctored. Others, such as the NHS supported Babylon GP in Hand, allowed patients living outside their geographic area to register. Babylon's unique selling point was based on remote consultations via smartphones. Their target customers were the technology savvy young who were less likely to have a serious condition and were less wedded to the traditional family-doctor paradigm.

NHS doctors were ambivalent in their views of such services. Some decried the eroding of Bevan's 'free at the point of care' vision and had a visceral antipathy to the enabling of the wealthy privileged to bypass the lengthy waiting lists that the rest of the populace endured. Other, pragmatic doctors, welcomed anything that might take the pressure off their perpetually full surgeries. Patients who could afford private healthcare were a boon to any GP practice and could be easily referred on!

Regardless of where they were seen, the relationship between patient and doctor had to be built on trust in knowing that the doctor will always act in the patient's best interests. The dynamics of that relationship have varied over time. In 1948, that trust was absolute, in more recent times, less so. That loss of trust and faith has occurred for several reasons, not all of them exclusive to the medical profession.

1.3.3 Public Opinion

Have public opinion and the individual's view of the medical profession changed over time? Anecdotally, the answer would be 'yes, and for the worse.' Healthcare professionals would claim that the previous covenant of mutual respect between user and provider has diminished to non-existence. With one voice, they would claim that the public is more demanding, more impatient, more abusive. Patients would bemoan the insurmountable barriers to accessing healthcare and the fragmented nature of receiving it. The elderly hark back to a utopian era of the GP as a family friend; the young see a public servant who should be available at a time and place of their choosing.

Several surveys sought to gauge public opinion and act as proxies for how patients view their doctor. The respected Ipsos MORI Veracity Index,[9] which has surveyed the British public annually since 1983, on its trust in key professions, has consistently placed doctors and nurses at the top of the list, politicians and journalists at the bottom.

The Care Quality Commission uses feedback, crude methods, such as the NHS Friends and Family Test, and web-based sites such as NHS Choices, but the samples are small and meaningless.

---

[9] www.ipsos.com/ipsos-mori/en-uk/ipsos-mori-veracity-index-2020-trust-in-professions

A proxy for public opinion on the profession might be the level of complaints filed. Official collection and analysis of written complaints have only been in place since 2004, when the Health and Social Care Information Centre (secondary care services) and Family Health Services (primary care) began collecting the information. NHS Digital publishes their report annually, with a detailed breakdown of the figures.[10] Complaints against GP practices rose by 77% between 2004–2016 but levelled off thereafter.

The number of written complaints against GPs remains encouragingly small when counted against the millions (307 million in 2018) of doctor-patient interactions. However, there is no room for complacency since the statistics are skewed by the entirely voluntary submission of data by CCGs and hospital trusts. A breakdown of the data suggests that the proportion of complaints relating to clinical areas, communication, and attitude had increased annually, accounting for over 50% of those made against doctors by 2017.

The GMC also collates data on complaints, euphemistically termed 'enquiries.' Total enquiries regarding a doctor's fitness to practice decreased from 9,624 to 8,573 and from members of the public from 6,572 to 5,677 between 2014–2018,[11] suggesting a stabilisation of the figures in light of the data from CCGs and hospitals.

Thus, for 2018 and excluding duplication, the public notified the GMC of less than 2% of registered doctors.

Of the 8,573 enquiries made in 2018, 6,258 were closed almost immediately, primarily for being outside the GMC's remit for investigation. Those deemed after initial triage to require further investigation by a case examiner numbered 1,208. Of these, 280 were referred to a tribunal, with 228 given advice or a warning. Ultimately, the GMC suspended 48 doctors from the Register, a total number representing less than 0.1% of all registered doctors. The figure led the GMC to state,

> the rise in complaints in recent years does not necessarily indicate increasing concerns about doctors' practice and, relative to the number of interactions between doctors and patients, the number of complaints is still very small.[12]

The GMC also noted some interesting demographic variations in the public enquiries. Doctors' age, sex, and country of medical qualification affected the number of complaints. Complainants were more often female patients aged 40 to 60 years. Patients tended to be more forgiving of doctors whom they had known for a long time, and the converse was also true. Doctors experienced more complaints earlier in their careers than later. The patient-doctor relationship was like

[10] https://digital.nhs.uk/data-and-information/publications/statistical/data-on-written-complaints-in-the-nhs/2020-21-quarter-3-and-quarter-4

[11] GMC fitness to practice statistics. 2018. www.gmc-uk.org/-/media/documents/fitness-to-practise-statistics-report-2018_pdf-80514861.pdf

[12] www.gmc-uk.org/-/media/documents/SOMEP_ES_web.pdf_53684201.pdf

any other, needing time to develop. Given that time, as in any marriage, both parties tended to mellow and become more tolerant and forgiving!

Both the data and their interpretation were often used by the press to drive articles that sold papers. The old newspaper maxim 'when a dog bites a man that is not a story, but when a man bites a dog, that's news' still prevailed.

Thus, correlating all the known data regarding GMC complaints one could extrapolate in a totally unscientific manner that the average complaint was levelled against elderly male GPs who had qualified overseas by middle-aged women regarding a clinical matter or, as a popular British tabloid with a fondness for alliteration might put it, male, foreign, family physician found fondling female's funbags.

Looking at the figures, there does seem to be a disconnect between genuine public opinion and the perceptions of the medical profession regarding the relationship between patient and doctor. This may be due to a simple facet of human nature, namely, that tragedy lingers in the mind longer than joy.

Realistically, doctors should attempt to maintain a sanguine, less morose view of the regard in which their patients hold them. That might be difficult to do when both the GMC and the legal profession estimate that a GP would be lucky to go through a 30-year career without being investigated at least twice by his or her own professional body.

Patients could also complain through the Patient Advice and Liaison Service (PALS).

PALS was announced in the NHS plan of 2000 and rolled out nationwide in 2002. It had an office in every primary care organisation and provided a ready resource and advice to anyone uncomfortable with the care that they may had from their local surgery or hospital trust. PALS[13] set out to:

- Be identifiable and accessible to patients, their carers, friends, and families
- Provide on the spot help, with the power to negotiate immediate solutions or speedy resolution of problems
- Act as a gateway to appropriate independent advice and advocacy support
- Provide accurate information to patients, carers, and families, about services and other health-related issues
- Act as a catalyst for change and improvement by providing information and feedback on problems arising and service gaps
- Operate within a local network with other PALS groups in their area and work across organisational boundaries
- Support NHS staff at all levels to develop a responsive culture

For 2017–2018, PALS received 94,637 written complaints regarding general practice. Of these, 17.7% related to clinical treatment, 14.8% to communication, and 11.3% to staff attitude/behaviour/values. The figures were slightly better than those for hospital and community health services, encouraging for primary care

---

13 www.nhs.uk/nhs-services/hospitals/what-is-pals-patient-advice-and-liaison-service/

where over 80% of doctor-patient interactions took place. From 1 November 2017 to 31 October 2018, there were 307 million such interactions.[14] Of these, 0.03% resulted in a written complaint to PALS.

The culture of complaints within medicine mimics that of society at large. In the austerity years following World War II, the population of the UK accepted the limited availability of goods and services. Expectations, apart from those related to queuing, were low. Yet, by and large, society muddled through, helped by a sense of unity in universal hardship. In the latter part of the 20th century, GPs continued to benefit from this residual post-war sentiment, as well as the high regard in which society held them. Complaints were either haughtily dismissed by an endemic hauteur within the profession or, more likely, managed sensitively and personally by the accused.

The formalisation of the complaint procedure in the GP contract of 2004[15] led to a cumbersome approach, with the practice manager in the lead. The legalistic, impersonal handling of the complaint, the early involvement of the medical defence union, and the introduction of an NHS Resolution team only seemed to further antagonise the litigant. Ultimately, what might have remained no more than a minor altercation ended up escalating into a GMC investigation with resulting anxiety, ill health, and extended sick leave for the medical practitioner. To avoid this fallout, doctors were encouraged to practise defensive medicine, their copious, time-consuming medical notes akin to the small print at the bottom of any insurance document. Patients may have felt better served when doctors focused less on protecting themselves and more on effectively managing health problems, although the two were not mutually exclusive.

The public's disinclination to complain may be further supported by the numbers who use NHS Choices,[16] a website set up in 2007 as a public portal for obtaining information on GP practices. Following continuing refinements since 2010, it included a facility for posting anonymous reviews of GP practices. The facility was rarely used by patients.

The population of the UK had infinitely greater access to medical information and misinformation in the 21st century than in the 20th. Typing 'headache' into an Internet search engine produces 251 million hits within 0.62 seconds. Patients can now look up their symptoms on the web and arrive at many life-shortening diagnoses. As with hypochondriacal first-year medical students, the ones that stick in the mind are those that have the most frightening outcomes. Hence, to the public at large, every headache is a brain tumour. The public no longer views the GP as the sole source of medical information, and thus, dependence on the GP is

[14] NHS digital appointments in general practice. Oct 2018. https://digital.nhs.uk/data-and-information/publications/statistical/appointments-in-general-practice/oct-2018

[15] NHS Choices. Feedback and complaints about the NHS in England. 2016. Accessed 13 Feb 2018 from www.nhs.uk/choiceintheNHS/Rightsandpledges/complaints/Pages/AboutNHScomplaints.aspx

[16] NHS Choices. Home page. Accessed 13 Feb 2018 from www.nhs.uk/pages/home.aspx

lessened. Media, traditional and electronic, needs feeding and grazes voraciously in medical pastures. Medical research, once exclusively published in specialist journals where it could be peer-reviewed and analysed, is increasingly found on the front page of a red-top tabloid. In any week, a paper could report that coffee caused cancer, coffee protected from cancer, and coffee had no effect whatsoever on cancer! Nowadays, the Internet performs the same function. Such stories create anxiety and confusion amongst patients and result in increased attendance at GP surgeries. They were and are irresponsible and potentially dangerous. COVID vaccine refusal based on stories on social media is only the latest example of looking to the media for medical information. The authors of such misinformation are never held to account; the health service is left to deal with the fallout.

Empowered by the information gained from varied, multiple sources, patients have become more inclined to question their doctor's decisions. Although understandable and welcome, this has led to a change in the dynamics of the relationship within the consultation, from that of parent-child to equal partners or, at the very least, teacher-student. Patients no longer wish to be patronised. In turn, doctors are happy to share information and decisions. To some degree, they had been doing so since the introduction of the NHS, through the desire to 'educate' the patient to be self-sufficient in managing minor illnesses. The reinforcement of verbal advice with accompanying leaflets had long been commonplace. The inclusion of patient information leaflets in drug packs following an EU directive in 2005 was a mixed blessing, tending to raise as many concerns as it alleviated. The etymology for adherence to advice moved from compliance to concordance and was more effective for doing so.

1.3.4 UK's Demography

The population of the UK increased by a third, from 50 million in 1948 to over 66 million in 2019. People were living longer, healthier lives. Life expectancy in 2019 was 79 years for men and 83 years for women. In 1948, the equivalent figures were 66 and 71, respectively. The improvements in morbidity and mortality were multifactorial, but a sizeable contributory factor has been the universal access to medical care that the NHS provides, at the forefront of which was general practice.

However, the definition of what constitutes a healthy life has become more nuanced. People are living longer but often with many controlled ailments on the way, each requiring continuous medication and supervision.

Doctors' attitudes towards ageing have also changed. In the 1970s, a patient came under the care of the geriatric department if aged over 65 years. By the 1990s, this had risen to 70 years, and beyond the millennium, if still considered a factor at all, to 75. The pejorative term 'geriatric' has been eradicated from the medical dictionary, replaced by 'the elderly.'

The early NHS was rationed both in resources and in interventions that it could offer patients. Many of the classes of drugs in common use today have only been marketed since the 1960s. Life-prolonging interventions, such as coronary artery bypass and stents, organ transplant, chemo and radiotherapy, only became commonplace in the last quarter of the 20th century. Renal dialysis was limited to the under-55s until the 1980s. Public expectations of a cure for every ill in the early decades of the NHS were low, and acceptance was high of the inevitability of decline in vigour with age. Although the term had yet to be coined, ageism was an inevitable and natural consequence of the limited options available. A woman developing heart failure due to mitral incompetence secondary to rheumatic fever in childhood (since consigned to a medical footnote alongside the plague) would be considered a candidate for palliative care. The early years of the NHS were not a good time to be ill.

Matters improved from the late 1950s, with the expansion of resources available to manage disease. The UK population was living longer but doing so required ever more medical support. Disease prevention and management, with its associated polypharmacy, became ubiquitous. Age is no longer a factor in the treatment of patients; quantity of life now sits alongside quality. News stories of hip-joint replacements in patients past their centenary have become commonplace. However, such stories come at a price. The sums of money required to provide universal healthcare for a bigger population with increased longevity and increasingly complex medical conditions place an ever-greater strain on an NHS budget that, in turn, requires an ever-greater share of gross national product.

A thoughtful paper on the ethos and ethics of treating the elderly was published in the *BMJ* in 2007.[17] In it, the authors posited that the medical measures that prolonged life in the elderly, preventive therapies, simply changed the cause of their death. They felt that doctors were driven to prescribe by three factors: an emphasis on single rather than multiple disease outcomes, sensitivity about age discrimination, and pressure from drug companies and research innovations. The authors felt that, at the very least, doctors were negligent in providing information for the patient to make an informed decision on selecting one form of death over another. For patients who had already exceeded average life expectancy, death was relatively imminent and inevitable. The quality of those remaining years was what was important or, to quote Philippe Pinel (1745–1826), a French physician whom many consider the father of modern psychiatry.

> It is an art of no little importance to administer medicines properly, but it is an art of much greater and more difficult acquisition to know when to suspend or altogether to omit them.[18]

---

17 Mangin D, Sweeney K, Heath I. Preventive health care in elderly people needs rethinking. BMJ. 2007 Aug 11;335(7614):285–7. doi: 10.1136/bmj.39241.630741.BE1. PMID: 17690369; PMCID: PMC1941858.

18 Pinel P. *Traité Médico-philosophique sur l'aliénation mentale ou la manie*. Paris. [Medicophilosophical treatise on mental alienation or mania]. Translated by Hickish G, Healy D, Charland L. 2008.

Finally, two groups of patients, at the extreme ends of demand for medical services, deserve a special mention: the 'heart sink' and doctors themselves. 'Heart sink' patients, a term denoting repeated attendance with disparate symptoms of indeterminate aetiology resistant to any medical intervention, are often the bane of any GP surgery, through no fault of their own. The terminology has changed over time. Historically considered hypochondriacs and, of late, medically unexplained physical symptoms (MUPS), such patients cause immense frustration, due to their frequent attendance and monopolisation of limited resources. Yet, clinicians direct the frustration they feel at themselves more often than at the patient. A doctor's vocation is to make people better, to eliminate the symptoms of disease, a course of action that is often simply not feasible, given the nature of MUPS. The symptoms may be physical, but the underlying causes are frequently social and psychosocial, elements over which the patient has limited control or capacity to change and the doctor even less. There is no malice in the doctor's opinion of these patients. Any irritation is a reflex reaction directed at his or her own helplessness in helping others. Quite simply, it is a sense of inadequacy and failure. Nevertheless, doctors need to retain their professionalism, quelling such feelings of impotence when presented with a patient with MUPS. After all, they are just as likely to develop a life-threatening condition as any other member of the public.

At the opposite end of the spectrum, doctors, also fall ill but rarely seek medical attention from their colleagues. They are prey to the same medical, mental and social ailments as those that afflict their patients. However, the way that they respond to their illness differs. They tend to underplay their symptoms and are reluctant to seek help from others. There is a cultural reluctance to admitting to weakness. This long-recognised problem within the medical profession has contributory factors, such as poor insight into the condition, poor recognition of the impact the condition had on their performance and patient safety, poor and often self-management of their condition, poor (though much improved) access to appropriate medical and mental health resources, fear of referral to a disciplinary body and loss of livelihood, job, and income. In short, doctors tend to cleave too closely to the biblical proverb, 'physician heal thyself.'[19]

The above points are tragically illustrated in the suicide rate amongst doctors, reported in the UK as two to five times greater than that of the equivalent population.

In recognition of this dire situation, NHS England produced an excellent document in 2020, detailing the various resources available to support struggling doctors.[20]

1.3.5 The Consultation

The interaction between patient and doctor, the 'consultation,' has a single and simple unity of purpose. One party, the 'patient,' has a problem; the other, the 'doctor,' attempts to solve it. All the ripples of subsequent management radiate

---

[19] The Bible Luke 4:23.

[20] https://gpcpd.heiw.wales/assets/Post-Covid/ResourcesNHSERCGP.pdf

from that initial pebble of a problem hitting the water of primary care. General practice differs from nearly all hospital specialties, apart from A&E, in never knowing how big that pebble will be.

The motion regarding whether general practice qualifies as a specialty subject within the broad spectrum of medicine has been repeatedly debated since the 18th century. The title 'general' practice has not helped, with its implied definition of a broader rather than a specialised field of knowledge. Acceptance of general practice as a medical discipline with its own specialised needs and skills began to focus, in the 1970s, on areas where those needs differed from those required in hospitals. Until the introduction of more innovative undergraduate teaching in the 2000s, medical education had been exclusively directed at disease management. The basic tenets underpinning doctor-patient interaction in hospital, broadly defined as the 'clerking' of the patient, included eliciting the presenting complaint, a broad history, an examination, investigations and subsequent management of the condition. This applied to both general and specialist disciplines, with variable weight put on the various elements of the process. For example, in primary care, the main (and often only) requirement was the verbal discourse of the history itself; in hospital, the examination and investigations had greater prominence. Naturally, this differing approach reflected the milieu in which general practice operated, where the patients arrived 'unfiltered,' often with psychosocial problems relating to deprivation. The length of the consultation was limited. In essence, in primary care, clerking was a shorthand history. The converse was true in hospitals where time allowed for the acquisition of the maximum amount of information potentially relevant to the presenting symptoms. Clerking in hospital evaluated the acute presentation or one-off problem, a systems-based rather than a holistic approach to disease management. Subsequent interactions between hospital clinician and patient, whether on an inpatient or outpatient basis, would be brief and referred at length to the documented clerked history. The patient was seen as the vessel of pathology rather than an individual with complex ideas, concerns, beliefs, and expectations. Although doctors entering general practice had been taught and raised in this system, once in practice, they soon recognised its shortcomings in primary care. Primary and secondary differed in other ways; the limited time of any consultation (5–10 minutes, compared to 30+ minutes for clerking); the means and need to make a diagnosis and management plan spread out over many consultations; familiarity with patients, their environment, family, and social circumstances; and the psychology of the individual. The recognition of these fundamental differences in the doctor-patient interaction in primary and secondary care led to an explosion of research and publications on the subject of 'consultation analysis,' the one currently in vogue being the Calgary-Cambridge model.

In the 1970s, the authors of texts on the doctor-patient interaction, Balint, Byrne, Long, Pendleton, and Neighbour, acquired minor cult-like status within the medical education establishment. Chapter 8, 'Education and Training,' discusses their work in further detail.

The academic obsession with consultation analysis frankly bemused long-established practising doctors, who generally viewed the whole exercise as an overcomplication of a simple interaction, a conversation between two individuals to acquire information in a timely manner. Certainly, before the emphasis GP vocational training placed on the subject, many GPs felt that doctors given the same basic set of social and professional tools could thereafter use, discard, or add to them, over time. They felt that the doctor-patient interaction was intuitive rather than definable through science or psychology, and their communication skills would naturally improve in the course of time. Those doctors who attempted to incorporate advice, such as Ideas, Concerns, and Expectations (ICE), in their own consultations quickly gave up on the idea after being repeatedly rebuffed in response to their question, 'What do YOU think is wrong with you?' with 'I don't know, Doctor. That's why I've come to see you!'

So, what is the consultation?[21]

Pendleton describes the consultation as 'the central act of medicine' that 'deserves to be understood. It is clearly central to the doctor-patient transaction relationship.'[22]

I certainly have no issue with this definition, though I would prefer the term 'interaction' to 'transaction,' regarding the subsequent relationship between the two parties. The latter suggests some form of negotiation. Though this undoubtedly takes place, it is the broader verbal and non-verbal communication, encompassing as it does all the nuances and interplay of communication that creates a relationship from which both parties, but particularly the patient, benefit. Interaction is a less threatening interplay between individuals, less adversarial than transaction.

The consultation as the basis of general practice has evolved over the years. Many factors have contributed to changes in consultation style, content, and length. In the 1950s, patients rarely had booked appointments and were accustomed to queueing to see the doctor. A GP could see upward of 50 patients a day. Consultation times were limited as a consequence. The clinical notes arising from a consultation, written on a Lloyd George card, were brief, pithy, and reflected only the doctor's perspective.

The 1960s and 1970s saw the introduction of booked appointment times, with each patient allocated five minutes. Today, the QOF and the increasingly complex co-morbidities of an ageing population demand a minimum of ten minutes, with some arguing that 20–30 minutes would be more appropriate.

To coin a modern cliché, general practice is a people-skills business. As such, the art (and, some would say, science) of communication is the core within which lies the heart, empathy, the ability to understand another person's feelings as if they were one's own. Is empathy innate or can it be acquired? Patients certainly are quick to recognise and respond when it is present. If absent in some students, the teaching of it may often suffice. Doctors must be consummate actors. The character that they play at work can bear little resemblance to that at home. Like

[21] Tidy C. Consultation analysis. 2014. Accessed 4 Oct 2018 from www.patient.co.uk/doctor/Consultation-Analysis.htm

[22] Pendleton D, et al. *The Consultation: An Approach to Learning and Teaching.* Oxford: Oxford University Press, 1984.

all good professionals, they grow into the part as they repeatedly perform the same play. Thus, empathy becomes more natural with age and the experiences gathered throughout life.

When asked, patients still set great store by the relationships nurtured over decades with the aged curmudgeon who had supported them through their major life events. To them, his or her ability to communicate and empathise was far more important than the clinical knowledge that resided in their gnarled cranium.

The post-war generation of doctors, predominantly male and Anglo-Saxon, tended to adopt a paternalistic attitude towards their charges. Having been left to their own devices for their entire careers with no peer scrutiny, most retired having never had any knowledge or interest in the mechanics of the consultation. Were they in some way remiss for adopting this laissez-faire attitude? Had their patients suffered due to their ignorance? No research or data covers the subject, but it is highly likely that the standard of care of their patients was no different from subsequent generations who underwent more rigorous training on the subject.

Societies change. Attitudes acceptable in the 1970s and 1980s are today deemed to be, at best, ignorant and primitive and, at worst, callous and discriminatory. The public is more demanding and inclined to complain when a service fails to meet expectations. To address these issues, interactions between doctors and the public needed optimisation, and since the 1970s, the use of consultation analysis has gone some way towards addressing this. However, the in-depth reflection required made such analysis impractical in a busy GP surgery. That does not mean that it does not take place. GPs ruminate, especially on 'dysfunctional' consultations, although any lessons learned also depend on the other party contributing to the consultation, the patient.

So, how can a GP's performance be assessed? One way is through patients; after all, they are the consumer in this caring equation. National and local patient surveys largely focus on the doctor-patient interface. Thankfully, the number of complaints as a surrogate marker of quality has always been relatively low. Though reassuring, most complaints in primary care still cover issues with communication.

The GMC's Disciplinary Committee report, covering the 8,546 complaints in all clinical disciplines for 2017,[23] identified four areas of failure relating to communication:

1. Providing a patient with appropriate and timely information
2. Listening to the patient
3. Keeping colleagues informed/share appropriate level of information
4. Working in partnership or collaboratively with patient/family or carers[24]

---

[23] Fitness to practice statistics. 2017. www.gmc-uk.org/-/media/documents/fitness-to-practise-statistics-report-2017_pdf-76024327.p

[24] Understanding communication failures involving doctors. GMC, 4 Nov 2019. www.gmc-uk.org/-/media/documents/communication-complaint-types-and-contributory-factors-report_pdf-80571206.pdf

The persistent prevalence of communication issues after so many years of focusing on the problem remains a cause for concern. Productivity enhancements that have taken place over time might provide an explanation. High-quality human interactions appear to be inversely proportional to increased technological connectivity. Emails, texts, phones, even video calls increasingly intrude on meaningful face-to-face human interaction. A distracted, stressed doctor can easily be confused with an uninterested one.

Short consultations can still achieve important objectives.[25] One study in the UK in 2004 found that whilst the average consultation length was eight minutes, only an additional minute was required to improve the quality of care in patients with complex psychosocial problems.[26] One minute with a focused doctor is better than ten minutes with a distracted one.

Patients continue to express dissatisfaction with the time spent with their GP. Although increasing the length of consultations can improve this, improving the way time is spent within the consultation may be more realistic.[27]

1.4 SUMMARY

The dictionary definition of the word 'patient' is a person who is seeking and receiving medical treatment. Every person living in the United Kingdom is a potential patient.

From cradle to grave, everyone, regardless of age, sex, race, socioeconomic group, or creed, will see a doctor at some time in their life. When they do, they expect one thing above all others, understanding; that the person in front of them is attuned to their concerns and dedicated to alleviating them. The main attribute we desire from our Good Samaritan is empathy; to be, in psychological terminology, an active, engaged listener. The foundation of every consultation is built on empathy. Of course, that empathy is further enabled if doctors possess it personal experience of similar events in their own lives. A doctor who is a parent will be more sympathetic to a parent presenting with a sick child.

What else do patients require of their family practitioner? To be seen quickly, at a time of their choosing, by a doctor they know and trust, who has ample time to discuss their issues, competence in managing their problems, and humility in knowing their own limitations and when to refer the patient to a more learned

[25] Deveugele M, Derese A, De Bacquer D, van den Brink-Muinen A, Bensing J, De Maeseneer J. Consultation in general practice: a standard operating procedure? Patient Educ Couns. 2004 Aug;54(2):227–33. doi: 10.1016/S0738-3991(03)00239-8. PMID: 15288919.

[26] Howie JG, Heaney DJ, Maxwell M, Walker JJ, Freeman GK, Rai H. Quality at general practice consultations: cross sectional survey. BMJ. 1999 Sep 18;319(7212):738–43. doi: 10.1136/bmj.319.7212.738. PMID: 10487999; PMCID: PMC28226.

[27] Ogden J, Bavalia K, Bull M, Frankum S, Goldie C, Gosslau M, Jones A, Kumar S, Vasant K. 'I want more time with my doctor': a quantitative study of time and the consultation. Fam Pract. 2004 Oct;21(5):479–83. doi: 10.1093/fampra/cmh502. PMID: 15367468.

authority. In the absence of any other trusted source, they seek guidance on disparate issues around family, community, work, poverty, housing, and many other non-clinical matters. Perhaps unrealistically, all expect to feel 'better' after seeing a doctor. To a degree, all these attributes have been implicit during various periods of the NHS, but all depended on the individual GP, in himself or herself as varied as the patients.

Simple actions go a long way. A sign on a door stating 'only one problem per appointment' raises hackles, is counterproductive, and is an immediate irritant to a patient who may have waited up to three weeks to get that appointment. Abruptly closing a consultation during a list of complaints is frankly discourteous and sometimes dangerous. In times of stress, GPs may perceive patients as an inconvenience, an irritant. If so, they should take the time to reflect on the substantial barriers, booking an appointment, taking time off work, travel, that person has had to overcome to be seen. Despite their doctor's jaundiced perceptions, people do not lightly choose to be ill!

On the other hand, simple actions, such as a condolence card to the bereaved relatives of a recently deceased patient, can go much further in enhancing the reputation of the doctor and practice than any 'outstanding' Care Quality Commission (CQC) report.

The acronym used in consultation training, ICE, represents the doctor's intent in exploring a patient's Ideas, Concerns, and Expectations. The balance amongst the three elements of this triad naturally varies with the individual, but also the lifetime of the NHS. For example, in the mid-20th century, the prevalence of infectious diseases, viral and bacterial, and the limited pharmacopoeia available to treat them, dominated patients' ICE. Later that century, the dominant influence moved to cardiovascular disease. By the 21st century, cancer and mental health had come to the fore. Medical advances in managing these conditions simultaneously raised and disappointed patient expectations of a cure for all ills. A perennially cash-starved national health service, free at the point of care, inevitably leads to unbridled demand that resources can never match. Frustratingly, everything a patient expects from primary care can never be met.

So why are patients not storming the barricades and demanding a better service? Why do they continue to regard the service, their doctors and nurses, so highly? The NHS England GP Patient Survey, with a return of over three-quarters of a million questionnaires, reported four in five responders as rating their overall experience of their GP practice as good or very good.[28] Surely these findings counter all that one reads in the press or hears in casual conversation with friends and neighbours. How does one explain the disparity in perceptions? The answer might lie in the consultation, the face-to-face interaction with the healthcare professional. In those few precious minutes, a patient must be entirely convinced that the person they are seeing is totally focused on their problems, that they share concerns and frustrations. In short, the doctor exhibits a degree of empathy

---

[28] NHS GP patient survey. 2019. www.england.nhs.uk/statistics/2019/07/11/gp-patient-survey-2019/

seldom found in any other human interaction, and for that, patients are truly grateful and willing to overlook everything else.

In 1948, the population of the UK was universally thankful for the free healthcare that the government had provided through the NHS. That legacy, the esteem in which they held both the institution and its workers, lingers to this day. Doctors should stay mindful of the goodwill in which their patients hold them and avoid the siren lure of complacency.

The relationship between patient and doctor, and the resultant continuity of care, are the bedrock on which general practice is built. Sadly, that bond has weakened over the lifetime of the NHS. The presence of the family physician as an accepted part of the family is unlikely to survive far into the 21st century. Whether society will mourn that loss depends on future generations of GPs.

2

The Practice Team

An orchestra playing in harmony

2.1 INTRODUCTION

The practice team involved in delivering primary medical services to the community has evolved[1] and expanded greatly over the lifetime of the NHS. The focus of this chapter is on the personnel working on the front line. Later chapters cover the strategic organisation, remote administration, and management of primary care in general.

At the inception of the NHS in 1948, the core and, indeed, the sole member of the practice team was, quite simply, the doctor. The doctor opened the door, kept the appointment book, treated the patient, dispensed the medication, wrote referral letters, and kept the accounts. In short, he was a one-man band; female medical practitioners were exceedingly rare in those days.

However, with the passage of time, that lonely role became impractical. As with a star in space, the gravitational pull of the doctor gradually drew in subsidiary planets and eventually created a universe of individuals forever orbiting in a symbiotic relationship. The first to enter the practice orbit was the housekeeper.

2.2 THE SPOUSE/HOUSEKEEPER

The first member to join the practice team was the doctor's wife or, if not a spouse, a housekeeper. In the post-war era, a general practice, indeed any medical practice, was almost entirely a male preserve, many doctors having been demobbed from the medical services of the armed forces following the end of World War II. Mindful of the workload and stresses placed in their charge by a demanding public that was only just adjusting to the novelty of free healthcare, the housekeeper acted as gatekeeper for the gatekeeper, a role that quickly became synonymous with the title, 'dragon.'

---

[1] Goodwin N, Dixon A, Poole T, et al. *Improving the Quality of Care in General Practice*. 2011. www.kingsfund.org.uk/sites/default/files/field/field_related_document/gp-inquiry-report-evolving-role-nature-2mar11.pdf

DOI: 10.1201/9781003256465-2

The duties of the spouse/housekeeper were multifunctional. They encompassed the mundane, ensuring that the house/surgery was kept clean and tidy, befitting a doctor's residence, to the specialised such as filtering contacts with patients, managing the appointments book, and filing the medical records. Depending on previous training and experience, many took on additional responsibilities, such as nursing and dispensing medicines. Family life ran in parallel with and was often compromised by the work. Anecdotal tales describe GP families going years without a holiday, children sent off to relatives in the summer. The work was all-consuming.

Over the following decades, doctors were encouraged to congregate in ever larger groups. The role of the omnipresent housekeeper expanded, becoming unmanageable for a single person. The number, titles and duties of support staff increased. The DH, abetted by the doctor's union, the British Medical Association (BMA), facilitated the increase in manpower by introducing in the 1966 GP contract, partial reimbursement of practice staff costs, thus allaying any concerns doctors may have harboured that money spent on staff was coming directly from the mouths of their children.

The first employee, the housekeeper, was joined by the second, the receptionist.

2.3 THE RECEPTIONIST

The receptionist took over all administrative duties, including the initial interaction with patients, booking appointments, managing correspondence, secretarial work, filing, making the doctor's coffee, and any other non-clinical requests that came her way. Then, as now, the job was unfairly regarded as menial and never accorded the respect it deserved. Stuck at the interface between patient and doctor, the calm and dependable receptionist was the butt of the ire of both. For that privilege, she (and without exception, the role was exclusive to women) was paid the minimum wage. No qualifications were required. Training was and largely remains non-existent, with new recruits expected to learn on the job. It was a hugely undervalued role, and those that remained in it did so as a vocation, rather than a job.

As the administrative team expanded, the receptionist with the longest experience segued into the informal role of senior receptionist. There, she was expected to take on some management functions, such as organising the working roster for staff, many of whom worked part-time, managing sickness absences, keeping the holiday diary, and ensuring that the practice administration ran smoothly. With time, she was also tasked with the thankless undertaking of securing a locum for unplanned GP absences. Craven GPs, knowing the difficulty, were happy to relinquish that task under the pretense that it was non-clinical and, thus, beneath them.

It was the receptionist's lot to remain forever undervalued. On the one hand, her employer, the doctor, held her responsible for his or her personal workload, especially unscheduled interruptions, whilst the patients regarded her as a sullen barrier whose sole purpose was to obstruct their access to a doctor. The patients' views were summarised in one of the rare studies looking into the role of the receptionist, aptly entitled 'There is a good reason why GP receptionists are so grumpy!'[2]

> There is a stereotype of GP receptionists as dragons behind a desk—unsmiling individuals with a curt manner and an apparent determination to be anything but helpful.

If the GP was the gateway to the NHS, the receptionist was the rather stiff latch on that gate.

The author went on to describe a typical scenario where the receptionist would be dealing with a queue of people with different needs and expectations, waiting to see the doctor, whilst the phone was constantly ringing with other patients, likely to be unwell and frustrated at having to wait so long, wanting to speak to the receptionist. Despite these pressures, the receptionist was expected to suppress her own emotions by adopting a detached manner, remaining professional and helpful throughout. Their apparent indifference was a shield against becoming emotionally exhausted.

By the 21st century, the role of receptionist had been put on a more professional footing. Name tags and uniforms were introduced. They received formal training, and certificates in conflict resolution and acting as a chaperone. Most receptionists would have been happy to swap any training for a little courtesy and kindness.

The receptionist was the shop front for the practice. A good practice was often only a reflection of its helpful and sympathetic reception staff. In short, the receptionist deserved all the support she could get.

2.4 THE MEDICAL SECRETARY

The next addition to the practice team was someone who could converse with hospital consultants and manage the paperwork resulting from such conversations. A step above the humble receptionist, the secretary acted as liaison officer, handling more complex interactions with patients and the hospital. Communication improved as neatly typed letters replaced handwritten referrals in undecipherable script.

Gradually, the role of the secretary also expanded to include bookkeeping and finance. Some even took on the role of writing out the repeat prescriptions on the FP10s,[3] although the doctor still needed to check and sign them.

In 1990, fundholding further expanded the role of the secretary, whose duties now encompassed the leviathan task of managing the reams of paper that the purchaser-provider paradigm generated.

---

[2] Ward J. There is a good reason why GP receptionists are so grumpy. Mail Online, 3 Jan 2012. https://www.dailymail.co.uk/health/article-2081457/There-good-reason-GP-receptionists-grumpy.html

[3] FP10s are the standard NHS prescription forms.

Just in case the secretaries were finding the role unchallenging, the early 2000s added the Choice and Book initiative. Intended to facilitate the process of booking hospital appointments, it also offered the patient the choice of where and when they wished to be seen. In practice, the IT software was cumbersome, waiting lists remained long, patients remained frustrated. All it succeeded in doing was transferring the booking process from secondary to primary care, who, in turn, chose to add the task to the burden already undertaken by the secretary.

At first, the secretary shared some receptionist duties with their counterparts at the front desk, but as the role expanded, they moved into their own dedicated space, becoming the 'medical secretary.' Tensions developed between the two, with the general administration staff perceiving the secretary as having unwarranted ideas of grandeur. The GP, or more commonly his spouse, now had to include personnel management as part of their brief.

2.5 THE FILING CLERK/DATA-INPUTTER

The role of filing clerk never existed in name as such; the filing of the decrepit Lloyd George envelopes was always part of the receptionist's basic duties.

The adoption of computerised medical records and the move towards a paper-lite and ultimately paper-free practice created the new role of data-inputter. Initially, this was not raw data but scanned documents, whether faxes from out-of-hours providers, letters from outpatient clinics, hospital inpatient discharge summaries, laboratory reports, or anything relating to a patient that had come in as hard copy. This work had to be done promptly to avoid an unmanageable backlog and allow contemporaneous access by the clinician.

The tasks later included the highlighting of vital information prior to scanning, one that placed an unsupported responsibility on an employee with no medical training. Otherwise, the tedious and repetitive role was surprisingly popular with employees, providing a respite from patient contact!

2.6 THE PRACTICE MANAGER

As group practice became established, the array of elements required for the delivery of a modern health service became too time-consuming for the GP or his spouse to manage. By the 1980s, the need for a manager to administer the practice became an imperative. Initially, most practices seamlessly moved the senior receptionist into the role, allocating a title and little else. As is often the case in any organisation, promotion from within a group led to tensions between those promoted and the erstwhile colleagues left behind, not an easy dynamic to manage. Some were instinctively adept at personnel management, others were not, and the latter compromised harmony within the team. Nevertheless, general practice was moving inexorably away from the haphazard and amateurish family concern and towards an increasingly commercial enterprise. Doctors were palpably incapable of overseeing this expansion while simultaneously coping with developments in their clinical duties, especially the increasing transfer of work from secondary to primary care. Fundholding practices led the way to recognising the need for a dedicated business and finance specialist. Thus, the role of qualified practice manager was born, requiring the external recruitment of individuals with the prerequisite expertise.

There was no shortage of applicants. The NHS was going through one of its periodic upheavals. Middle managers within the lower echelons of the administrative structure, the Family Practitioners' Committee and Family Health Services Authority, were being made redundant. They soon found a welcoming home in general practice, as indeed did unlucky bank managers caught in a similar upheaval in the financial sector. GPs had an embarrassment of choices. New recruits tended to be male, the first of that sex (apart from the doctor) to join the practice team. By 2012, the number of men that general practices employed had markedly increased.[4]

This new breed of manager was better trained and qualified but did not necessarily understand the milieu in which general practice operated. Strategic decisions were still firmly in the hands of the partners. General practice was neither a commercial business nor a public service in thrall to bureaucracy. However, the influx of skills from outside of the inward-looking world of primary care did benefit the practice. Outsiders brought in new ideas. They were more familiar with the utility of computerisation, especially in managing accounts, payroll, and invoicing. The influx of men, especially high-status ones from banking, presented challenges to an all-female staff with generally low self-esteem. The partners also had to adjust to an individual likely to be more knowledgeable about certain aspects of their business than they were. Competent appointees could address and defuse such concerns. Those less confident in their abilities focused on the paperwork and hid in their offices.

Many appointees settled smoothly into the role, but others found it difficult to adapt to the hectic environment of a workplace under constant pressure. Turnover was rapid in the early years. Those managers in fundholding practices, dealing with complex activities such as contract negotiations between purchaser and provider, installing and running IT systems, and liaising with external agencies, were particularly stressed by the job. Partners were only too keen to delegate such responsibilities provided the bottom line on the accounts continued to rise.

The role of practice manager was indispensable by the 21st century, by which time GPs had absolved themselves entirely of the day-to-day operation of the practice, retaining only strategic decision-making. Some practice managers became equity holders, sharing partnership profits. Many were on substantial salaries, depending on the practice size. Others became board members on the clinical commissioning group (CCG).

One group was not entirely happy with the practice manager's rise in status, sessional doctors. Doctors were a proud bunch, bridling at reporting to a

---

[4] National Careers Service. GP practice manager. 2017. Accessed 7 Oct 2021 from https://nationalcareersservice.direct.gov.uk/advice/planning/jobprofiles/Pages/gppracticemanager.aspx#tabsctl00_m_g_d4df449d_0624_4d6f_a3ba_b73501ce66d5_HostWebPart-1

non-peer. Traditionally, they had operated within a medical hierarchy, but the culture in primary care was only following that which had preceded it in secondary care. Doctors were adjusting to becoming employees like the rest of the practice team.

2.7 THE PRACTICE NURSE

The practice clinical team expanded in parallel with the administrative staff. Central reimbursement of staff costs allowed for the recruitment of nurses to assist GPs in providing clinical care, such as dressing wounds, childhood vaccinations, and cervical cytology. In due course, the nurse's role developed further into phlebotomy, electrocardiograms (ECG), and spirometry, before moving to new patient assessments, chronic disease, asthma, chronic obstructive pulmonary disease, diabetes, epilepsy management, contraception, and health promotion. A patient denied access to a doctor saw the more approachable practice nurse. Receptionists in particular welcomed a less intimidating conduit for their demanding patients. On-site throughout the day, the nurse was often the sole resource that the receptionist could turn to for medical advice. Thankfully, most recruits were highly capable, experienced nurses previously employed in either the local hospital or district.

The increase in the number of nurses in general practice accelerated following the budgetary flexibility of the 2004 GP contract. GP practices employed 2,166 more nurses in 2013 than they had a decade earlier, with a female to male ratio of 3:1. By 2017, nearly 16,000 full-time equivalent (FTE) nurses worked in general practice,[5] compared to 33,100 FTE GPs.

In turn, the increasing responsibilities of the practice nurse led to the evolution of the role, in stages, to nurse practitioner and advanced nurse practitioner.

2.8 THE NURSE PRACTITIONER

The continuing need to meet ever-increasing public demand within a constrained budget led GP principals to explore innovative means of delivering services. Many presentations in any surgery were minor and self-limiting, and a less-qualified practitioner could probably manage them. GPs were also mindful that nurses were cheaper to employ than doctors. Driven as much by fiscal concerns as workload, experienced nurses seemed to provide a solution. Practice nurses retrained for the role, eager to introduce some variety into their workload.

At first, patients were reluctant to see anyone but their doctor. However, ease of access overcame such concerns, and by 2020, a nurse practitioner's clinic could include anyone over two years old with a 'minor' illness, in fact much of what a qualified doctor normally saw!

Whilst the nurse practitioner could perform many of the doctor's functions, there remained one glaring absence: the prescribing of drugs. The hurdle was overcome by completing a community practitioner nurse prescribing course that

---

[5] https://digital.nhs.uk/news/2018/statistics-show-change-in-nhs-workforce-over-time

allowed access to a limited British National Formulary (BNF) Nurse Prescriber Formulary. Those nurses looking for further challenges needed to become advanced nurse practitioners.

2.9 THE ADVANCED NURSE PRACTITIONER

A supercharged nurse practitioner, the advanced nurse practitioner, had a higher level of postgraduate training, up to master's degree level, and access, excluding controlled drugs, to the British National Formulary used by licensed doctors.

Advanced nurse practitioners were expected to see any patient, undertake a history and physical examination, arrive at a differential diagnosis, request investigations, prescribe, refer patients to an appropriate specialist in the practice or hospital, and arrange onward management. In other words, an advanced nurse practitioner functioned as a doctor, barring certification of death and managing maternity, the result of a turf war with midwives!

2.10 THE PHYSICIAN ASSOCIATE (PREVIOUSLY PHYSICIAN ASSISTANT)

Originating in the United States in 1965, the role of physician's associate crossed the Atlantic in the 2010s and became a faculty of the Royal College of Physicians in 2015.

Candidates for the post had to have a primary degree and specialty diploma or a master's degree. Such courses, developed and overseen by the Faculty of Physician Associates, numbered fewer than 50 across the UK by 2019. As with the advanced nurse practitioner, the physician associate undertook all duties of a qualified doctor but remained supervised by and answerable to the GP.

2.11 THE HEALTHCARE ASSISTANT (HCA)

The role of HCA was a further illustration of primary care developing services to conveniently meet patients' needs. Initially, the HCA took over phlebotomy duties, previously done by the GP and then the nurse, as these became both remote and limited in secondary care. In due course, the role expanded to include much of what the practice nurse had traditionally done, including ECGs, spirometry, and simple wound care.

2.12 THE PHARMACIST/PHARMACY TECHNICIAN

Some GP practices, invariably rural, had long contained an in-house dispensary that was intimately integrated with the management of patients. Those that did not were denied the expertise of a pharmacist, relying instead on liaising with the local commercial chemist.

The role of the in-house pharmacist, often shared between practices, became more common as GP practices cooperated in larger groupings, a federation or latterly a primary care network.

The duties of the pharmacist came under the broad heading of medicines management: repeat medication reviews, consultations for drug side effects and interactions, converting prescribed expensive drugs to cheaper bioequivalent generics, drug budget reviews, transferring information from hospital discharge summaries and monitoring some simple conditions, such as uncomplicated hypertension and diabetes. Pharmacists also gave injections, the annual influenza or, during the pandemic, COVID-19 vaccines.

The pharmacy technician worked under the direction of the pharmacist in dispensing drugs, reviewing repeat prescriptions, stock management, storage of drugs and vaccines, sales of over-the-counter medication, and responding to patient queries.

Although not technically a member of staff, some surgeries had robotic dispensaries that could accept electronic prescriptions and, without any human help, sort, label, stack, retrieve labels, and dispense medication, as well as keep stock and reorder from a wholesaler. They were hypnotically entertaining to watch in full flow but automation rarely resulted in reduced headcount.

2.13 THE PHYSIOTHERAPIST

As with the pharmacist, practices shared the in-house physiotherapist, more common as GP practices cooperated in larger groupings.

The role centred on the rapid assessment and management of acute musculoskeletal conditions, sprains, tendinitis, backache or arthritis, for which they provided more immediate access than the long waiting times previously offered by secondary care. Initially, they could only take doctors' referrals, but over time, they too became more independent, allowing for direct patient access. The benefits to patients and doctors were immediate and immense.

2.14 THE SOCIAL PRESCRIBER

The NHS Long-Term Plan of 2019[6] promoted the role of the social prescriber in primary care, as providing patients with:

> choice and control over the way their care is planned and delivered, based on 'what matters' to them and their individual strengths and needs. This happens within a system that makes the most of the expertise, capacity, and potential of people, families, and communities in delivering better outcomes and experiences. Personalised care takes a whole-system approach, integrating services around the person. It is an all-age model, from maternity and childhood, through to end of life, encompassing both mental and physical health support.

---

[6] www.england.nhs.uk/publication/social-prescribing-and-community-based-support-summary-guide/

This represents a new relationship between people, profession-als, and the health and care system. It provides a positive shift in power and decision-making that enables people to feel informed, have a voice, be heard and be connected to each other and their communities.

Unusually in the NHS, the grandiose waffle was not misplaced; social prescribers became a helpful, time-saving resource for GPs, allowing rapid and informed access to such areas as statutory state benefits, in which doctors had no training and little interest. In addition, the post had the added benefit of 100% funding by NHS England.

2.15 THE CLEANER

Last, but certainly not least, the cleaner. The nature of GP practices as buildings filled with infectious people between the hours of 8.00 a.m. and 7.00 p.m. made the role of the cleaner vital in maintaining the safety of all occupants.

Notwithstanding the antisocial hours, due to the primary use of the building, cleaners were often the most overlooked and worst paid members of the practice. Apart from keeping the building clean, the cleaner also supplied another vital function, gossip. Living in the community and tuned in to chatter regarding the practice, they provided invaluable feedback on a practice's reputation in the community. Sadly, GPs lost that information, once cleaning services were outsourced to commercial providers in the 1990s.

2.16 CORPORATE IMAGE

In the 1980s, practices began introducing staff uniforms, to present a profes-sional corporate image to the public. Initially, staff members baulked at the idea, especially when asked to personally pay for their uniforms, becoming more ame-nable when their employers took on that charge. In the meantime, the sartorial travel direction for their employers was moving in the opposite direction. The dress code for male doctors went from the three-piece suit, denoting paternalism, respect, and gravitas, through the casual jacket, shirt, and tie, welcoming and accessible, to a casual open-neck shirt, short sleeves, and chinos, relaxed, friendly, infection-aware. Women GPs similarly traversed fashion styles from twinset and pearls to colourful blouse and slacks. To a degree, these changes reflected those in other spheres of society and the move away from the formal to the relaxed. Both sexes flirted with white coats, conveying professional parity with hospital consul-tants, but these were quickly discarded as pretentious.

The costs to employ a full staff complement to run an efficient general practice were and are considerable. Salaries for staff vary, from the UK living wage for a cleaner and receptionist, to £50,000 per annum for a practice manager or a physi-cian's associate.

A non-dispensing practice of 10,000 patients and five partners would need, in full-time equivalents, a minimum of one practice manager, two secretaries, one data-input clerk, six receptionists, two practice nurses, one healthcare assistant, and one cleaner, amounting to a payroll of around £320,000, excluding employer National Insurance and pension contributions. With 70% reimbursement by the NHS, this would still leave a deficit of £96,000, to be accounted for through the partnership profits, not a trivial sum.

2.17 THE DOCTOR

Finally, the sun around which all planets orbited, the doctor.

The primary aim of founding the NHS in 1948 was to allow British citizens free and easy access to one commodity, the doctor, and more specifically, the general practitioner. All subsequent healthcare provision flowed from that access. The GP, based in the local community, was the gatekeeper of the NHS. Access was open to all, every hour of every day of the year. Patients could not be turned away. There was no cap on demand. Not knowing when and who was going to come through the consulting room door made the GP's day both daunting and stimulating in equal measure. That uncertainty, along with the freedom of the independent contractor status, attracted a certain kind of individual, confident but mindful of their ignorance, open-minded and non-judgemental, able to deal with uncertainty, and most importantly, with a genuine concern for the welfare of their fellow man. In other words, medicine, and general practice in particular, arose from a vocation.

As the title implies, GPs are generalists. No other medical specialty offers the opportunity to treat any condition from cradle to grave; pregnant mothers, their babies, spotty adolescents, injured athletes, menopausal women, the frail and demented elderly; from mental illness to endocrine diseases to cancer. A GP's knowledge is broad but not deep. They know how and when to intervene, through prevention, treatment, education, and referral, and, importantly, when not to intervene!

In 1948, a GP's duties were clearly defined: see ill people and make them better. Over the following seven decades, those duties have expanded and become more complex. The fundamentals have remained the same, but the requirements and means for achieving that initial aim have changed in line with society's expectations. All General Practitioners, except for a few assistants, were GP principals, independently contracted to the NHS to provide a comprehensive primary healthcare service. Seven decades later, many GPs were employees identified as Salaried, Sessional, Registrar, and Retainer. Nevertheless, the front-line responsibility for delivering healthcare to the nation remained with the GP principal, or 'Partner.' To coin a phrase, the buck most definitely stopped with the GP partner.

2.18 THE GP PRINCIPAL/PARTNER

In 1948, the generally accepted definition of a GP principal was any qualified medical practitioner independently contracted to the NHS. In 1981, after the introduction of mandatory postgraduate training, that definition became 'a vocationally-trained GP in the UK with full GMC registration and contracted by a local health authority or health board to provide General Medical Services to patients without supervision.'[7]

A non-principal differed by being an employee of either a GP principal or primary care organisation, academic institution, locum agency, or another medical services provider.

General practice initially attracted individuals with certain character traits. Broadly speaking, these included a sense of fierce independence, strong work ethic, reluctance to rely on others, intolerance of weakness or dissent, and often, ironically for a job in which human interaction was paramount, an innate inability to work with others. These traits, at the fore in early generations of GPs working in the NHS, led them to choose general practice over a career in the hierarchical, restricted, and regimented environment of secondary care.

As the practice team expanded, one can imagine that having to work with others would seem quite daunting. Many GPs chose not to do so, either by remaining as single-handed practitioners or else by entering a loose confederation where doctors operated independently but under the same roof as their erstwhile colleagues.

The embryonic general practice, with its nucleus of GP plus one other, had its drawbacks, but the doctor easily understood it. Duties were clearly defined, with the doctor left to undertake all clinical and financial responsibilities by the other's absorption of all other tasks. It was a relationship that had one boss. The 1960s upended all that had gone before, as individual practitioners were induced by that most seductive of carrots, money, to combine with other colleagues in group practices. Doctors had to adjust to working with others, ideally in a collegial manner. Clinical responsibilities for patient lists remained personal, but partners had to share the management of staff and the increasingly complex finances. Some doctors managed this transition better than others. However, it was by no means uncommon to find that one authoritarian individual might dominate a partnership, often by virtue of longevity, and to dictate strategy and operations to the others. Relinquishing power as the NHS evolved was to prove a significant challenge to some doctors.

The GP principal's position remained secure and unchallenged at the pinnacle of the hierarchical pyramid. He took little interest in the general administration of the practice, provided surgeries were not overbooked and patients were uncomplaining. He garnered the credit for the smooth running of a practice; any failings fell on lesser beings. The clinical team was headed by the senior partner, the best acting as a benign, paternalistic figure.

Doctors within a group practice spent most of their day in their consulting room, venturing forth only for coffee, the allocation of home visits, writing repeat prescriptions, or informal clinical meetings. These brief interactions provided opportunities for social bonding, venting of spleen, and discussion of complex cases. More formal general management and clinical meetings took place on a weekly or monthly basis, often shoehorned into lunchtime with sandwiches provided by a drug company, in return for a brief presentation of their wares. Formal

---

[7] Medical Dictionary. Definition of GP principal. Accessed 7 Oct 2021 from https://medical-dictionary.thefreedictionary.com/GP+principal

business meetings to discuss the annual accounts took place once or twice a year, invariably at a partner's home. Apart from these infrequent occasions and perhaps an educational meeting at the local postgraduate centre (oiled by the attached bar), there were few opportunities to mix with one's peers. It was an unexpectedly lonely job, one that became paradoxically lonelier as practices grew in size.

GP partners were supportive and forgiving of each other. The ethos of autonomy made criticism of a colleague's performance difficult. Unsafe habits, such as alcoholism, were noted but swept under the carpet until they became too obvious to ignore. The relationship could be a repressed one, where irritations were contained, and grievances were allowed to foment. Whistleblowing was unheard of.

Until the late 20th century, the GMC's operations were relatively peripheral to the lives of most doctors and patients. Periodically, the press reported on a salacious misconduct case, which usually involved drugs, alcohol, and/or inappropriate sexual liaisons. Complaints were relatively few, with only a handful of hearings by the Professional Conduct Committee (PCC) each year.[8]

Adjusting to working with medical colleagues may have been difficult, but working with an ever-expanding practice team was more so. Communication between members remained limited. There was a professional affinity with the practice nurse, who needed to be flattered since she took on an increasing part of the clinical burden. The senior receptionist or practice manager might attend practice meetings but was otherwise expected to report only on matters of urgency. The medical secretary acted as personal assistant and, thus, had greater access. All other staff were acknowledged but generally, unforgivably, ignored.

The picture painted may seem a bleak one, but it certainly applied to many GP practices, often without the partners realising what took place outside of their consulting room. Of course, there were equally many exemplars of happy practices, driven by free and open communication between all.

The introduction of the practice manager in the late 20th century increased the isolation inherent in the GP's job. Once the role became established, GPs tended to withdraw completely from all aspects of the day-to-day running of the practice, sometimes with unexpected and unwelcome consequences, including fraud. Notorious cases of embezzlement were periodically reported in the regional newspapers and over the past decade, individual cases have included significant sums of money of over half a million pounds.[9,10,11] The stories behind

8 CIVITAS. The general medical council: fit to practise? 2014. Accessed 7 Oct 2021 from www.civitas.org.uk/pdf/GMCFittoPractise.pdf

9 www.ipswichstar.co.uk/news/ipswich-practice-manager-accused-of-stealing-264-000-from-her-2764246

10 www.manchestereveningnews.co.uk/news/greater-manchester-news/jailed-stockport-practice-manager-who-3158399

11 www.manchestereveningnews.co.uk/news/greater-manchester-news/gp-surgery-manager-jailed-calculated-16566955

the headlines were uniformly banal. The practice manager had total control of the practice finances, had personal problems, the fraud spanned many years and there was no financial oversight by the partners. Such extreme examples of fraud made good stories but were rare. They provided a salutary warning of the consequences of GP partners relinquishing aspects of their job, enticed into focusing solely on clinical duties and forgetting that they were also running a business.

The proportion of GP principals in primary care has shrunk over time. The onerous responsibilities of managing patients' problems hindered by increasing bureaucracy and scrutiny were cited as significant contributory factors in the decrease. As smaller practices amalgamated with bigger ones, partners took the opportunity to retire early, enabling salaried GPs to replace them.

2.19 THE SALARIED (SESSIONAL) GP

The role of the salaried or sessional GP within a practice only became widespread following the 1997 GP contract and the creation of PMS. The move accelerated following the contract of 2004. The expansion of salaried posts resulted from a single trigger; the switch of the basic practice allowance from individual GP principal to the practice as a whole. It made economic sense to replace an equity-sharing partner with an employee on a lower salary. A surrogate marker, jobs advertised in the *British Medical Journal*, showed an almost total absence of advertisements for partners in the decade following the 2004 contract. Meanwhile, doctors entering general practice, increasingly women, were wary of the full-time commitment of a partnership and were seeking more flexible working conditions instead. The trade-off was lack of tenure and reduced income.

GP principals now had to adjust to supervising colleagues who were equally qualified to practice medicine. Some took to doing so in a formative, constructive manner; others, not to belabour the point, mistreated their colleagues much as their predecessors had abused 'assistants with a view'[12] in earlier times. Tensions developed between the two groups, fed by poor communication and misconceptions of the relative roles.

Salaried doctors were aggrieved that they were earning around 50% of what a partner earnt, despite seemingly doing the bulk of the clinical work. Partners felt that salaried colleagues were lucky to have a defined structure to their day with no administrative responsibilities. Meetings between the two to address such issues were rare in a perpetually busy workplace. Resentment was allowed to fester.

Patients also had a nuanced view of the salaried doctor or locum. They trusted their familiar family GP but were unsure about the seemingly less-qualified salaried doctor and downright wary of the unknown locum. Patients were more

---

[12] A reprehensible practice where a GP Principal would take on a salaried doctor at a reduced rate of pay by enticing them with informal promises of partnership after a set period of time, e.g. 1–2 years. Sadly, they then found excuses, such as inadequate performance, to either extend that period or dismiss that doctor, only to repeat the process with their replacement.

likely to complain about non-principals. Over time, the reaction of patients could lead to an erosion of confidence and self-esteem in the peripatetic physician, resulting in a genuine belief that they were less worthy than their exalted colleagues.

Comparison of the roles of GP principal and salaried GP:

GP Principal	Salaried GP[13]
• Self-employed	• Employed
• Partnership agreement	• Contract of employment
• Autonomous	• Supervised
• Shared partnership profits	• Fixed income
• Income >£100,000 per annum	• Income <£70,000 per annum
• Open-ended day	• Defined day
• Not bound (until 2020) by the European Working Time Directive, EWTD	• Bound (until 2020) by the EWTD
• Answerable to partners	• Answerable to practice manager
• Concerned about Quality and Outcomes Framework (QOF) income	• Unconcerned about QOF income
• Concerned about Care Quality	• Unconcerned about
• Commission inspections	• Care Quality Commission inspections
• Precedence for holidays	• Negotiated holidays
• Time off in lieu of business meetings, etc.	• No business meetings
• Seniority allowance	• No seniority allowance

Prior to the 21st century, salaried doctors were employed on a gentleman's agreement and rarely had a formal contract of employment.[14]

The significant disparity in income between GP partners and salaried doctors decreased over the years, in response to supply and demand. By 2020, the BMA estimated that an average income for a full-time salaried GP was £90,000, the partner's £105,000.

The role of the salaried doctor should not be confused with that of a locum doctor, despite both working under the umbrella heading of 'sessional GP.' Locums had an itinerant existence, employed by a practice at short notice and for a limited period. As such, the availability of work and, therefore, income, varied widely. In return, the role provided variety, flexibility, experience prior to a long-term commitment, and an avenue for clinical practice for the recently retired. There were disadvantages: isolation, few employment rights, excessive travelling, and difficulties meeting the requirements of appraisal and revalidation.

---

[13] www.bma.org.uk/media/2901/bma-salaried-gp-handbook-july-2020.pdf

[14] www.bma.org.uk/pay-and-contracts/contracts/salaried-gp-contract/sessional-and-locum-gp-contract-guidance

Locums advertised their services independently through the primary care organisation, Local Medical Committee, National Association of Sessional GPs, or a commercial agency. The BMA provided invaluable advice for those doctors drawn to locum work.[15]

Remuneration reflected the instability of the workload, depending on whether it was a buyer's or seller's market, with rates commanding between £75 to £100 per hour or around £700 a day.

2.20 PARTNERSHIP DYNAMICS

In the early years of general practice, incoming partners were often known or recommended to incumbents. The advertising of vacancies was often unnecessary. Doctors, notoriously parsimonious, baulked at paying the substantial fee for an advertisement in the *BMJ*. Interviews were conducted over a pint in the pub; the shortlist of candidates by a dinner with the partners and their spouses. The opinion of the senior partner's wife could make or break any deal. The success of a candidate was based on subjective views rather than objective evidence, although any additional fee-earning qualifications or skills would be more highly regarded. Tacit in the process was that any appointment would be for life. If ever a scenario screamed out for pre-employment psychometric testing, this was it. The 'old boys' network' reigned supreme.

By and large, the process of appointing a new partner worked surprisingly well, and partnerships moved forward contentedly and efficiently. Partners became firm friends, with their respective families closely intertwined through the following generations. This harmonious idyll prevailed particularly throughout the settled decades from 1966 to 1986, often called the 'golden years' of general practice.

The partnership dynamic began to come under pressure following the contract of 1990, which was more prescriptive than previous contracts, regarding the role of a GP. Some doctors were more receptive to change and innovation than others. The move towards a financial- and productivity-driven general practice business model appealed to doctors who felt constrained by their clinical tasks alone. Major DH initiatives, such as fundholding in the 1990s, pitting practice against practice, caused heated debates within partnerships. Doctors were forced to make strategic decisions that had never arisen in the first 40 years of the NHS. Consensus and unanimity varied between partnerships. Those outvoted could become withdrawn and resentful. The phrase 'it's nothing personal' became accepted in the lexicon of partnership decision-making. Doctors had never been trained in conflict resolution.

Medicine was a scientific discipline informed by evidence. Doctors, conservative in nature, were resistant to new ideas until they had been proven. They were uncomfortable with change, and change was coming at a time of increasing workload and fewer opportunities for the partners to meet.

---

[15] www.bma.org.uk/pay-and-contracts/contracts/salaried-gp-contract/bma-locum-practice-agreement

The basis on which partnerships formed also changed. The elopement to Gretna Green was replaced by dating sites and prenuptial agreements. The vagaries of workforce shortages resulted in partners being taken on from desperation rather than by choice. That workforce was also becoming more mobile. The cost of buying into a practice was prohibitive and increasingly rejected. The concept of a job for life was no longer credible.

Although GPs cite the burden of workload, bureaucracy, and annual appraisal as the main causes of discontent within the profession, the major cause of stress that led to partnerships dissolving was friction between the partners. Doctors were less sympathetic and empathic to their colleagues than they were to their patients.

The common triggers of interpersonal clashes ranged from workload to ill health.

Workload:

- Doctors doing more surgeries than others
- Doctors finishing surgery early and dashing off-site
- Doctors grabbing one home visit and leaving the other 20 to share out between the others
- Doctors not signing repeat prescriptions
- Doctors withdrawing from non-clinical work (for example, insurance medicals)
- Should the practice enter a local enhanced service?

Holidays:

- Doctors grabbing school holiday slots without discussion
- Doctors wishing to book time off for the same dates

Income:

- Unequal 'parity' share of practice profits
- Disagreement of what was included in practice income and what was not
- Uneven share of practice dispensary income

Numbers of patients seen:

- Should a doctor who has a slow consultation style be allowed to see fewer patients than one with a faster style?
- Should all surgeries have the same number of patients booked in?
- Is each doctor seeing their fair share of extras?
- Responding to DH/PCT/CCG initiatives
- Does a doctor overprescribe?
- Does a doctor over-investigate?
- Does a doctor over-refer?

Character clashes:

- Sometimes people just do not get on!

Property ownership:

- Who owns the premises?
- How is the income from cost/notional rent distributed?
- Is the rent fair to the non-equity partners?
- Who is responsible for the upkeep of the premises?
- Who owns the in-house pharmacy?

External jobs/income:

- Does an external job (for example, GP with a special interest) remove the doctor from the surgery?
- Should income from such work be shared or kept by the individual doing that work?

Maternity leave:

- How long is she going to take?
- How many more pregnancies is she going to have?
- Who will pay for a locum?

Ill health:

- Is the doctor really ill?
- How long is the doctor going to be off work?
- What are we going to do about locums?
- Who is going to pay for a locum?
- How are we going to cope with the extra work?
- Is the GP a drug-addled alcoholic?

Many of the above issues were covered in an excellent article published in *BMJ Careers* in 2013.[16]

Despite all the pitfalls inherent in a small group of strong-minded individuals working in close proximity in a highly pressured environment, GP partnerships were remarkably stable. The partnership model remained pivotal in the delivery of healthcare to the population of the UK and, despite the diminishing number of GP principles, were still integral to the successful roll-out of primary care networks in 2020.

---

16 Taylor R. How to prevent GP partnerships breaking down. BMJ. 2013;346:f1346. Accessed 7 Oct 2021 from http://careers.bmj.com/careers/advice/view-article.html?id=20011203

2.21 SUMMARY

Seventy years of the NHS have seen the role of the GP move from solitary busker to conductor of an orchestra where each section must play harmoniously if the result is not to be a discordant cacophony. A successful GP practice works as a team.

The culture of any practice is set by the GP partners. A happy and efficient surgery is apparent as soon as one approaches the reception desk. Simple acts of courtesy, such as a greeting in the morning, a thank you, an acknowledgement of work well done, have an inestimably greater impact on elevating morale than any annual appraisal of staff members or patient surveys.

The role of the GP has had to evolve to encompass the need to work with colleagues from a wide range of backgrounds. Each member of the team has been appointed to lessen the doctor's workload. They have succeeded in doing so by removing many of the onerous duties of administration, finance, liaison, and even clinical, leaving the doctors to focus on what they were trained to do, treat patients. As such, any doctor should be eternally grateful. Nevertheless, the gains made by spreading the work have continued to be overwhelmed by the increase in volume of work. The appetite for medical care is insatiable. Primary care has no option but to continue to try to satiate it.

The total workforce in the primary care sector stood at 150,000 in 2021.[17] In 1948, that workforce was overwhelmingly medical; 70 years later, doctors made up barely 24%, 36,000, of the total. Administrative and non-clinical roles numbered 70,000.

The numbers working in primary care have increased but so have the size of the practices in which they work. The evolution of practices from single to group to networks has resulted in a larger workforce employed under one management, disrupting team cohesion, and fracturing the link with the local community it serves. The importance of strong interpersonal relationships has been reduced to an irrelevance. The vocational element of all roles has diminished. Scaling up general practice may well bring benefits, but at a cost.

Doctors have also had to relinquish some of their cherished autonomy. Partnerships have evolved with some members moving into strategic executive roles whilst others remain focused purely on the clinical. Friction can arise between the two, hampered by an increasingly itinerant medical workforce with no say in anything bar the patient in front of them.

Regardless of change, primary care has and will always provide an exemplary service to the citizens of the UK. GPs are used to adapting and making the best of the prevailing circumstances. Teams working in GP surgeries have always remained primarily focused on meeting the healthcare concerns of their patients. Respect, courtesy, and kindness can overcome all hurdles.

---

[17] www.nuffieldtrust.org.uk/news-item/what-does-the-gp-workforce-look-like-now

3

The Working Week

As it was in the beginning, is now, and ever shall be, work without end.
(Apologies to *The Anglican Book of Common Prayer*)

3.1 INTRODUCTION

Has a GP's working week changed over the past 70 years? The simple answer is no, or at least, very little. A time-travelling doctor from the 1950s could still walk into a GP practice on any given Monday morning in 2020, out again on a Friday afternoon, and not feel at all out of place. Why? Because, to date, GPs continue to function under the central precept that underpins their existence: seeing patients. Everything was and still is organised around this kernel of activity. The other elements of general practice, the business, administration, information technology, maintenance of medical knowledge, outside interests, and additional income streams have always been bolted onto the lattice of the clinical surgeries that take place every weekday of the year.

So, what constitutes the pattern of the average working week for full-time GP principals? How many hours do they work? How many patients do they see? How are duties allocated? How is the time apportioned to the clinical/administrative/educational requirements of a GP? The answers to these questions are more opaque than one might expect, primarily because of the self-employed status of the GP and consequent presumption of autonomy. In theory, GPs can do whatever they like! But of course, in practice, this is not so.

Prior to the 2004 GMS contract and the sea of change it brought about, GPs were individually contracted to provide round-the-clock care for their patients for every day of the year. This obligation was loosened somewhat in the 1966 GMS contract that allowed some flexibility in managing how they chose to administer this onerous charge. A single-handed GP working in isolation in a rural community, geographically remote from any other practice, would have little choice but to continue to provide an isolated, personal, and comprehensive cover for his patients. On the other hand, a colleague in a more populated area had the option of sharing the workload, especially for out-of-hours and holidays, with nearby practices, GP deputising services, or OOH cooperatives. However, regardless of their previous individual circumstance, the GMS 2004 contract provided the

DOI: 10.1201/9781003256465-3

first significant reprieve from the general practice daily 24-hour commitment, in place for over half a century.

Set times for direct patient contact, 'surgeries,' or 'sessions' structure the week. Despite no clear definition of what a session entails, the consensus is a 3.5-hour period that includes seeing patients on-site and dealing with the accompanying paperwork. Each weekday is split into two half-day sessions. Theoretically, a full-time GP principal undertakes ten sessions in a week; in fact, this is rarely so. Most do eight or nine sessions. The deficit ostensibly allows GP partners time to deal with the other aspects of general practice, such as administration and training. However, the half and sometimes whole day was traditionally subsumed into periods for rest and recreation, to compensate for night-time and weekend work. How GPs spent that time was entirely down to the individual; typical activities ranged from hobbies; golf, sailing, and stamp collecting, to work-related; catching up on medical journals, scrutinising the accounts, or, inexplicably for an overworked and stressed professional, supplementing income through locum work at another practice! Certainly, whatever one did during this time, it was tacitly accepted that it should rarely be spent on practice premises. It was protected time that GPs could use in any way they wished.

The length of the working day has remained constant over the lifetime of the NHS, set at 8.00 a.m. to 7.00 p.m. The doors of the surgery would be open between those hours, although in later years, some practices would close for lunch to 'allow staff to catch up.'

The average day was organised around a morning and an evening, or rather, a late afternoon surgery. Morning surgery began at 8.30 or 9.00 a.m. and ran for three hours. Afternoon surgery began at 4.00 p.m. and ran for a slightly shorter period.

The composition of appointments within a session varied little over the years. From 1950–1975, patients were allocated, on average, five minutes for an appointment. This time gradually increased to seven and a half minutes, and by the turn of the millennium, it was ten, even a heady fifteen minutes. The increase in length of the consultation responded to patients' expectations, increasing complexity of patients' conditions accompanying increased longevity, chronic disease management, preventive medicine, the threat of litigation, and counter-intuitively, computerisation. In the early years of the NHS, the time limitation on the consultations matched the physical limitations, with the cramped space of the Lloyd George record card discouraging any more than the most cursory record-keeping.

A doctor would expect to see around 18 booked appointments in the morning and 15 in the evening. Any 'extras' that urgently needed to be seen would be added to that day's number. The total number seen varied from day to day and could double in times of extra demand, such as winter. Mondays and Fridays were always busy, due to holding back from and in anticipation of the weekend. On any day, it was rare for a surgery not to be fully booked.

The variety of acute presentations at a GP clinic has remained constant over the decades. A (by no means comprehensive) list of physical presenting symptoms included (chronologically by age) crying, pyrexia, diarrhoea and vomiting, earache, sore throat, rash, acne, contraception, conception, headache, backache, dyspepsia, bleeding from various orifices, menopause, fatigue, joint pain, and frailty. Mental health symptoms included failure to meet developmental milestones; behavioural problems; self-harming; anxiety; depression; physical, emotional, or sexual abuse; and dementia. Whilst presenting symptoms changed little over time, their prevalence has, with mental health and dementia coming to the fore. Staple chronic conditions, hypertension, diabetes, asthma, chronic obstructive pulmonary disease (COPD), and epilepsy were interspersed amongst the acute presentations. In later years, prescription reviews joined the list.[1,2]

The morning session would end with a coffee, some administrative tasks that included referral letters, prescription signing, and telephone calls, and the distribution of home visits that had been requested during the morning. The number of home visits varied from day to day and practice to practice, but they tended to be greater on Mondays. The only constant was calls to residential and nursing homes, which by and large remained steady throughout the week.

Over the decades, patients were weaned away from expecting a home visit. Certainly, in the early years of the NHS, tradition and received wisdom still governed patients' expectations, so, for example, a child with a high temperature was to be kept in bed; thus, a doctor's opinion could only be gained by a home visit. It was difficult convincing a worried parent that exposure to fresh air would not jeopardise their child's well-being. Anxious parents asked to attend the surgery could become quite irate and abusive. Almost imperceptibly, parental attitudes changed as GPs sensitively but remorselessly pursued a policy of patient education facilitated by continuity of care and the application of 'best practice.'

Changes in the pattern of home visits from 1970 to 2020:

Home Visits	1970	2020
Child with a high temperature	Almost always	Rarely
Child with vomiting	Often	Rarely
Acute back pain	Often	Rarely
Chest pain	Almost always	Never. Call 999
Stroke	Almost always	Never. Call 999
Residential/nursing home	Infrequent	Frequent
Urinary retention	Almost always	Direct to Accident & Emergency
Psychotic episode	Often	Sometimes. Community Mental Health Team
Vaginal bleeding in first trimester	Often	Rarely. Midwife or maternity unit
Intra-natal and post-partum care	Frequent	Never
Patients in hospital	Sometimes	Rarely

[1] Cooke G, Valenti L, Glasziou P, Britt H. Common general practice presentations and publication frequency. Aust Fam Physician. 2013 Jan–Feb;42(1–2):65–8. PMID: 23529466.

[2] Ten most common conditions seen by GPs Harry Brown British Journal of Family Medicine, 6 July 2019. www.bjfm.co.uk/ten-most-common-conditions-seen-by-gps

The choice of whether or not a home visit was warranted rested with the doctor; social conditions informed such decisions as much as the clinical. The doctor's intuition of the circumstances regarding the request also played no small part.

In the early years of the NHS, transport links were poor. Few households had cars. There were five million cars in the UK in 1960, compared to 40 million in 2020. Telephones at home were just as rare. Even by 1970, only a third of households had a telephone line. As a result, doctors often maintained lengthy lists of patients whom they visited on a regular basis; more often the elderly with chronic conditions, such as chronic obstructive pulmonary disease or osteoarthritis, due as much to social as to medical concerns. The pressure of time management and the dubious benefits that arose from such visits gradually put paid to such practices, so that by the late 1980s, they had become a rarity, especially in group practice. It became incumbent upon a newly appointed GP partner to cull the lengthy list of home visits inherited from a retiring partner. Some did so more enthusiastically than others, much to the chagrin of both patients and sometimes colleagues.

Anecdotal tales surrounding home visits included a single-handed village GP who, after the Christmas Day service, would partake of a wee dram with the vicar before walking home to his turkey dinner. On the way, he would pop in to one or two parishioners and share a sherry with them. After some years, the vicar, having noted this, asked the doctor why he chose to visit some but not others on his Christmas walks. The wise old doctor replied that the ones he visited were the ones who would not live to see another Christmas. They may not have known it, but he was bidding them a final farewell. Another related to a man who had been bedbound for 30 years; his incarceration had originated in the 1960s when he had developed acute abdominal pain. His patrician doctor advised he should stay in his bed until the doctor returned to tell him otherwise. The doctor never returned and retired soon afterwards, leaving illegible records that his recently qualified replacement could not decipher. He continued the visits. Both patient and subsequent doctors, too respectful of the original doctor's advice, colluded in the status quo until the patient died of a pulmonary embolism at the age of 70. A post-mortem revealed no pathology apart from a DVT, much to the distress of his family who felt that their lives had been martyred to a fictitious illness.

The time taken for home visits varied according to their number and complexity. A significant complicating factor would be an illness requiring hospital admission that could often take hours to arrange. On such occasions, the doctor could forget any prospect of lunch.

Urgent callouts could also occur during morning surgery whilst a doctor was still responsible for patients registered on his or her personal list. As a rule, as of midday, urgent requests from patients would be passed to the on-call partner. Should a call come in about a patient with chest pain, then the doctor would drop everything, terminate the consultation underway and immediately attend the patient off-site. This created yet more pressure on the doctor who, on the one hand, was trying to focus on delivering appropriate care to the patient at home whilst, on the other, was distracted by thoughts of patients piling up at the surgery. The latter would still expect to be seen. These pressures tested the integrity of the practice team; invariably and ideally, his partners would chip in and slot those waiting patients into their already full surgeries. Similar pressures arose in the delivery of maternity services, especially labour, resulting in GPs willingly relinquishing such care to midwives when the latter became more assertive in defining their role. However, the GP was still called upon where the insertion of an intravenous drip, episiotomy, or forceps delivery was required.

Writing up the notes on a home visit would be done retrospectively on the Lloyd George cards scattered around the footwell of the doctor's car.

The first half of the day's work would ordinarily be completed by 2.00 p.m., allowing a reasonable gap in the day during which doctors, most of whom lived either in or within a short distance of the surgery, could unwind at home before returning to the fray for the evening session. The doctor on call for the day was expected to keep in touch with the receptionists but not necessarily be present at the surgery. They also had a booked evening surgery which, depending on the partners' generosity, might contain gaps for patients requiring an urgent appointment.

The afternoon break could also be filled with other tasks, for example private work, such as insurance medical reports, or other time-consuming activities, such as minor surgery. Many GPs ran an antenatal or child health clinic in the slot between the morning and evening surgeries.

The evening session was a more relaxed affair for the doctors not on call. A fixed number of patients were booked, and complications, such as urgent admission to hospital, were rare.

The last appointment would be for 6.00 p.m., and the doctor could expect to head home an hour later. Surgery doors would close at 7.00 p.m., and the on-call doctor was left to manage any further requests until 8.00 a.m. the following day when the routine would be repeated.

3.2 OUT-OF-HOURS

The out-of-hours workload varied. The evening might bring in some calls around minor conditions, especially in children, many of which could be managed over the telephone. As a rule, patients were reluctant to phone a doctor after midnight, and calls after this time would trigger alarm bells, with a home visit the rule rather than the exception. Rarely did an on-call doctor have an undisturbed night's sleep. In practice, it was difficult to sleep soundly in the knowledge that they could be roused at any time. Naturally, this also affected the doctor's spouse, who would not only be disturbed by the sporadic ringing of the phone but would need to remain vigilant after the doctor had left, to answer any additional calls. Often, a nocturnal home visit was more expedient than lying awake in bed mulling over potentially serious symptoms. Nobody enjoyed a night on call.

Doctors could claim a nominal fee from the FHSA (£17.50 in 1990) for each face-to-face consultation that took place between 11.00 p.m. and 7.00 a.m. Plumbers were charging £30 at that time for a similar service. The derisory sum did not compensate for, but at least recognised, the stress inherent in these nocturnal requests. Paltry as it was, the fee still acted as an incentive to postpone an evening request for a home visit until after 11.00 p.m.

The doctor who had been on call during the night was still expected to undertake a normal morning surgery the following day. In fact, the expectation would be to continue with a normal day's duties, though many practices would factor in a half-day off after an on-call session. Such a move was prudent. The doctor was unlikely to function efficiently or, more importantly, safely after a poor night's sleep.

The on-call roster for each doctor followed the same pattern each week, only varying if a partner was away. Then, another doctor would double up on duties to cover that absence. Friction between partners would arise if anyone was thought to be abusing this arrangement by taking excessive annual leave or sickness absence for a minor ailment. A culture of endurance was encouraged; absenteeism on health grounds was extremely low.

The practice would close for the week at 7.00 p.m. on a Friday evening. The weekend would be covered by the on-call partner from that time until 8.00 a.m. Monday morning, a total of 61 unbroken hours. Most practices tried to relieve some of the pressure by having a restricted surgery on Saturday morning, where an additional doctor and skeleton staff would attempt to lessen the impending burden. In due course and recognition of the onerous burden, many practices chose to either split the weekend days internally or enter into an informal relationship with other local surgeries. The benefits of collaboration included fewer weekends on call; the drawbacks were that they would be extremely busy! In part, the changes reflected the increased patient demand over the decades.

3.3 ANNUAL LEAVE

The time allotted for annual leave, generally set at six weeks, was consistent across most practices. One week for 'study' leave was added to that number. It was considered good form to take leave in weeks rather than days. However, since the nature of the GP's role was one of a self-employed individual running his own business, many partners did not take their full allocation of annual leave. There was a strong ethos in partnerships that elevated the duties to the practice above everything else. The understanding was based on reciprocity and guilt; if you were away, then those remaining had to do extra work, and vice versa.

3.4 EDUCATION MEETINGS

Extracurricular educational meetings took place quite frequently and were almost exclusively sponsored and funded by the pharmaceutical industry. Sales representatives, 'reps,' arranged meetings and conferences that took place at the local postgraduate centre, practice, or restaurant. Industry funding was generous, and cheque books were always open to pay the bill at the end of yet another agreeable meal. Did they secure any extra influence or business because of this practice, subsequently all but outlawed by the Association of British Pharmaceuticals Industry? It might be naïve to think not; British GPs were far too cynical, educated, and independent, but it would be hard to make the case in light of a sophisticated industry that was unlikely to spend its marketing budget for no commercial return.

Attendance at educational meetings was sporadic and dictated by the topic of the meeting. Pharmaceutical companies, having invested heavily in developing a drug, would ensure that they had recognised names willing to endorse its qualities over and above those of their competitors. These 'unbiased' experts were used to spice up a dry subject and entice GPs to attend. Yet, often, the presentations were repetitive, mimicking those of competitors, and campaigns running over years would inevitably lead to meeting fatigue and a consequent drop in the numbers attending. That was particularly so in the 1980s and 1990s, with the introduction of more beta-blockers, calcium channel blockers, ACE inhibitors, and statins. Subsequent decades saw attendance at local meetings drop off significantly until only a handful of die-hard GPs would attend, even when the venue was a Michelin-starred restaurant.

The structure of the working week remained largely unchanged until the general roll-out of computerisation in the 1990s. Computers were and remain paradoxically labour-intensive, resulting in doctors lingering longer in their consulting rooms. Computers allowed for electronic messaging, cutting down on face-to-face interaction. GPs within a practice began seeing less of one another. The increase in the average consulting time compounded the isolation. Surgeries became longer and gaps between, shorter. Lunch became a sandwich eaten in the surgery rather than a hot meal at home.

3.5 WEEKLY WORKLOAD

Managing patients involved more than just the face-to-face consultation in the surgery. Innumerable collateral activities included reviewing pathology results, reading correspondence, writing prescriptions, and responding to primary care organisation (PCO) directives, to name but a few. GPs found the bureaucracy increasingly burdensome. Data inputting became an increasingly significant part of the job. In particular, the voracious appetite for data required for the QOF was both disrupting and time-consuming in any consultation. The demands of QOF remained a distraction despite being passed, in part, to the administrative team. GPs in the 21st century continued to cite bureaucracy in general and QOF in particular[3] as contributory factors in lowering morale.

The working practices of fellow healthcare professionals were also changing. Nowhere was this more evident than in midwifery where GPs effectively and happily surrendered all care for pregnancy to midwives, including intrapartum and the dreaded episiotomies. Paramedics were being added to ambulances, and the definition of 'emergency' was expanded and diluted. Some practices had a paramedic embedded on-site, to undertake urgent home visits. People with chest pain or stroke symptoms were advised to call 999 rather than their GP. Disruptions of booked surgeries fell dramatically, reducing one area of potential GP stress.

---

[3] Owen K, Hopkins T, Shortland T, Dale J. GP retention in the UK: a worsening crisis. Findings from a cross-sectional survey. BMJ Open. 2019 Feb 27;9(2):e026048. doi: 10.1136/bmjopen-2018-026048. PMID: 30814114; PMCID: PMC6398901.

Table 1.1 Summarises some of the changes that took place in the activities of the typical working week over five decades.

1970	2020
5-minute appointments	10–15-minute appointments
Surgeries disrupted by emergency calls	Surgeries less likely to be disrupted by emergency calls
GPs called to chest pain	Call 999
GPs called to strokes	Call 999
Paper investigation results unlinked from patient notes	Electronic investigation results automatically linked to patient records
Calls for residential/nursing homes rare	Calls for residential/nursing homes common
No QOF or similar data inputting	QOF or similar data inputting
Maternity care at any time	No maternity care
Phlebotomy by GP	Phlebotomist
Chronic disease management by GP	Chronic disease management by nurse
Childhood vaccinations by GP	Childhood vaccinations by nurse
Cervical cytology screening by GP	Cervical cytology screening by nurse
Hospital visits by GP	Hospital visits rarely done
Palliative care by GP	Shared with district nurses, Macmillan nurses, and hospice
No CQC	Compliance with CQC inspections
No revalidation	Compliance with annual appraisals for revalidation

Rules dictating that GPs should live within a short radius of the practice premises were relaxed, leading to doctors commuting to their workplace from ever-greater distances. This made going home at midday impractical, making the day much like that in any workplace, albeit a tad longer since it still covered 11 hours from 8.00 a.m. to 7.00 p.m.

By 2020, in-house and locality-based education meetings had all but disappeared, as had drug reps visiting GP surgeries. The latter had become an irritant as the free time a GP had in any day became progressively squeezed.

However, the number of formal practice meetings in any one month increased, in response to many demands, including frequent changes to clinical protocols and care plans, changes to referral criteria, PCO initiatives and communications, significant-event and complaint audits, and multidisciplinary team meetings covering care of the elderly, palliative care, and deaths. Most such meetings still took place over lunch, but practices increasingly ring-fenced time, periodically closing their doors to routine consultations.

The single change that had the greatest impact on the GP working week was the removal of 24/7 responsibility for patient care that was part of the seminal

GMS contract of 2004. At a stroke (and albeit theoretically), a GP's weekly hours were reduced by two-thirds from 168 to 55. Although the contract went live in April of that year, the portion passing responsibility for OOH to other providers was delayed by six months, to allow external provisions to be placed. Primary care trusts were charged with the responsibility of creating an OOH service, often from scratch, because many GP cooperatives had chosen to disband. Service specifications were rushed through, new commercial players in the field submitted tenders, and within six months, all GPs choosing to do so could reclaim a significant portion of their lives for the loss of less than 6% of their income. Most GPs could not sign the cheque fast enough. They felt liberated from arguably the most onerous part of their working life. Older, jaded doctors contemplating retirement postponed plans to do so, temporarily staving off a manpower shortage that was threatening the very viability of primary care in the UK. Happy days were here again, but for how long?

3.6 SUMMARY

The structure of a GP's working week may not have changed since 1948, but the intensity certainly has. GPs may see much the same number of patients each day, but the work related to those patients has expanded greatly.

By 2019, general practice morale had sunk to a new low. When asked why this is so, GPs commonly cited the extra burdens of bureaucracy and the removal of autonomy that were the unforeseen consequences of the 2004 GP contract. The need to provide evidence of work undertaken and the increased scrutiny by both the public and professional bodies all added to the pressures of the day. They felt that the soul of family practice had been sold for a figurative handful of silver. But were these activities as onerous as reported?

Although QOF requires time-consuming vigilance in undertaking certain prescribed data inputting, such as blood pressure monitoring or smoking advice, many of these tasks were delegated to nurses and administrative staff, greatly assisted by increasingly sophisticate clinical software that allows for automated data capture. Computerisation has facilitated other administrative activities, such as monitoring correspondence, investigations, internal messaging, and issuing prescriptions, making them safer, slicker, and more efficient than before. Arguably, modern voice recognition and other dictation systems have speeded up the referral process although doctors must now check and comply with a referral algorithm before dictating a letter.

National Service Frameworks set out guidance on managing medical conditions, and this has undoubtedly had an impact on autonomy and the doctor's sense of self-worth. The need to justify everything to an ever-intrusive PCO generates a need to spend more time on administration and less in clinical practice.

The requirements of General Medical Council doctor revalidation and CQC compliance are perceived as a burden that adds little to improving patient services. Many GPs view these requirements as a distraction from a doctor's core duties. Yet, apart from the infrequent CQC inspections, they take little time out of the working week.

National and local initiatives or 'schemes' extending surgery hours into the evenings and weekends are generally voluntary; if undertaken at all, they are not too burdensome when partners split them up.

GPs also cite the increasing complexity of clinical practice as a further contributor to early burnout. They have tried to adapt by increasing consultation times, but this has inevitably led to longer surgeries with less downtime in between. The introduction of telephone triage and consultations, with talk of adding teleconsulting, such as Skype or Zoom, to the scenario, in the expectation that the change in practice will save time, and improve productivity, have proven to be a mirage. The technology merely increases the number of patients seen.

Dealing with patients and their illnesses is both demanding and exhausting, and there is a limit to how many interactions a doctor can manage before they seize up mentally. GPs in 2020 are dealing with up to 50 patients on any given day. Such numbers are not only unsustainable but also potentially dangerous.

An overlooked factor contributing to GP stress is the isolation inherent in the role. Despite human interactions numbering in the hundreds every week, the role of a GP is a lonely one. Opportunities to meet and offload with colleagues are limited. Established GPs are reluctant to sit in on each other's surgeries, losing a golden opportunity to both learn from and support each other. The collegiate nature of small-group practice has given way to the anonymity and threat of censure in large primary care networks. GPs in large group practices are as isolated now as they were in single-handed practices in 1948. Sadly, the social side of partnership has all but disappeared, to the detriment of all.

The basics of a GP's working week never changed. What has changed is the intensity. As the new millennium became established, the workload became ever more arduous as the twin evils of increasing patient demand and decreasing GP workforce numbers began to lead to a crumbling of the primary care edifice.

The overriding counterpoint to many of the negative issues raised here is that of a clearly defined, albeit long working week, shorn of out-of-hours, night, and weekend responsibilities. The stress associated with out-of-hours work cannot be overstated. It was a significant contributor to burnout and early retirement.

Doctors entering general practice since 2004 have had a markedly different working experience than their predecessors. It might even be mischievously suggested that this cohort of doctors has been allowed to indulge in what initially attracted them to a career in medicine, that is, the luxury of time to actually practise medicine!

Yet, fundamentally, the timetable of the working week has remained unchanged since the beginning of the NHS. Every day is intense and stressful. There is no such thing as a quiet day. Every generation feels that it has had to work harder than the one before. There is a timeless consistency about general practice that transcends generations.

And what of our time-travelling GP from 1948? Given a six-month refresher course and some IT training, they would surely find little problem settling into our 'modern' GP practices. After all, the basis of the job remains as it always was, seeing patients.

4

Out-of-Hours

For the night is dark and full of terrors.

(George R R Martin)

4.1 INTRODUCTION

'Out-of-hours' almost deserves a whole book to itself since it played such a signifi-cant part, both temporal and emotional, in the GP's life.

For the first two decades after the founding of the NHS, the term 'out-of-hours' (OOH) was unrecognised by GPs who were individually contracted to provide medical services for their patients 24 hours a day, 7 days a week, 365 days a year. The GP contract of 1966 introduced recognition of OOH with the introduction of payments for medical services outside of the 'normal' day. The term also covered weekend, bank, and festive holidays. Thereafter, OOH remained an onerous part of the GP's workload until the GP contract of 2004 removed the responsibility for arranging for that cover. Indeed, the burden of year-round medical provision and its contribution to GP burnout, low morale, and early retirement was argu-ably the prime reason for a new understanding between the profession and the government, the 2004 contract.

Up to the first major renegotiation of the GP contract in 1966, most GPs worked independently as sole practitioners running their own surgeries, often out of their homes, and looking after lists numbering more than 3,000 patients. The individual doctor organised their daily routine. The recognition of a defined 'day' that would start around 8.00 a.m. and finish around 7.00 p.m., during which the doctor would run surgeries, undertake home visits, deal with emergencies, deliver babies, visit patients at home, and complete any administrative tasks, left the night for responding to urgent and emergency calls.

Since many practices were run from the doctor's residence, there was consid-erable blurring of the boundaries between work and family life. The latter gave way to the demands of the former. Conscious of the doctor's devotion to their care and well-being, most patients were respectful and considerate in making demands on their doctor, a member of the community with whom they closely identified. They only called on their doctor when they felt they absolutely had to.

DOI: 10.1201/9781003256465-4

Yet, this rose-tinted view of the stoical labourer of 'olde' England, collectively doffing his cap to the venerable physician, was likely to have been the stuff of sentimental fiction; in practice, following the creation of the NHS, the service almost collapsed within the year due to the huge demands made on it.

Access to free medical services led to a surge in demand from a long-suffering population that no longer saw a fiscal need to endure any symptoms of ill health, no matter how minor. A review of clinical records kept by an Essex country GP in 1965, revealed entries peppered with frustration. Phrases such as 'trivial case only needing a little common sense!' liberally covered each page. Patients' petty demands irritated doctors then as they do now.

Few houses had a telephone. Doctors may have had one, but many of their patients did not. Thus, the only way that patients could contact their doctor was in person, by turning up at the surgery.

Transport was limited. Few people had cars, and most were dependent on public transport or, more likely, their own two feet. For the same reasons, home visits were much more common and often routine, especially for children, older patients, and the chronically infirm.

The combinations of these factors led many GPs to reside within their communities and have a clearly defined geographic practice area in which their patients lived.

A detailed and moving account of the life of a GP, Dr David Geddes-Brown, in the 1960s is well worth a read.[1]

Even before the introduction of the 1966 GP contract and its encouragement to form group practices, GPs were collaborating to provide cover for each other, to release some recreational time. Initially, informal liaisons between neighbouring practices would allow a *quid pro quo* arrangement in which a doctor would pass over limited responsibility for his patients for a defined period. Thus, the occasional weekday afternoon and night off became a reality, allowing the doctor to be able to truly rest without fear of being disturbed. This, in turn, led to the glacially slow relaxation of the Presbyterian work ethic that drove most doctors at that time, much to the relief of their families. In due course, doctors began to cherish this time off so that few demurred when, 40 years later, they witnessed the introduction of the 'office hours' working week.

Prior to 1963, when collecting official data on manpower began, fewer than 29% of medical students were female.[2] GPs were thus predominately male, likely working from one location, their home, a modest Victorian edifice where the consulting room was a converted front room, complete with desk, examination couch, privacy screen, and shelves covered in dusty manuals and apothecary bottles. Another part of the house, often a section adjoining the kitchen, may have been converted into a rudimentary pharmacy for dispensing pills, potions, and

[1] www.dailymail.co.uk/news/article-2385735/80-patients-day-27-home-visits-On-night—The-humbling-diary-GP-different-age.html

[2] Jefferson L, Bloor K, Maynard A. Women in medicine: historical perspectives and recent trends. Br Med Bull. 2015 Jun;114(1):5–15. doi: 10.1093/bmb/ldv007. Epub 2015 Mar 8. PMID: 25755293.

lotions. The dispenser? Probably the spouse. The receptionist? Almost definitely the spouse. The administrator? The doctor!

The spouse dealt with phone calls and attending patients waiting patiently to be seen. Patients trudged to the surgery during open times, gave their name to the receptionist, and joined others in the queue waiting to see the doctor. The lucky ones might even have had a chair to sit on. The wait was invariably long. Eventually, their name was called, and they were ushered through the door for their five minutes with the doctor. The wait may have been even longer than usual when the doctor had been called out to an emergency. Those patients left in the waiting area did not complain. There was a tacit understanding that others might have a greater need of the doctor's time than they did. Nevertheless, they waited until the doctor's return. And thus, the day continued until the early evening when the doors finally closed.

The expectation that an emergency call might come in at any time only added to the stress arising from a previously busy day. The normal routines of family life, playing with the children, meals, sleep, took place in the knowledge that a knock on the door or a phone call could derail them at any time. An elderly man with chest pain? A young woman in labour? A child with croup? Anything could happen, so the doctor had to remain alert. Trouble-free nights did not necessarily lead to a trouble-free mind. The one constant was that whatever the evening and night brought, the following day would commence as it always did, proceeding along its predetermined path.

Individual doctors adjusted to these nocturnal pressures as best they could. Some snatched moments of relaxation, perhaps aided by a tot of whisky, between calls; others remained on high alert throughout. No matter how they coped, the OOH nightmare was an accepted part of the doctor's life. Many GPs had served in the armed forces during the World War II and were accustomed to the privations of military service. All had previously trained in unforgiving, unsupported hospital jobs with onerous rotas and 80-hour shifts and they were used to sacrificing their sleep to work. However, such working conditions did have repercussions on their own health. Life expectancy of GPs was lower than their peers in other professions, such as dentists, lawyers, bankers. Doctors were more likely to succumb to heart attacks, strokes, alcoholism, and suicide. The noble Dr Geddes-Browne died aged 63 years.[3]

Working from home did allow the doctor some time with his family. Whilst it meant that family and work were inextricably entwined, there was room for the doctor to switch smoothly from one to the other. Slack periods during surgery hours allowed the GP to retire to the kitchen for a cup of tea, a read of the newspaper, and, likely, a smoke. Since the doctor's home was in the practice area, home visits were within a short distance and could be completed with minimum disruption to the doctor's day. Arguably, time was used more efficiently.

3 Geddes-Brown L. Spectator: Leslie Geddes-Brown on the NHS. Country Life, 7 Aug 2013. Accessed 7 Oct 2021 from www.countrylife.co.uk/comment-and-opinion/spectator/spectator-leslie-geddes-brown-on-the-nhs-6136

My first experience of general practice was for just such a practice. I had just completed my year's preregistration house jobs in the summer of 1976, and I had moved to London whilst awaiting a job abroad. I applied to an advertisement in the *BMJ* that a single-handed GP in Kew had placed, seeking a locum for two weeks of holiday cover. I was invited for an interview. A caricature of a wizened and wise hospital consultant, resplendent in a solemn grey three-piece suit, greeted me in the fusty parlour of a splendid Georgian house. We spent ten minutes in general polite conversation. No questions regarding skills or experience were asked. I was shown around the 'surgery,' a lounge with French doors that opened out onto an overgrown garden. We shook hands and I started the next day. His formidably built housekeeper *cum* receptionist fussed around me, making sure I was not bothered by any unnecessary trivia whilst constantly plying me with tea and cake. My surgeries tended to be underbooked because patients were generally happier waiting for the 'real' doctor to return from his well-deserved rest. I spent the nights sleeping on a lavishly upholstered examination couch in the consulting room. Night calls were few. The ubiquitous Mrs F answered the telephone and, if a visit was requested, would wake me with a hot drink before sending me on my way. It was a most genteel introduction to general practice and, in addition, one that paid handsomely well for a recently qualified doctor! Nevertheless, my anxieties regarding the quality of the care I was providing and even more so the thought of being called out at night made me feel that it was money well earned. I almost exploded with relief when Dr W finally returned to take up the reins.

The on-call arrangements I experienced in the mid-1970s were typical for a single-handed practice. After 'hours,' a human being, the doctor or his spouse, had to answer the telephone. The process for a patient gaining access to a doctor was both simple and direct.

A decade later, telephone answering machines had replaced the redoubtable Mrs F, a replacement not without its own problems. Issues arose as to who would record the message, what it would say, the clarity of the instructions, the responsibility for turning the machine on in the evening and off the following morning. Monday mornings could be eerily quiet if patients rang in only to be greeted by the information that 'the surgery is now closed.'

From solitary practitioners moving to a loose arrangement with like-minded local colleagues, to the formal development of group practice that the 1966 GP contract encouraged and accelerated, doctors were slowly sharing OOH care, allowing protected time in the week when the doctor could genuinely switch off and relax with the family. Taking a weekday afternoon off became standard practice. In-house rosters for night-time and weekend work became the norm. Doctors accepted being busier when they were on call, in return for periods when they could freely relax. Nevertheless, anticipation of an impending weekend or bank holiday on call was met with increasing dread as the days approached.

Being on call not only affected the doctor but also the family. The doctor was self-centered, anxious, paranoid, and ill-tempered. As far as it existed, communication between members of the family was limited and terse. The children learned to keep out of the way of adults on such days. In the era before mobile phones, the spouse and, therefore, the children were confined to the house to answer the phone. In winter, this might have been acceptable, but on a hot summer's day, the family felt imprisoned. The situation marginally improved with the arrival of cordless phones in the 1980s. They extended the cordon sanitaire from the confines of the house, to include the garden. Their introduction saved many a marriage. The nights remained as disrupted for the spouse as for the partner. Invariably, a call from a patient would come in whilst the doctor was already out on another call. The doctor had to keep loose change about their person and be ready to phone home from a public call box, to save a journey in and then back out again. Nobody rested.

The evolution in telecommunications slowly made the routine more bearable. Supplementary landlines by the bed, phones with long cords, cordless and wireless phones, pagers, mobile phones the size and cost of a Luis Vuitton trunk, smartphones, all contributed to eventually making the spouse redundant and allowing the patient to contact the doctor directly, no matter where they each might be.

Each practice developed its own way of dealing with the OOH burden. Working together was better than working alone, though the option was not available to all. Single-handed and rural GPs often had to continue managing by themselves.

Practices in cities also had the option of subcontracting the OOH duties to deputising services, which came into being in the late 1960s. Deputising services[4] were commercially run companies, not contracted to the NHS, that for a substantial fee offered to cover any GP who wished to have some time off work. Despite their cover, individual GPs remained legally liable for the care of patients on their list. Although the costs of the service were significant, many inner-city GPs with large patient lists felt that the financial hit to their income outweighed that to their sanity. The availability of a deputising service also allowed some flexibility for cover if a GP needed time off at short notice, for ill health or family commitments. Fees in the Red Book[5] for night visits continued to be paid to the patient's GP and contributed to offsetting the costs of the deputising service.

Deputising services were based on the concept of a single site with a sizeable administration backing up clinicians responsible for both triaging calls and dealing with clinical problems. Many of the clinicians were local GPs, familiar with the area, looking to defray the cost of their own use of the service. Extra capacity came from junior hospital doctors looking for a little additional cash. The role was not an easy one. A service could cover a wide geographic area and a large population.

The use of commercial deputising services decreased following the NHS (Primary Care) Act 1997 that encouraged and funded the creation of GP

---

[4] https://api.parliament.uk/historic-hansard/commons/1977/jan/19/general-practitioners-deputising-services

[5] The Statement of Fees and Allowances by which GPs were paid for services provided under the General Medical Services (GMS) contract up to 2004.

out-of-hours cooperatives. Though structured and manned similarly to their private-sector forebears, local GPs managed and ran the cooperatives on a not-for-profit basis.

The definition of what constituted a night-time consultation remained remarkably constant throughout the lifetime of the NHS. The hours varied slightly but were essentially those from 7.00 p.m. to 7.00 a.m. A fee could only be claimed for face-to-face contact, not for telephone advice, an incentive more attractive to a deputising service than to an exhausted GP. The fee for a visit after 11 p.m. was £17 in 1990, equivalent to £40 in 2020. By 2004, the average income per GP from OOH fees was estimated at around £6,000 per annum, and this sum was deducted from the income of those opting out of OOH duties, following the GMS contract of that year. Commercial providers were subsequently invited to tender for providing OOH services, with the understanding that existing money would fund their services, the £6,000 plus £3,000 per GP that had previously funded OOH provision under GP cooperatives. The tenders proved to be wildly optimistic, and many providers struggled to meet their contractual costs.

Part of the reason why commercial providers had always struggled with meeting the demands of the OOH provision lay in their treatment of the patient as the customer, a person with a pricetag attached. That view ran contrary to what had existed in general practice, where the patient was regarded as a partner in the management of their condition. One of the mantras of general practice at that time was 'educating the patient.' It was thought positive and negative reinforcement could modify patient behaviour, to an extent to which they could manage minor symptoms, at least overnight, thus reducing demands on the service. Positive messaging included safety-netting and reassurance, should symptoms deteriorate. Negative messaging could include an explanation, delivered in a somewhat tetchy tone, that a sore throat would sort itself out within days and did not require antibiotics. But educating the patient required a consistent approach that was not provided in the early years following GPs self-imposed removal from OOH care. The numbers seen out-of-hours, rising before 2004, exploded thereafter.

A Derbyshire GP wrote in the *Times* newspaper:

> Even in my own practice in a small town nobody can explain to me why with a static population with 100% child immunisation the out of hours call rate went from six or seven per week in 1985 when I joined the practice to over 10 times that number in some weeks in 2004.[6]

Few partnerships had leeway for a morning off after a night's duty. The doctor was expected to get on with it, regardless of how tired or sleepy they might be. This was not entirely in the best interest of patients but remained the only practical way of dealing with daytime demand.

---

6 http://peterenglish.blogspot.com/2013/04/peter-holden-responding-to-times.html

What medical conditions would a doctor likely see at night? They varied from the trivial to life threatening. The doctor had to be very confident of the diagnosis to reject any call. Ultimately, it was less troubling seeing a patient than relying on the spoken word alone.

Ambulances were never called, nor was a patient ever admitted to hospital without first having an assessment by a GP. If the GP receptionist appeared to be a barrier to primary care, she was a free pass compared to a sleepy junior house officer who would pour derision on any suggestion that a patient would be admitted on history alone. Everyone had to be seen. The common causes for any call-out included distressed babies, pyrexia, diarrhoea and vomiting, sore throat, earache, pain in any area, bleeding from any source, urinary retention, stroke, and falls. GPs were also responsible for obstetric care, including prescribing strong analgesics, inserting intravenous drips, suturing episiotomies, and complex deliveries, all of which could result in many night-time hours attending a woman in labour. It is easy to see how this constant mental and physical demand could stoke a fatigue that would consume the constitution of even the most robust doctor.

By 1990, any lingering benefits of the 1966 contract had faded, and morale within the profession was once more at a low ebb. Newly graduated doctors no longer viewed general practice as a viable career option. In recognition of the precarious state of GP recruitment, the DH made some minor changes to the Statement of Fees and Allowance, broadening payments for items of service for OOH work and, in 1996, adding a sum of £3,000 per doctor per annum for the development of new OOH initiatives, foremost of which were the GP Cooperative.

4.2 GP COOPERATIVES

GP cooperatives had already been informally established in some parts of the country prior to the NHS Act of 1997, and the message coming out of them was highly encouraging. As the name suggested, cooperatives were founded on the principle of cooperation between local practices, to spread the workload of OOH care. Individual cooperatives varied in size depending on locality, with the largest covering populations of more than 50,000. They were entirely managed and manned by local GPs. Although not mandatory, practices tended to join as a unit, with the proviso that individual partners could opt-out if they chose to do so.

Various models of funding were used. The most common was based on patient numbers, with a practice paying a pro-rata sum per patient for all OOH cover. Since this could be a sizeable sum of money, doctors would be expected to recoup most of the outlay through undertaking paid clinical sessions for the cooperative. The model was an early example of a 'circular economy.' The choice was left to the individual doctor to balance the overall costs against the desire to be relieved of OOH work. Young principals with mortgages and school fees chose to do extra sessions; older doctors with fiscal burdens behind them prioritised undisturbed nights. These market forces led to a service that was generally well staffed throughout the year, including weekends and bank holidays. Since doctors tend to be a parsimonious bunch, clinical sessions were almost exclusively manned by local practitioners, bringing with them the advantages of knowing patients, locality and hospitals, continuity of care, peer benchmarking, and mutual support; all rather neat and tidy.

The administrative structure of the cooperative had to expand to deal with the intricacies of managing many doctors and tens of thousands of patients. Some became limited companies with a board of directors, a full-time secretary, and finance officer. Some operated out of existing surgery buildings, but most moved into rented offices with easy patient access. Nurses were hired to triage calls and deal with minor problems. Drivers were employed to chauffeur leased cars equipped with blue lights and decorated with the cooperative logo. In short, whereas a doctor and his wife had previously run an OOH service using a private, self-purchased mobile phone and car, undertaking the same work now required a hugely expanded and expensive infrastructure. Despite the increased costs, most cooperatives managed to balance their books, and some were indeed profitable, paying dividends to their shareholders, the local contributing GPs. Cooperatives became an example of practical Marxism operating in a capitalist society.

Cooperatives had other unexpected benefits. Since doctors from different practices had to work together, cross-fertilisation of ideas could lead to practice improvements. The week became more structured, with clearly defined periods of work and leisure. Spouses and children were liberated. A doctor at 'work,' whether during day or night, was out of the house, allowing family life to proceed peacefully without them. Equally, when the doctor was at home, they were likely to be rested and, therefore, easier to live with. Morale improved greatly.

This was genuine shift work, as practised in factories since the industrial age, and doctors took to it with alacrity. Shifts were defined, short, and often in the sociable company of colleagues. Doctors chauffeured to home visits could focus purely on the details of the medical case at hand. They carried an array of drugs and equipment, such as oxygen cylinders, parenteral fluids, and defibrillators, luxuries unheard of when operating alone. Some cooperative hubs were adjacent to hospital A&E departments, allowing a closer integration of emergency services and further breaking down of barriers between primary and secondary care. GPs fondly reminisce about these years as the golden age of OOH care. Sadly, it was not to last.

In addition to routine patient off-site care, a significant number of selfless doctors also provided emergency cover in liaison with the ambulance service. They acted as an enhanced 'first responder,' attending road traffic accidents in their locality, frequently arriving at the scene before an ambulance. They were highly trained, comprehensively equipped, and skilled in enacting procedures, such as tracheal intubation and deep vein cannulation.

The service was voluntary, their attendance unpaid. Why did they do it? Undoubtedly, out of a sense of public duty, but many also claimed to enjoy a deep sense of satisfaction from using their skills in life-or-death situations, something that rarely took place in their daytime job. The role was regarded uncharitably by the volunteer's partners since 'emergency' calls often belied the definition, leaving them to see extra patients whilst the Samaritan was away.

4.3 THE CARSON REPORT 2000[7]

The developments and conversation surrounding out-of-hours medical services and the introduction of the national NHS Direct service in 1998 arose from the appointment of Dr David Carson, Head of Primary Care Strategy and Performance at East London and the City Health Authority, to head a commission to advise on the future of all urgent and emergency care. The commission reported in 2000 and made 22 recommendations, the core proposal being an integrated emergency service with a single point of contact, NHS Direct.

The Carson Report proposed a new model of integrated out-of-hours provision, commissioned by PCTs, at the heart of which were ease of access for

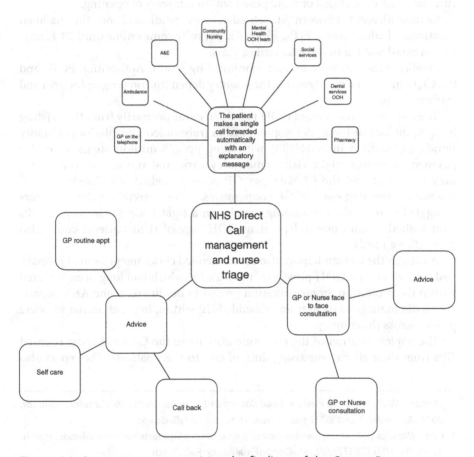

Figure 4.1 Organogram summarising the findings of the Carson Report.

[7] Department of Health. Raising standards for patients new partnerships in out-of-hours care. An independent review of GP out-of-hours services in England. 2000. The Carson Report is longer in print, but the recommendations can be accessed at: https://www.thewholesystem.co.uk/wp-content/uploads/2014/07/leedsoohrecs.pdf

patients, seamless information exchange amongst service providers, high-quality standards and control, flexible staffing, and adequate funding. To their credit, PCTs were quick to act and commissioned OOH services within six months of the ink drying on the 2004 GMS contract absolving GPs from their 24-hour duty of care. Patient access was not only improved through a central phone-line, initially NHS Direct, which became 111 in 2010, but also by the creation and expansion of Primary Care Centres: 230 walk-in centres[8] (or 369 urgent care centres)[9] and Darzi centres.[10] Local GPs welcomed any initiative that would alleviate the pressure on their surgeries but were baffled as to why these extra resources had not been allocated directly to those best able to manage them, themselves! Their reservations were confirmed. The additional centres proved to be expensive to run and most were closed or repurposed within ten years of opening.

Communication between stakeholders was predicated on the national Electronic Health Record, EHR, which did not fully come online until 2018, relying on email and fax in the intervening years.

Quality standards were set and monitored by Health Authorities, PCTs, and the CQC and varied widely across the country depending on geographic area and staffing levels.[11]

The funding of the revised OOH provision came primarily from the existing budget, the out-of-hours development fund (rebranded Out-of-Hours Quality Fund); £92 million in 2004/2005 with a top-up £28 million, items of service payments covering night visits, emergency care, and immediate and necessary treatment and the £3,000+ per GP principal which previously covered the annual running costs of GP cooperatives.[12] Commercial service providers struggled to meet the demanding metrics on a tight budget. Meanwhile, GPs who wished to continue independent OOH care of their patients could also access these funds.

Although the Carson Report also recommended closer integration of primary and secondary care OOH provision, the logic for which had long been accepted within the profession, implementation proved to be elusive. Some A&E departments did manage to include an embedded GP within, but such initiatives were patchy across the country.

The implementation of the recommendations in the Carson Report released GPs from their all-encompassing duty of care to their patients. The report also

8 Monitor. *Walk-In Centre Review: Final Report and Recommendations*. London: Monitor, 2014. Accessed 7 Oct 2021 from https://tinyurl.com/y8adqvpz

9 https://assets.publishing.service.gov.uk/government/uploads/system/uploads/attachment_data/file/283778/WalkInCentreFinalReportFeb14.pdf

10 Darzi centres: an expensive luxury the UK can no longer afford? BMJ. 2010;341:c6287. doi: 10.1136/bmj.c6287 (Published 8 Nov 2010).

11 www.nao.org.uk/report/hours-gp-services-england-2/

12 House of Commons Health Committee. GP Out-of-Hours Services Fifth Report of Session 2003–04 Volume 1. https://statesassembly.gov.je/scrutinyreviewresearches/2006/38359-10396-552006.pdf

informed the negotiations leading up to the GMS contract in 2004, which gave GPs the ability to opt-out of personal OOH service provision for the bargain price of £6,000 per annum, a sum more than offset by the 40% rise in income from meeting the targets set in QOF. Dr Eric Rose, a GP and member of the General Practitioners Committee of the BMA, wrote an insider's detailed account of these discussions and how the BMA negotiators, in effect, outwitted their DH counterparts by arriving at an OOH solution so advantageous to the profession.[13]

PCTs were tasked on short notice to set up an OOH service from scratch. Specifications were quickly written and invitations for tender sent out. Successful bidders included commercial providers; Harmoni (now Care UK),[14] IC24,[15] and Virgin Care;[16] NHS providers; ambulance trusts; and not-for-profit pre-existing cooperatives. Staffing the service proved to be problematic. Having offloaded the most onerous aspect of their working lives, GPs were naturally reluctant to pick up the load, particularly for a faceless corporation. The sessional pay may have been better than before but was not, of itself, incentive enough to encourage mass recruitment. Commercial providers had to resort to more imaginative use of resources, resulting in the employment of other healthcare professionals, such as nurses and paramedics, as well as doctors from the European Union. IT, in the form of health management algorithms, was deployed to assist clinicians. However, chronic understaffing remained unresolved.

Patient access to OOH services became disjointed and confused. Whereas previously a patient had only to ring their surgery, there was now a plethora of options: 999, 111, NHS Direct, walk-in centre, and OOH medical centre. The only constant was the obligatory wait before they were connected to a clinician. Eventually, patients gave up and, instead, used the one constant that had been left unaffected by all the recent changes, the one place guaranteed to be open, where they could always see a doctor, the local A&E department. Ironically, recently introduced NHS targets, such as the four-hour wait to be seen in A&E, made the latter even more accessible and attractive, compared to OOH centres.

The numbers attending A&E departments shot up in the first year after GPs relinquished OOH duties, rising from an annual 14 million in 2003/2004 to 17 million in 2004/2005. Eleven years later the number had reached 23 million.[17,18]

Meanwhile, the service provided by commercial OOH companies continued to deteriorate.

[13] Rose E. *The True History of GP Out of Hours Services. A Better NHS.* 10 May 2013. Accessed 7 Oct 2021 from https://abetternhs.net/2013/05/10/true-history/.

[14] www.careuk.com/

[15] www.ic24.org.uk/

[16] https://virgincare.co.uk/

[17] www.england.nhs.uk/statistics/wp-content/uploads/sites/2/2017/06/Monthly-AE-Report-April-17.pdf

[18] www.kingsfund.org.uk/blog/2013/04/are-accident-and-emergency-attendances-increasing

Studies evaluating patients' experiences reported that commercial providers were falling some way short of patients' expectations.[19] Patient satisfaction with their not-for-profit or NHS counterparts was higher. Companies responsible to their shareholders found it difficult to run a profitable service and pay a dividend on the tightly regulated income of around £8 per head of population. Or, to quote Dr Peter Holden, a General Practitioners Committee negotiator:

> Not-for-profit, John Lewis-type co-ops are the way to do out-of-hours. If you are insisting on a dividend, there's only so much money to run the service.[20]

GPs had even less confidence in NHS Direct, which was often dismissed as 'NHS Direct to your own doctor.' Morning surgeries became filled with patients with minor ailments who had been told to see their doctor immediately by NHS Direct. Initially, communications between OOH providers and GP surgeries were poor, resulting in requests for a patient to be seen that day arriving either later in the week or not at all.

By the 2020s, OOH provisions had become even more fragmented. Some doughty GPs were still caring for their own patients; traditional GP cooperatives still operated in some urban areas whilst social enterprises, hybrid private-public ventures, covered nearly 50% of the UK population.[21] Social enterprises, often GP federations,[22] worked well because they were organised from the bottom up. The social enterprise model of delivering OOH care proved to be successful for reasons that included strong communications with their GP stakeholders, uniform IT systems across all sites, respect and higher pay for its sessional clinicians, and not being held hostage to shareholder dividends. They were a prime example of how local providers, given the freedom to innovate, could best provide local solutions.

4.4 SUMMARY

The definition and details of the term 'medical services' have been a contentious subject at every GP contract negotiation since the founding of the NHS. However, the principle of a GP's 24/7, including organising and providing OOH care, for

---

[19] Barry HE, Campbell JL, Asprey A, Richards SH. The use of patient experience survey data by out-of-hours primary care services: a qualitative interview study. BMJ Qual Saf. 2016 Nov;25(11):851–9. doi: 10.1136/bmjqs-2015-003963. Epub 2015 Oct 21. PMID: 26490004; PMCID: PMC5136714.

[20] www.pulsetoday.co.uk/news/urgent-care/not-for-profit-gp-providers-cheaper-and-rated-higher-than-private-out-of-hours-firms/

[21] GP co-operatives mutate into out-of-hours social enterprises The Guardian, 20 Sep 2013. www.theguardian.com/social-enterprise-network/2013/sep/20/gp-co-operatives-out-of-hours-social-enterprise

[22] https://suffolkfed.org.uk/

patients was never questioned until the turn of the millennium; when it was, summarily, abolished!

Since 2004, debate has raged, at times heated, both in the public domain and within the profession, as to whether that decision should be reversed. So far, front-line clinicians have strongly resisted such a move, but some concessions, such as the introduction of extended-hours evening and weekend surgeries, have been made to placate the more hawkish administrators at Richmond House.[23]

The principle that all OOH care should be unified, or at the very least coordinated, remains sound, but its implementation has been flawed. Any failures, such as they are, can be blamed on the lack of an overall strategic plan, haphazard forward planning, and repeated NHS reorganisations. All these elements contributed to the initial confusion and chaotic roll-out of OOH provision following the 2004 GP contract.

PCTs were rushed into the tendering process for the provision of OOH services, which had to be functioning by 1 October 2004. Some PCTs negotiated with and co-opted pre-existing GP cooperatives, whilst others, wedded to the philosophy that the private sector was needed to bring fresh rigour into the public domain, chose commercial providers. Many winning bids came from businesses with no previous experience in healthcare management. Often these bidders seemed to be naively unaware of the constraints that a cash-strapped NHS contract would place on their future profitability and, thus, shareholder returns. Many providers subsequently gave up their contract due to financial losses or had their contract terminated due to poor service provision.

Around 40,000 GP principals were practising in the UK in 2004. Each had the option of giving up £6,000 of their annual income to opt-out of the provision of OOH services. If the £3,000 per GP principal allocated to GP cooperatives and the £92 million OOH development grant were included, then the total budget available for the provision of OOH services for a UK population of 60 million people amounted to around £450 million, or £7.50 per head! A small sum indeed, 5% of the overall budget for the NHS of £90 billion at that time. GPs had previously managed this financial sleight of hand on an even tighter budget but had only succeeded in doing so through a combination of martyred stoicism, an ethos of public service, and simply because they had to. In return, both their health and morale suffered. Had their efforts been better recognised and rewarded at the time, they might not have pushed so hard for the removal of OOH from their NHS contract. The fiasco of a fragmented and inadequate service in the following years only confirmed that a golden opportunity had been allowed to pass.

Despite no longer being directly involved, GPs remained committed to the welfare of their patients after hours. They recognised the faults in the new system and, although not wishing to return to the old, nevertheless reminisced about the days when GP cooperatives were as close to an ideal of marrying the aspirations of doctors and patients as had existed at any time within the NHS. Influential voices, such as that of Professor Clare Gerada, former chairperson of the Royal

---

[23] Government address of the Department of Health and Social Care.

College of General Practitioners, were pressing for the return of a hybrid OOH service, combining the best elements of GP cooperatives and private sector IT and call handling.[24] Such views gained considerable traction within the profession, and through the formation of social enterprises, provided OOH cover for over half the population of England and Wales by 2020.

In the final analysis, no data thus far have demonstrated a link between the partial removal of round-the-clock care by GPs and its replacement by a variety of OOH providers as adversely impacting morbidity or mortality. As a whole, the citizens of the UK have remained remarkably resilient and uncomplaining.

Doctors entering general practice after 2004 have not had to endure the obligatory panic of a night-time call or absence from the family on a Christmas Day. Their job may be less exciting but more sustainable than their predecessors. It is heartening to know that patients' health has not been compromised by the removal of OOH responsibility from GPs. That any doctor currently working in primary care would support reinstatement is highly unlikely.

---

[24] Davies M. Gerada: future GPs should take back OOH care. 2013. Accessed 7 Oct 2021 from www.pulsetoday.co.uk/news/urgent-care/gerada-future-gps-should-take-back-ooh-care/. See also another detailed account by Dr Peter Holden: Holden PJP. General practice to blame? eGPlearning, 30 Apr 2013. Accessed 7 Oct 2021 from http://egplearning.co.uk/ramblings/general-practice-to-blame/.

5

Information Management and Technology

Anything you can do; IT can do better.

(Apologies to Irving Berlin)

5.1 INTRODUCTION

The NHS differs from most healthcare systems around the world in having primary care as the first port of call for every person seeking medical advice. Thereafter, their medical records remain with their registered practice unless their personal circumstances change, for example, moving house. Both patient and doctor benefit from continuity of care, only possible if supported by a time-line of recorded interactions kept in one place. The system of record-keeping is fundamental to the provision of the holistic care. For the best part of a century, the main and, indeed, only form of medical record-keeping for a general practitioner was the Lloyd George card.[1]

5.2 MEDICAL RECORDS

Lloyd George records were introduced following the National Insurance Act 1911. They were widely used by health boards and private doctors prior to the founda-tion of the NHS in 1948. With more pressing issues at stake, they were retained under the NHS and remained in common use until the end of the millennium. Marginally bigger than a seaside postcard, they consisted of a beige card covered in closely spaced lines, red for men, blue for women. A summary card prefaced the bundle. All recorded information, including hospital correspondence, labora-tory results, and imaging reports, were kept in a slightly more robust envelope. The bulging package was subsequently stacked, like soldiers on parade, on basic bookshelves covering the walls behind the reception desk.

---

[1] https://peopleshistorynhs.org/museumobjects/lloyd-george-envelope/

DOI: 10.1201/9781003256465-5

To a degree, the paucity of space to record details was emblematic of the type of medicine carried out in the early 20th century, when medical knowledge was limited, patients' expectations low, access to investigations and therapeutics restricted, and consultation times short. For these reasons, entries tended to be concise and pithy. The use of space-saving acronyms, 'TATT' for 'tired all the time' or 'FLK' for 'funny looking kid,' covered much in a small space. Common presentations, such as 'sore throat,' and their treatment, 'penicillin,' would be entered in cryptic form, such as 'ST. Pen,' with no additional detail regarding the history, examination, or dosage of the drug prescribed. Safety-netting was something only seen at the circus.

The cramped space encouraged a scrawled, indecipherable script on a par with that of Leonardo da Vinci's notebook. The doctor's handwriting became a byword for illegible script, a cliché lingering to this day.

The Lloyd George envelopes, quite adequate for the newborn, gained weight and girth with time, mirroring the humans to whom they related. Letters from hospital consultants arrived in A5 and A4 format, to be folded like intricate origami and stuffed into the envelope. Esoteric debates raged and inconclusive research undertaken as to whether such letters should be folded inwards with their writing concealed or outwards for visual accessibility. Investigations, whether laboratory or radiography, had their own reports. Should they be buried in the general hospital literature or folded separately? Information was filed according to source rather than collated according to purpose.[2]

Above all, the principle that nothing could be discarded reigned supreme. Envelopes became morbidly obese, spawning additional envelopes for the chronically ill, each bound to its companion by thick rubber bands or sellotape. Prizing a sheet from such a record was akin to a dentist extracting a wisdom tooth using only fingernails. Yet, this system prevailed until the 21st century and only the universal adoption of computerised records finally laid it to rest.

Desktop computers were introduced into general practice in the 1980s and in common usage by 2000. They became a necessity after 2004, when elements within the GMS contract, such as the QOF, could only be managed and remunerated using information technology. Most GP practices were either 'paper-lite' or totally digital by the end of that decade.

The task of digitising the written medical records was Sisyphean in nature,[3] requiring literally thousands of man-hours. Inevitably, there was some leakage of data. Because doctors were unsure how great this would become, they kept legacy paper records as a backup.

Prior to computerisation, academic GPs had recognised the limitations of Lloyd George cards. In the 1960s, there was a strong move to adopt A4 records that could be encased in a folder-like cover, similar to the hospital files. Arguably logical and easier to use, the idea never gained traction with most GPs, due partly

---

[2] Ed Bruce Levy. Medical records in practice: guidance for general practitioners. BMJ. 1996 Nov 16;313(7067):1270–1.

[3] Denoting a task that can never be completed.

to cost but mostly to lethargy, and the legacy system persisted. Where adopted, the dual approach inevitably led to further data loss when a patient changed practice.

The Lloyd George format allowed for a summary card at the front of the file, which was rarely used before the 1990 GP contract that introduced financial incentives for the management of chronic diseases, such as asthma and diabetes. Thereafter it was used for recording the significant medical events in a patient's history. Documenting such events remained patchy, as did the interpretation of what constituted a major event. Some doctors dutifully included every sore throat, whilst others omitted life-changing operations. The summary itself became ever longer and ceased to function in the true sense of that word. Additional formats were needed to act as disease registers. Primitive, 'easily' interrogated databases using punched cards[4] were added to the record system. The drive to tabulate became unstoppable. It was all rather messy. Computers arrived just in time to satiate this data-collecting frenzy.

The computerisation of primary care lagged that of such commercial sectors as finance and retail, due to the lack of an investment to drive change. Adoption in hospitals[5] and subsequent IT developments were even slower, with providers only moving to Windows systems in the first decade of the 21st century.

Early commercial entrants into the field of GP computerisation included AAH-Meditel,[6] EMIS,[7] VAMP,[8] GPASS,[9] with EMIS and VAMP dominating the field.

The current widely used EMIS Web was built on the popular EMIS software which, before the upgrade, was entirely keystroke-driven. EMIS Web, along with SystemOne and VAMP Vision, were a revelation in the organisation of medical information; seeking to electronically emulate the doctor's cognitive processes in handling a typical consultation. All the software systems allowed for the input of free text whilst guiding the user towards set headings and Read[10]/SNOMED codes.

---

4   www.ibm.com/ibm/history/ibm100/us/en/icons/punchcard/

5   Benson T. Why British GPs use computers and hospital doctors do not. Proc AMIA Symp. 2001:42–6. PMID: 11825153; PMCID: PMC2243530. Benson T. Why general practitioners use computers and hospital doctors do not–Part 1: incentives. BMJ. 2002 Nov 9;325(7372):1086–9. doi: 10.1136/bmj.325.7372.1086. PMID: 12424171; PMCID: PMC131190

6   Acquired by Torex in 1999, BMJ. 2002;325:1086.

7   Egton Medical Information Systems.

8   Value-Added Medical Products.

9   General Practice Administration System for Scotland.

10 Read Codes use a co-dependent hierarchy where each code has a parent code up to a maximum of four other characters, each representing a diagnosis, process of care, or medication. SNOMED codes, on the other hand, give a unique 'concept ID' to every clinical term
    https://digital.nhs.uk/services/terminology-and-classifications/read-codes
    https://digital.nhs.uk/services/terminology-and-classifications/snomed-ct

Yet, despite the software's sophistication, the applications remained comparatively cumbersome and, for many doctors, more time-consuming than the old handwritten record. However, they were vastly superior for legibility and data interrogation.

The irony of 'efficient' computerisation has been the pressure put on the limited time of an average consultation. There is a feeling amongst doctors that the purpose of the consultation has shifted from managing the patient's problems to validating the process of patient management, through a traceable audit trail. Whereas a request for a laboratory test could be quickly written on a paper form, an identical action took much longer electronically. The former had the disadvantage that it could be mislaid in the system; the latter, the advantage that it could be followed throughout its journey to laboratory and back. The NHS Choose and Book (C&B) programme, introduced in 2005 as part of the National Programme for IT (NPfIT), was equally cumbersome and irritating.

5.3 CHOOSE AND BOOK

Despite its basis on sound principles of patient choice, C&B was intended for routine outpatient referrals; emergency and acute referrals continued to be handwritten and addressed to the recipient clinician and cancer referrals passed through archaic fax machines, thought to be more direct and secure than the Internet. The C&B software was meant to be the stormtrooper that would demonstrate once and for all the utility of the flagship NPfIT policy, Connecting for Health (CFH). CFH aspired to connect and integrate all NHS providers through an NHS 'spine,' a centralised hub of patient records easily accessible to all healthcare professionals. Initially, C&B only highlighted subsequent issues within CFH, including slow broadband, system outages, lengthy lists of providers, and outdated information. These became so innumerable that they eventually led to the termination of the enterprise, at great cost to the taxpayer. However, C&B endured although the original purpose, a hospital booking whilst the patient was seeing the doctor, was rapidly replaced by the pre-existing process, an appointment made through the medical secretary.

C&B was added to the list of well-intentioned but counterproductive DH initiatives that sought to enhance consumer choice whilst neglecting the basics of healthcare provision. What patients really wanted was rapid access to specialist clinics at their local hospital. What they got was a flashy, complicated booking system for a service that was hamstrung through inadequate funding and limited resources. The former was an extravagant fig leaf to cover up the failings of the latter. Nevertheless, having allocated £100 million over three years to overcome resistance from GPs and hospital consultants, the DH was hardly likely to backtrack. In return, primary care was left with a cumbersome process, driven by politics, requiring extra resources, and managed through primary rather than secondary care, a scenario frequently repeated throughout the history of general practice in the UK.

C&B survived in its original format for ten years until its replacement by the NHS e-Referral Service, ERS[11] in 2015. The new system was a marginal improvement,

---

[11] www.nhs.uk/using-the-nhs/nhs-services/hospitals/nhs-e-referral-service/

although, by that time, access to hospital clinics had become even more limited, partly due to the CCG drive to limit referrals.

5.4 E-PRESCRIBING

One area where computerisation did have a beneficial impact on GP workload and patient satisfaction, was the issuing of prescriptions, specifically repeat medications. To provide some perspective, from 1948 and for the following 40 years, prescriptions were entirely handwritten, usually by the doctor, on a standard form, the FP10. The task itself was not onerous in the early decades of the NHS when the list of prescribed medications was small, but it became increasingly so as treatable conditions and the drugs to treat them became more numerous. In England, 456 million prescription items were dispensed in the community in 1994,[12] rising to over 1 billion per annum 25 years later. By 2020, a GP with a list size of 2,000 people would expect to issue around 150 prescription items, acute and repeat, every working day, clearly an unsustainable task without the aid of IT.

Prior to computerisation, the process for patients requesting a repeat prescription was archaic. They had to submit a request in writing, at the surgery, wait up to 72 hours for the prescription to be issued, then take it to the chemist for the drug to be dispensed. Patients and GPs owed a debt of gratitude for alleviating this cumbersome process to the visionary doctors of Exeter who, in the 1970s, pioneered the use of computers in general practice and, more specifically, developed the FP10(comp) prescription form. The FP10(comp), double the width of the standard FP10 form in order to feed the inkjet tractor printers of the time, was divided into two halves. The left-hand side was identical to the previous FP10, the right contained the patient's details, list of repeat medications, and space for messages, such as details of the annual influenza vaccine programme or dates of surgery closure.

In an obtuse understanding of reverse psychology, the DH was at first reluctant to sanction the use of computer-generated prescriptions because it feared that the ease of prescribing would generate a boom in items prescribed! However, to its credit, it recognised the utility and improved safety inherent in the system and sanctioned its use of the FP10-(comp) across the NHS in 1981, predating by many years the use of similar systems in Europe and the USA.

5.5 COMPUTERISATION IN PRACTICE

Drs John Preece and Bradshaw Smith, Exeter GPs, can justly claim to have been the joint godfathers of computing in primary care. Their surgery was the first in the world to pilot the use of a desktop, real-time GP computer system. Patients' details were kept on a mainframe server in Croydon, connected by a telephone landline to a slave terminal in the surgery, a system almost identical to that proposed 40 years later under the National Programme for IT (NPfIT). The partners

---

[12] https://files.digital.nhs.uk/publicationimport/pub01xxx/pub01237/pres-disp-com-eng-1994-2004-rep.pdf

collaborated with IBM, which invested £250,000 in the project, in the hope that success in Devon would persuade the NHS to roll out its systems across the rest of the country. They succeeded in their first aim, only to see their British rival, International Computers Limited (ICL), pick up the DH contract for that roll-out!

Dr Leo Fogarty has written an eloquent personal account of computerisation in general practice that is well worth reading.[13]

Despite the pioneering work of Preece and Bradshaw Smith, the widespread use of computers in primary care did not take place until ten years later. Price drove the delay. The computer systems of the 1970s were expensive. GPs could not afford the initial outlay and were reluctant to commit to the ongoing running costs. Early providers of GP systems, AAH-Meditel and VAMP, sought to overcome such hesitancy by introducing novel commercial arrangements which, in effect, were the first to recognise the monetary value of patient data. The company would provide the hardware, including the main server and a terminal on every desk, ongoing running costs, and training, in return for anonymised prescribing data. It was a compelling offer at the time, one that would have been ethically unacceptable 20 years later when the public had become increasingly concerned regarding data protection.

After a lead time for initial data entry of patients' personal and medical details, practices entering an agreement contracted to allow providers to mine the data for prescribing trends, selling that information on to the pharmaceutical industry. The contract contained targets and stringent quality standards covering data entry, to ensure that the data were comprehensive and robust. But the contract wording was vague and ultimately not legally binding. The viability of the business model proved to be financially unsound, and, eventually, such contracts were discontinued, due to the poor quality of the data, data protection regulations, rapidly falling IT costs, and GP disquiet with the Faustian pact. All collaborations were discontinued within five years, reverting to a traditional purchaser/provider model.

Nevertheless, the short-lived partnership between practices and their IT suppliers did accelerate the use of computers in primary care, as well as highlighting the drawbacks in their use. The main server was the size of a washing machine and needed to be housed in its own room. Frequent backups had to be done using floppy discs, taking up most of a weekend and requiring off-site storage, usually in the boot of the doctor's car. Green-screen VDUs, printers, and clunky keyboards left little room on the desk for its historic occupants, the mercury sphygmomanometer, stethoscope, and auroscope. Patients and doctors alike focused more on the equipment than on the matter at hand. The consulting room became rather cluttered.

The computer had an insatiable appetite for data. Thousands of man-hours went into feeding in the patient's details, name, address, date of birth, then on

---

[13] Fogarty L. Primary care informatics development: one view through the miasma. J Info Prim Care. 1997; 2–11. Accessed 7 Oct 2021 from www.primis.nottingham.ac.uk/informatics/jan97/jan2.htm

to the summary of past medical history and current and repeat medications. Naturally, not all the information contained in the Lloyd George envelope could be transferred, and there was little desire to do so since the rationale for the new system was clear: clean data, easily accessible to all users. The minutiae of a patient's medical history no longer resided in the doctor's head. Any clinician could become familiar with the fine detail in the time it took the patient to walk from the waiting to the consulting room. The link between family doctor and patient had been loosened.

The computer became the third person in the room. The doctor could no longer focus purely on the patient but now had to also heed the presence of a somewhat demanding interloper. The facility for medical checks in the software led to frequent prompts and pop-ups appearing in any consultation. The patient's agenda was being hijacked by untimely requests to undertake a medication review, check immunisation status, book a cervical test, record a blood pressure reading, or give advice on smoking and diet. In short, reduced to the role of a functionary, the doctor no longer had charge of the consultation. It was all somewhat irritating and viscerally humiliating. Nevertheless, the doctor who ignored the prompts would likely later regret doing so. The suggestions relating to QOF contributed to practice income, and repeated omissions were likely to result in sanctions from the practice manager or more compliant partners. A prescription issued contrary to the guidance from the software could potentially lead to rare side effects and a lawyer questioning why the doctor acted contrary to that advice. Even acting on the prompts was likely to lead the perceptive patient to question whether such actions were in their interest or the doctor's. Beneficence and non-maleficence, key principles of medical ethics, were no longer implicit in the doctor-patient relationship.

Apologists for the software alerts argued that their presence protected the patient and ultimately the doctor. The argument for prescribing would have been hard to refute, had it not been contradicted by NHS data showing annual increases in the number of iatrogenic events. A study published in the *Journal Economic Evaluation of Health and Care Interventions*[14] estimated that in 2017, there were 237 million medication errors in England, 66 million of which were potentially clinically significant. Of these, 47 million (71%) originated in primary care, with hospital admission and mortality resulting in 627 cases. Although these figures represented a small percentage of the 1 billion prescriptions issued annually in primary care, they were nevertheless surprisingly high when every issued prescription was electronically safety-netted.

Despite their initial misgivings, GPs as a whole, including those with calloused index fingers, took to computerisation in primary care with varying degrees of enthusiasm. Of course, computers came as second nature to the younger cohorts of doctors entering general practice. The wizened elderly liked playing with the new toy but fondly reminisced about a bygone era when they could scribble in

---

[14] Accessed 7 Oct 2021 from www.bpsassessment.com/wp-content/uploads/2020/06/1.-Prevalence-and-economic-burden-of-medication-errors-in-the-NHS-in-England-1.pdf

the notes and did not have eye strain. All recognised that the advantages of comprehensive, clear, accessible medical records far outweighed the drawbacks. For those doctors of an academic bent, the availability of easily interrogatable data provided a wonderful resource for research and a significant contribution to best practice.[15]

Running in parallel with the computerisation of primary care, the national IT programme was getting underway.

5.6 CONNECTING FOR HEALTH (CFH)

Whilst micro-computerisation was proceeding apace in primary care, separately and simultaneously, secondary care was also employing computerisation. The logic for allowing both sectors of the NHS to communicate with each other and share information was irrefutable. To address this aspiration, CFH was born on April Fool's Day 2005, the spawn of the DH and NHS Information Authority. The original estimate that CFH would cost £2.3 billion proved to be wildly optimistic. The project was ditched eight years later, the cost having risen to £13 billion.

An inherently cynical group, doctors were nevertheless sorry to witness the demise of CFH. The vision of seamless electronic communication between all healthcare providers was enticing, but in truth, from the beginning, CFH was never a 'national' programme. The government of the day, recognising what a vast and unmanageable beast it would become, decided to break up the project into five geographic areas covering the country. Requests for tenders were posted, and the private sector applied in numbers. Fujitsu, Accenture, and British Telecom were duly contracted to deliver the dream. Established experts in the field, such as EMIS, whose systems covered 50% of GP surgeries, were excluded from tendering for the regional roles.

SystemOne, Vision, and Microtest Health became the approved NHS systems of choice.[16] EMIS was excluded, but practices could continue using their system at their own cost.

SystemOne was the first entrant into the NHS market to offer genuine connectivity between the disparate arms of health and social care, an invaluable asset to all users, doctors, midwives, district nurses, health visitors, and social workers, who could now access the patient's complete record electronically and remotely. SystemOne was also the first to offer GPs Personal Data Services (PDS) tablets for recording home visits, a time-saving tool that has been an asset in improving safer patient care. More popular electronic tablets have since replaced them. By 2020, SystemOne was in use in over 7,000 NHS organisations, including 2,600 GP Practices.

[15] Hobbs R. Is primary care research important and relevant to GPs? Br J Gen Pract. 2019 Aug 29;69(686):424–5. doi: 10.3399/bjgp19X705149. PMID: 31467002; PMCID: PMC6715475.

[16] Gold S. NHS connecting for health's biggest 20 suppliers, 2010–11. The Guardian, 11 Oct 2011. Accessed 7 Oct 2021 from www.theguardian.com/healthcare-network/2011/oct/11/nhs-connecting-for-health-supplier-profiles

Meantime, EMIS (now EMIS Health) continued to maintain a sizeable market share in primary care computing. In part, this was due to the axiom 'local knowledge provides good solutions.' Both founders, Peter Sowerby and David Stables, full-time GPs and self-taught computer programmers, developed the user-friendly system in the 1980s.

EMIS retained and expanded a loyal following of users and, by 2020, was the software of choice in over 9,000 GP practices across the UK, with a strong presence in pharmacies, hospices, and community and secondary care. The company logo strapline, 'written by doctors, for doctors,' had never been more apposite.

SystemOne and EMIS Web have a duopoly of IT clinical systems, for which they received £77 million from the NHS in 2018. A third provider, Practice Systems (INPS) Ltd Vision (evolved from VAMP), operated exclusively in Wales.

The financial sums that the NPfIT/CFH programmes involved were astronomical, but the deliverables inherent in the names, 'national' and 'connected,' proved unachievable.

In 2007, part of CFH's remit was broken off and, under the title GP Systems of Choice (GPSoC), allowed GPs greater autonomy in choosing the clinical system to which they wished to upgrade. GPSoC would provide the funds for the purchase and maintenance of these systems, but only with pre-existing approved commercial suppliers. In 2014, these included EMIS, SystemOne, and Vision.

Remarkably, despite providing 'free' money, 25% of GP practices declined GPSoC's overtures, choosing instead to remain stubbornly loyal to their pre-existing supplier.

Regardless of the origins of funding, computerisation in primary care accelerated and the technology improved. Over a five-year period from 2005, systems moved from rather basic and bland clinical records and prescription issuing to a more visually engaging Windows framework that provided seamless communication between practices and segments of secondary care, such as laboratories.

Patients could now book and cancel GP appointments online, order repeat prescriptions, send secure messages, view their medical records (within limits, of course), and update their personal details. Meanwhile, waiting room automated check-in, electronic referrals to secondary care, email from other healthcare providers, electronic remote prescribing, and computer tablets for home visits enhanced practice administration.

GPSoC was replaced in 2020 by the GP IT Futures (GPITF) programme, which pithily described itself as 'a critical enabler for taking primary care towards the requirements set out in the NHS Long-Term Plan, five-year framework for GP contract reform and the Digital, Data and Technology Vision.'[17]

GPITF still allowed CCGs, PCNs, federations, and GP practices to choose their IT system from a list of approved providers that included EMIS and SystemOne, as well as new entrants specialising in the field of online, video, and remote consultations. All these centrally funded additional services were now cost-free to GP practices.

---

17 Future GP IT systems and services. https://digital.nhs.uk/services/gp-it-futures-systems

GPFIT aspired to finally complete the vision, set out 15 years previously, of providing seamless connectivity and operability between all parts of the NHS, including patients, and furthering advances in the use of apps on smartphones and tablets to increase the volume of remote, online patient interactions. Also hidden in its stated vision was the slightly Orwellian aim of enabling comparison of workload and clinical outcomes, in other words, if one was inclined towards conspiracy theories, GP productivity.

Those working in primary care now had a huge and varied palette of tools available to them. Recent consultations, previous medical history, current drug therapy, linked conditions, linked drugs, allergies, drug interactions, hospital correspondence, and countless other functions were all present at the click of a mouse. Laboratory investigations were on a doctor's monitor screen within 24 hours of giving a blood sample. Hospital discharge letters no longer suffered the vagaries of the post. Out-of-hours providers slept soundly in the knowledge that their reports would be present on the GP's screen as they logged on in the morning. Electronic prescribing with repeat prescriptions directed to pharmacists not only dispensed with the arduous prescription signing ceremony but also with the potential for mislaying FP10s as they made their way around a surgery.

Other aspects of a GP's workload have also been simplified. Recording diagnoses, drugs, and many other aspects of the consultation are automatically READ coded and, as such, can be quickly interrogated. Data searches allow for rapid access to patient groups for improved chronic disease management or compliance with Medicines and Healthcare products Regulatory Agency (MHRA) alerts. Quality improvement activity, such as QOF, would be impossible without the sophisticated software. The production of the annual report on practice activity and payments has been almost completely automated.

The practice intranet allows for electronic communication between staff that could be immediately actioned and audited. There was even a discrete panic button in every room to reassure staff in a turbulent world of frustrated patients. Google aids the doctor in confirming their diagnosis or learning about the latest popularised medical acronym. Patient advice leaflets on any medical condition are readily available for instant printing. The desktop monitor became so indispensable that often an extra one had to be added.

Despite their utility in the doctor's consulting room, GP systems were still not fully integrated with the systems used in other parts of the NHS. There was no single patient database that could be used by all healthcare providers. A central hub for clinical records, the Summary Care Record, was needed.

5.7 SUMMARY CARE RECORD (SCR)

The Summary Care Record[18] was a centralised silo or 'spine' of essential medical information that all health and social care providers could access. Secure access was guaranteed; only those carrying an NHS Smartcard could log in to the

---

[18] https://digital.nhs.uk/services/summary-care-records-scr

system. The logic for such a system may have been irrefutable to the profession, but the public demurred. An increasingly suspicious society needed reassurance that the personal data would be secure, confidential, and not used for any other purpose, bar medical, without their consent. A public information campaign, a hefty information pack containing an NHS Care Record Guarantee,[19] was posted to over 42 million people to address these concerns. Most households consigned the pack, unopen, to the bin. Eventually, in 2010, every citizen of the UK was automatically enrolled on the SCR, unless they chose, in writing, to opt-out.[20]

The cost of gaining the public's support for the SCR? In a written parliamentary answer in 2009, the health minister at the time said that nearly £100 million had been spent, with a further £50 million projected. The same hapless minister also put the cost of producing each public information pack at £13.59,[21] which, if true, meant that some printing firm was taking the government for an almighty ride! The sums quoted excluded the time and resources spent by primary care trusts, Clinical Commissioning Groups, and GPs in persuading the public of the utility of the project. The information held on the SCR went on to include:

- Name, address, date of birth, gender, and NHS number
- Medications (acute and repeat)
- Allergies
- Adverse reactions
- Reason for medication
- Significant medical history
- Anticipatory care information (such as information about the management of long-term conditions)
- Communication preferences
- End-of-life care information
- Immunisations

Potentially sensitive coded items specifically related to *in vitro* fertilisation, sexually transmitted diseases, termination of pregnancy, and gender reassignment were automatically excluded unless the patient requested otherwise.

By 2013, over 24 million SCRs had been created across England. However, SCRs are due to be phased out in 2024, to be replaced by more detailed, 'richer' Local Health and Care Record Exemplars (LHCRE),[22] managed by NHS regions instead of NHS Digital.[23]

---

[19] http://systems.hscic.gov.uk/scr/library/crg.pdf

[20] http://systems.hscic.gov.uk/scr/library/optout.pdf

[21] Daily Hansard. Written answers. *Medical Records: Publicity*. Column 774W. 2010. Accessed 7 Oct 2021 from www.publications.parliament.uk/pa/cm200910/cmhansrd/cm100316/text/100316w0013.htm

[22] www.nhs.uk/using-the-nhs/nhs-services/hospitals/nhs-e-referral-service/

[23] Health Service Journal Summary care record to be replaced, says NHS digital chief. 28 Jan 2019. www.hsj.co.uk/technology-and-innovation/summary-care-record-to-be-replaced-says-nhs-digital-chief/7024274.article

Meanwhile, patients continued using low-tech methods to access information from their immediate healthcare provider, their GP surgery.

5.8 PRACTICE LEAFLETS AND WEBSITES

The 1948 NHS Act and the GMC banned GPs from advertising their services to recruit patients or to compete with other practices in their geographical area. The restrictions on advertising were only removed from the GMC's ethical guidelines 60 years later, in 2009.

However, practices still needed to apprise their patients, particularly those newly registered, of the practice details and services. Initially, this was done through word of mouth, but by the 1960s, printed formats, generically the 'practice leaflet,' had become the norm. Originally a single sheet of typewritten A4, the leaflet evolved to a professionally printed booklet and, finally, to a glossy website. The information contained also expanded from basic contact details and opening times to interactive formats containing a wealth of material on the practice and advice on health-related topics.

The Statement of Fees and Allowances (SFA), also colloquially known as the Red Book, had mandated that the practice leaflet be updated annually and that copies should be available to the Health Authority, every patient on the doctor's list, and really anyone who wanted one. Thus, huge numbers would be printed, with stacks left in waiting rooms where they would remain, dog-eared, yellowed, and ignored by most patients, who preferred to read ancient copies of the *Readers Digest* instead.

Information on the practice had to include surgery times, the appointment system, ways of obtaining non-urgent and urgent appointments, home visits, arrangements for when the doctor was not on-site, OOH, repeat prescriptions (and dispensing, if relevant), other services (child health, minor surgery, contraception, maternity), staff and their roles, patients' comments and complaints, map of practice boundary, details of disability access and whether the practice was a training one under the GP Vocational Training Regulation 1979 or taught undergraduate students.

Where there is money, an enterprising business is always only too willing to take it. No sooner had the PCT made practice booklets compulsory than commercial providers flooded GPs with offers to waive production and printing costs in return for advertising space in the booklet. At times, these adverts, for medical negligence law firms or local funeral directors, seemed misplaced. These concerns were overlooked as the niche providers also took on the responsibility for producing a Red Book-compliant booklet, thus releasing the uninterested practice from this onerous and time-consuming task.

In due course, similar commercial arrangements took place for placing televisions in waiting rooms, although the medically related programmes and adverts tended to be as boring and repetitive as a TV summer schedule. They may have been useful in disseminating medical information, but as with the booklets, most patients ignored both the TV and the advice. A tech-savvy public preferred to get their information from Google or social media platforms. The overall impact on health education was minimal.

Practice websites began to appear at the turn of the millennium and generally eschewed any overtly commercial input. Website builders blossomed everywhere; though pricey at first, they gradually came down in cost as competition increased, and the technology and software became cheaper. Pamphlets and websites ran in parallel for some years, but by the mid-2010s, the former had generally been made redundant.

5.9 SUMMARY

Safe healthcare provision is dependent on many factors, not the least being good medical records. Over the past 70 years, the infrastructure and quality of record-keeping have evolved, expanded, and improved. Clarity, accessibility, and transfer of information are all light-years better than they were in 1948. GP IT systems contain a wealth of material that not only provides for targeted and safe care for the individual but also elevates the quality of care for patient populations. Aggregated data mining allows improved diagnosis, treatment, productivity, research, and best practice in primary care. Checks and balances are in place, especially with prescribing software that should reduce the potential for iatrogenic misadventures.

After a slow start, primary care IT systems are now at the forefront of software development in the NHS. They address the progress of the entire patient journey, from booking an appointment with the GP to discharge from hospital. They ensure routine monitoring of chronic conditions, tabulating every metric. Patients are better cared for and safer than ever before. So, patients should be reassured that they are, at last, receiving the best care possible within a nationalised health service, right?

If you are a GP reading this chapter, try asking the next patient you see in your surgery what they think about the VDU and keyboard on your desk. Their response will probably not surprise you. The young will ignore your question because they will be concentrating on texting from their smartphone. The middle-aged will be sanguine regarding the matter. The elderly would complain that you are more interested in the screen than you are in them. Nevertheless, overall, patients increasingly accept that they must share their time with HAL.[24] But acceptance is not synonymous with contentment. There is an undercurrent of resentment at the way the computer has inserted itself in the interaction between patient and doctor. Patients are irritated by the doctor's eyes being constantly drawn towards a computer monitor. It is hard for them to distance that act from one of bored inattention. The result is that they lose faith in that doctor. The loss of intimate human connectivity, empathy, vital to the relationship, is hard to reclaim. Patients who feel ignored become aggrieved, less forgiving, and more inclined to complain vexatiously when a minor mishap in their care occurs. They feel relegated to a peripheral role within the consultation. Doctors are aware of this conundrum but not how to solve it.

---

[24] HAL 9000 is a sentient computer that controls the systems of the Discovery One spacecraft and interacts with the ship's crew in Arthur C Clarke's *Space Odyssey* series.

The above views are entirely subjective, reflecting those of front-line GPs and perhaps countering those of the few objective studies on the subject. A survey in a business magazine in the United States (2014) of 4,500 patients found that most people either preferred or were untroubled by their doctor using an EHR.[25] However, a US family physician, Dr Susan Kovan, wrote an impassioned piece in the *Boston Globe* in the same year, elegantly encapsulating how many doctors felt about the subject.[26] Her article included the following opinion from Dr David Blumenthal, US National Coordinator for Health Information Technology from 2009 to 2011:

> 'For physicians of a certain generation,' the current status of computers in medicine is 'a painful interlude in an important historic process.'

Paraphrased: computerisation was inevitable; learn to live with it; a view as likely to be espoused by doctors in Boston, Lincolnshire as it was by their US counterparts.

Currently, doctor and computer have a symbiotic relationship. How long that remains a partnership of equals remains to be seen. Patients have become inured to the benefits of smart technologies in accessing their doctor, a scenario accelerated by the COVID pandemic. As the number of face-to-face consultations diminishes, will GPs eventually be replaced by IBM's Watson[27] or Alphabet's DeepMind[28] and will patients mind? A sobering thought.

---

[25] McCormack M. Survey: do patients really care if you use your EHR in the exam room? 2014. Accessed 7 Oct 2021 from www.softwareadvice.com/resources/survey-do-patients-really-care-if-you-use-your-ehr-in-the-exam-room/

[26] Koven S. Doctors, patients, and computer screens. Boston Globe, 24 Feb 2014. Accessed 30 Apr 2018 from www.bostonglobe.com/lifestyle/health-wellness/2014/02/24/practice-doctors-patients-and-computer-screens/JMMYaCDtf3mnuQZGfkMVyL/story.html

[27] www.ibm.com/uk-en/watson-health

[28] https://deepmind.com/

6

Ailments and Diseases

The art of medicine consists in amusing the patient, while nature cures the disease.

(Voltaire)

6.1 INTRODUCTION

Why do people seek medical advice? In one word, fear. Everyone is familiar with and expects their body to function faultlessly from one day to the next. They become concerned when it fails to do so. The threshold for that concern varies between individuals; once reached, they seek reassurance; they visit their doctor.

The commonest acute presenting symptoms seen at a GP surgery are fever, cough, pain, fatigue, anxiety and depression; the causes, viral and bacterial infection, musculoskeletal, stress, and disenchantment with life. The rest of the doctor's clinic is taken up with ongoing management of chronic conditions, hypertension, diabetes, asthma, COPD. The evil intruder, cancer, is mercifully rare but ever lurking by the door. The clinician has to be ever vigilant in preventing it gaining entry. A study from Australia,[1] with a culture and demography comparable to the UK, suggested that a GP be familiar with up to 200 conditions. The World Health International Classification of Diseases[2] lists over 10,000! Occasionally the unexpected sneaks in; the symptoms may indeed have an underlying sinister cause.

The population of the UK prior to 1948 was inured to suffering due to the privations arising from two World Wars, limited healthcare provision, and cost. A consultation with a doctor was an action of last resort in combatting an illness. The overall health of the nation suffered as a result.

The founding of the NHS promised universal free healthcare according to need. The definition of need was diluted over the following decades; transmuting to want. Patients wanted reassurance. If that could not be safely provided then they wanted a cure, a return to their previous physical and mental state of well-being. Drugs became synonymous with cure, an illusion adopted by both parties

---

[1] www.racgp.org.au/download/Documents/AFP/2013/January/February/201301cooke.pdf

[2] The World Health. www.who.int/standards/classifications/classification-of-diseases

DOI: 10.1201/9781003256465-6

in the medical consultation. Patients were disappointed if they left the GP surgery without a prescription; a prescription was a quick and easy way for the doctor to usher them back out the door. But before they could do so they needed a diagnosis, or at least, the semblance of one.

A diagnosis is the culmination of the lifetime of learning a doctor accumulates in anatomy, physiology, and pathology as applied to the various biological systems, cardiovascular, respiratory, and so on, of the human body. Medical students are taught how to elicit a comprehensive history of symptoms and to distil the information into manageable nuggets. They learn by rote and use mnemonics; SOCRATES (Site, Onset, Character, Radiation, Association, Timing, Exacerbation, Severity) for pain and VITAMIN CD (Vascular, Infective, Traumatic, Autoimmune, Metabolic, Iatrogenic, Neoplastic, Congenital, Degenerative) for pathology. They graduate in an educational state of conscious incompetence. Five years later they become unconsciously competent GPs ready to meet all their patients' medical needs; mindful that they are treating the sentient organism, not individual organs.

6.2 THE MANAGEMENT OF DISEASE BY SYSTEM

The following section covers the changes that took place in the practice of medicine in primary care over the lifetime of the NHS. The most significant of those changes seem to have conveniently fallen during three periods, each covering approximately a third of the lifespan of the NHS: 1948–1975, 1976–1999, and 2000 onwards.

6.3 CARDIOVASCULAR

6.3.1 1948–1975

The introduction of effective antihypertensive agents,[3] diuretics, methyldopa, and beta-blockers occurred before there was a defined level of systolic and diastolic blood pressure above which a person was considered at risk. Medical consensus was that a diastolic blood pressure above 100 mm Hg was likely to be harmful, and treatment aimed to bring it below that level. Systolic blood pressure was considered too labile; its true significance as a contributing factor to cardiovascular (CV) disease not recognised until 1990. The treatment of hypertension gradually devolved from secondary to primary care over this period. The only equipment needed was a mercury sphygmomanometer and stethoscope.

The benefits of treating hypertension were seen in the UK cardiovascular mortality figures, which declined by 16% between 1961 and 1985 although some of

---

[3] Saklayen MG, Deshpande NV. Timeline of history of hypertension treatment. Front Cardiovasc Med. 2016 Feb 23;3:3. doi: 10.3389/fcvm.2016.00003. PMID: 26942184; PMCID: PMC4763852.

this may have also been due to increased public awareness of the danger of smoking to health.[4]

Primary care offered little to those with established CV conditions, such as strokes (cardiovascular accident, CVA) and myocardial infarction (MI). Cardiac enzyme blood tests were available to GPs, but the turnaround time for results was too long to inform a diagnosis outside of hospitals. A GP had to see acute myocardial events to administer intravenous diamorphine and cyclizine, before admission to hospital. MIs and CVAs were managed by prolonged bed rest in hospital. Once discharged home, the family doctor could only offer a sympathetic ear.

The management of cardiac arrhythmia, particularly atrial fibrillation, was through modifying heart rate and myocardial contractility, for which digoxin/digitoxin, commenced by GPs, were the sole agents. Disopyramide was used for ventricular arrhythmia. Anticoagulants were not part of the regime.

Digoxin, along with loop diuretics such as frusemide (furosemide), routinely prescribed with potassium supplements such as 'Slow-K,' were used to manage cardiac failure, the diagnosis of which was made entirely on history and clinical examination, with occasional recourse to chest X-ray.

Peripheral vascular insufficiency was also diagnosed solely by history and examination. There were no effective drugs licensed for treatment.

Hyperlipidaemia was being recognised as 'a bad thing,' and patients with very high cholesterol levels were advised to go on a low-fat diet. Diet had little impact on those levels, so drugs such as fibrates and cholestyramine were added. Both were unpalatable, ineffective, and had no impact on cardiovascular morbidity.

6.3.2 1976–1999

The association between certain risk factors and cardiovascular disease gained traction, and calculator-type tools were designed to quantify the risk. An influx of novel cardiovascular drugs, including ACE inhibitors, calcium channel blockers, and statins, fed into the increasing acceptance of preventive medicine. The statins, in particular, had a marked impact on CV morbidity and mortality, but for years their use remained limited due to cost. During this period, an average GP could expect to see at least one acute MI and CVA a month.

The management of hypertension now focused on reducing blood pressure to below 160/90, although this was age-dependent. An abnormal systolic pressure was calculated as above 100 plus the patient's age. Systolic pressure was given precedence over diastolic.

Thrombolytic agents for use in CVA were marketed, but these had to be injected intravenously and were available for hospital use only. Aspirin, oral, 300 mg was given to everyone with suspected MI as soon as they were seen.

---

[4] Trends in coronary heart disease, 1961–2011. British Heart Foundation. www.bhf.org.uk/informationsupport/publications/statistics/trends-in-coronary-heart-disease-1961-2011#

Some drugs, such as pentoxifylline (Trental), claimed to help symptoms of claudication but, in practice, showed few, if any, benefits.

ECG machines were finding their way into most GP practices, although capital costs restricted their universal presence. Many were funded by a mix of patient donations and drug company sponsorship. An ECG became a vital part of a GP's workup of any patient presenting with chest pain or irregular pulse. Echocardiography services for community access also became available for investigating cardiac failure. Concerns over mercury toxicity led to replacing traditional manometers with aneroid or electronic versions.

6.3.3 2000 Onwards

Previous decades had shown a marked reduction in the number of acute cardiovascular events. The reason was considered a vindication of the public health policy of prevention. The introduction of the Quality Outcomes Framework in 2004 included points for CV risk identification and management, to encourage GPs to be more vigilant in this field. Monetary incentives were unnecessary. Most practices achieved maximum points in the first year of QOF implementation simply because of their previous rigour in managing these conditions.

Protocols based on good clinical practice were being introduced for many conditions. Although meant to be advisory, in reality their use was obligatory; a doctor had to have sound reasons for not complying with their 'guidance.' In turn, protocols were informed by a variety of risk calculators, ischaemic heart disease, transient ischaemic attack, and deep vein thrombosis to name but a few.

A diagnosis of atrial fibrillation required immediate anticoagulation with warfarin and rapid referral to a hospital outpatient clinic.

Blood pressure deemed to be too high on repeated reading was defined as 140/90. By now, practice nurses were managing most hypertension and encouraged to take readings from both arms, as well as erect and supine.

Practices introduced automated manometers in their waiting rooms. Ambulatory BP monitoring was encouraged as the price for such machines dropped and they became widely available from any high street chemist. Every practice had to have a defibrillator and all staff had to be trained in its use. Annual cardiopulmonary resuscitation training became mandatory for all GPs and their staff.

An unexpected impact on GP workload arose from the public health campaigns highlighting the early symptoms of MI or stroke and advising people with such symptoms to call 999 immediately. Doctors now rarely saw such conditions in the community and callouts during surgery hours became extremely rare.

Sensitive laboratory tests for serum troponin levels in MI or blood natriuretic peptide (BNP) in heart failure remained primarily for use in hospitals, although they were slowly seeping out into community practice.

All the above measures, along with improved prosperity and lifestyle changes, especially smoking cessation, were rewarded by an 80% drop in deaths from heart and circulatory diseases in the UK between 1961 to 2017.[5]

---

[5] fwww.bhf.org.uk/what-we-do/our-research/heart-statistics

6.4 RESPIRATORY

6.4.1 1948–1975

Tuberculosis, lung cancer, asthma, and chronic bronchitis/emphysema were the major respiratory conditions affecting the adult population during this time. Signs of haemoptysis resulted in immediate referral to hospital. A wheezing child under the age of three had croup; over three, asthma.

The high prevalence of chronic bronchitis in the community was due to smoking, air pollution, and employment in dirty industries, such as coal mining. Chronic bronchitis was defined clinically as a productive cough, producing a small cup of sputum daily for a minimum of three months a year. Chronic bronchitics were described as 'blue bloaters,' cyanosed and oedematous; those with emphysema as 'pink puffers,' flushed and gasping for air. The diagnosis was made on clinical grounds, with the occasional aid of a chest X-ray. Spirometry was not available. Peak flow meters were uncommon in the immediate post-war period. Treatment was steam inhalation, oxygen, salbutamol, aminophylline, and antibiotics for infective exacerbations. GP home visits for respiratory distress were common.

The paucity of effective treatments for asthma was little better. Isoprenaline, as a metered-dose inhaler identical to the design still in use today, had been licensed in the UK in the mid-1960s, but the arrival of salbutamol in 1969, still the most widely used asthma drug to this day, was a genuine lifesaver. The efficacy and safety profile of the latter transformed the management of asthma, providing instant relief to patient and doctor alike.

Salbutamol was available in several formulations, including liquid, tablet, and nebulised solutions, but primarily as an inhaler, both meter-dose and breath-actuated. The meter-dose inhaler was a highly effective way of administering the drug, despite being irritatingly beyond the dexterity of many patients.

6.4.2 1976–1999

Salbutamol was good but had a short half-life. Salmeterol, a long-acting beta-adrenergic agonist (LABA), available from 1990, provided a useful adjunct in both the treatment of acute wheeze and the prevention of bronchospasm. Inhaled corticosteroids (ICS) were marketed and shown to be useful in both the prevention of and pulmonary destruction from chronic asthma. Inhalers combining a LABA and ICS, such as Seretide, were widely prescribed, overcoming the profession's antipathy to their high cost and drug combinations in general. GPs were inundated with a host of inhaler devices. Spacer devices and peak flow meters were issued to patients with asthma, and they were encouraged to keep a peak flow diary that was periodically reviewed by a clinician, increasingly a nurse. A step-by-step hierarchy of drug treatment was introduced. Patients were allowed to keep rescue courses of steroids and antibiotics at home for severe exacerbations.

The management of both chronic bronchitis and emphysema remained largely unchanged, apart from semantics; both were brought under the unifying banner of COPD. Cigarette smoking was in sharp decline, but this had little immediate impact on the prevalence of COPD.

A short-acting muscarinic antagonist, ipratropium, again by inhaler as pro-phylaxis therapy, was added to the GP's armamentarium, but it did not have the same dramatic impact on COPD that salbutamol had had on asthma.

6.4.3 2000 Onwards

The management of COPD, soon to be relabeled as chronic obstructive airways disease (COAD), became increasingly protocol-driven and was largely devolved to respiratory nurses.

All surgeries had a spirometer. COAD was no longer solely a clinical diagnosis but had become an equation: FEV1/FVC $\times$ 100 (Forced Expiratory Volume in 1 second, Forced Vital Capacity). If the sum was less than 70%, the patient had COAD. If not, they did not!

Tiotropium, via a once-daily inhaler, replaced ipratropium as the muscarinic receptor antagonist (LAMA) of choice.

Frustratingly, figures for morbidity and mortality for asthma and COAD remained stubbornly high. Those for the latter had diminished, but much of that was due to smoking cessation by the public, the closing down of the coal and other 'dirty' industries, and the enactment of health and safety legislation in the workplace. The story differed for asthma. Whether this was due to an increased prevalence of asthma, improved diagnosis, patient awareness, or poor medical management remained debatable. Annual mortality in England and Wales for asthma stabilised at around 1,300 from 2001 to 2018.[6]

Since the 1990s, the management of stable, chronic conditions, such as asthma and COPD, has shifted towards dedicated nurse-led clinics. A common refrain from doctors nowadays is that they feel increasingly deskilled in these areas. Addressing such shortfalls in knowledge through continuing professional devel-opment does not compensate for daily practice.

6.5 GASTRO-ENTEROLOGY

6.5.1 1948–1975

GPs had little recourse, apart from their clinical acumen, in diagnosing patients presenting with vomiting, diarrhoea, abdominal pain, abdominal mass, hemateme-sis, or melaena, nor did they have much in the way of treating such symptoms.

Faecal microbiology provided the first useful investigation in identifying symptoms with an infective origin. Barium meals and enemas became the imag-ing technology of choice in diagnosing pathology of the digestive tract, but these, of course, could only be performed in hospital. The first colonoscopy was per-formed in 1969, but it did not become widely used until the late 1970s.

---

[6] Deaths from Asthma England and Wales, 2001 to 2018 Asthma UK analysis ONS data.

The available drugs were primitive and included simple antacids, laxatives, and emetics. GPs felt helpless; their patients literally so.

6.5.2 1976–1999

The introduction of cimetidine, the first of the targeted H2-receptor agonists, revolutionised the management of upper gastrointestinal diseases, such as reflux oesophagitis and peptic ulcer. These conditions were predominantly treated in primary care. GPs trained as 'GP with special interest' (GPSI) in endoscopy procedures, such as gastroscopy and sigmoidoscopy, with some going on to provide gastroscopy services, in dedicated on-site suites, to their local medical community. Testing for *H. pylori* became available, and triple-therapy was introduced to eradicate the bacterium.

Targeted therapies, sulfasalazine, were introduced for inflammatory bowel diseases, with ongoing management in primary care following the confirmation of diagnosis.

Faecal occult blood (FOB), three samples taken on separate days, was the standard screening test for gastrointestinal (GI) bleeding and bowel cancer.

Jejunal biopsy, involving the patient swallowing a large metal capsule with a trap door (Crosby capsule) on the end of a length of string, was introduced to confirm the diagnosis of coeliac disease. Thankfully, the procedure was only performed in hospital.

6.5.3 2000 Onwards

Generally, little changed. Sadly, the number of GPs providing endoscopy services declined, the attraction of the role was buffeted by stringent health and safety measures, poor remuneration, and improved access to secondary care.

Faecal immunochemical tests (FIT) requiring one sample replaced FOB testing.

6.6 NEUROLOGY

Common presentations included meningitis, headache, migraine, transitory loss of consciousness, strokes, seizures, epilepsy, and sensory and movement disorders.

6.6.1 1948–1975

Meningitis remained a terrifying diagnosis with a high mortality rate.

The doctor had little to offer for any of the neurological presentations, apart from sympathy and reassurance. Headaches were treated with simple analgesics.

Epilepsy was controlled with phenobarbitone, phenytoin, and ethosuximide. All had side effects, the most significant being sedation and gum hyperplasia. Matters improved towards the late 1960s as sodium valproate and carbamazepine were introduced to the market.

Strokes were common, with catastrophic sequelae. Those who recovered from the initial event were left with profound disabilities. Rehabilitation through physiotherapy and occupational therapy was largely unavailable. Overall, GPs were left as helpless as their patients.

6.6.2 1976–1999

Meningitis still terrorised parents, and their GPs. Doctors carried penicillin and chloramphenicol in their emergency bag, ready to inject any child with the first signs of the disease prior to hospital admission. A public health programme taught parents the signs of a meningococcal rash.

Aspirin, paracetamol, and non-steroidal anti-inflammatory drugs (NSAIDs) remained the mainstay of treatment for acute headache.

The introduction of the triptans paralleled developments in the rational management of headaches. GPs increasingly accepted that the multifactorial origins of headaches required differing therapies. The entities of chronic headache syndromes and analgesic abuse gained purchase, as did the need for different drug classes to combat each type. Even the old warhorse, the tricyclic antidepressant amitriptyline, in low doses, gained a new lease of life in pain management. Headache diaries were encouraged. Expectations of what constituted a cure were lowered. None of these actions stopped headaches from being one of the most common presentations in general practice.

GPs were seeing fewer strokes, thanks to the improvements in lifestyle and more rigorous control of hypertension and hyperlipidaemia. Unfortunate patients succumbing to a stroke were no longer seen first by a GP but admitted via 999 straight to hospital, where thrombolytic therapies greatly improved the chance of a full recovery and minimal subsequent disability.

Newer drugs for the management of epilepsy, vigabatrin, lamotrigine, and gabapentin, were introduced with much fanfare. These were initially prescribed by a neurologist and, thereafter, monitored by the GP in the community.

GPs became highly adept at diagnosing complex neurological conditions, such as multiple sclerosis, motor neuron disease, and Parkinson's disease. Treatment for the latter was often initiated in primary care, with a patient only referred to a specialist should their symptoms remain refractory or side effects uncontrolled.

6.6.3 2000

The threat of meningitis receded following the introduction of HIB (haemophilus influenza B), pneumococcal, and meningococcal C vaccines to the infant immunisation programme. The last, introduced in 1999, had a dramatic effect on cases which fell by 50% within four years.[7]

---

[7] www.meningitis.org/getmedia/7a77a71e-4113-48f7-b0e6-eee01a64bfe5/Recent-epidemiology-of-meningococcal-disease-and-impact-of-immunisation-programmes-in-the-UK-Ray-Borrow

The management of epilepsy became part of QOF, requiring an annual review of patients with the condition.

As new drugs became available, patients were referred to specialist clinics at the first signs of Parkinson's disease. I vividly recall uncomfortable conversations with the embarrassed and distressed spouses of two previously mild-mannered, somewhat nondescript individuals, who had become addicted to online gambling and pornography. The gentlemen themselves were more blasé, convinced that they had found an activity that provided a modicum of relief from the ravages of Parkinson's. Thankfully, at least for their wives, their marriages were saved when their behaviour reverted to 'normal' on discontinuation of the drug.

Doctors were urged to refer any patient at the first sign of a movement disorder to a specialist clinic.

6.7 UROGENITAL

The common urogenital conditions presenting in general practice were, and remain, lower urinary tract infections, ureteric and bladder obstruction due to stones, or prostate and erectile dysfunction in men; stress/urge incontinence, pelvic pain, and non-menstrual vaginal bleeding in women.

6.7.1 1948–1975

Urinary tract infections were diagnosed clinically and treated blind with fluids thought to acidify the urine, mostly containing potassium citrate, and sulphonamide antibiotics.

Acute renal and ureteric colic were initially managed with pethidine or morphine analgesia, anticholinergic smooth-muscle relaxing drugs as hyoscine, and plenty of fluids. If this combination did not relieve symptoms, then the patient was referred to A&E.

Acute obstruction of the bladder neck by an enlarged prostate gland, at any time of the day or night, demanded urgent assessment and bladder catheterisation, providing instant and grateful relief. Invariably, patients went on to have an open prostatectomy performed by a general surgeon.

Women with stress incontinence (urge incontinence was not recognised as a distinct entity at that time) were basically told by their male doctors to 'get on with it.' There were no specific treatments for dysmenorrhoea, menorrhagia, or polymenorrhoea, although the combined oral contraceptive pill, increasingly prescribed, was found to serendipitously benefit these symptoms. Hysterectomies were routinely performed. Drugs such as mefenamic acid were marketed as an improvement on NSAIDs for relieving dysmenorrhoea, but this was not borne out in practice.

Doctors of the time carried out rectal and vaginal examinations as a matter of course. The word 'chaperone' had yet to enter the GP vernacular.

6.7.2 1976–1999

Urinary tract infections were diagnosed on a mid-stream sample of urine sent to the local microbiology department, with antibiotics prescribed following the results of culture and sensitivity.

Alpha-blockers drugs were introduced for the management of the symptoms of benign prostatic hypertrophy. GPs still catheterised patients, but district nurses also began taking on that task. The prostate-specific antigen test (PSA) was introduced in 1986 and, alongside digital rectal examination, used as a screening test for prostate cancer.

Hormone-containing intrauterine devices (IUD/IUCD) were used to manage menstrual problems, reducing hospital referrals and hysterectomies. These were inserted by any GP who had completed an obstetrics and gynaecology job within their GP vocational training schemes (VTS). Further training was not required.

Female patients were offered a chaperone if an intimate examination was being considered, but this was very much on a piecemeal basis. Any member of staff could act as a chaperone.

6.7.3 2000 Onwards

Samples for suspected urinary tract infections were only sent to a local laboratory after a dipstick test had been done in the surgery. The length of any antibiotic course was shortened from ten to three days in uncomplicated infections.

GPs rarely performed bladder catheterisations; patients went directly to hospital, and catheter changes were done by community nurses.

An unexpected consequence of the National Institute for Clinical Excellence (NICE) guidelines catapulted a significant proportion of the elderly population into a state of panic over their kidney function. It took years and innumerable blood tests before these fears were finally allayed in both patients and physicians.[8]

Sildenafil allowed doctors to treat erectile dysfunction in a far more acceptable manner than the bicycle pumps, needles, and, privately funded, psychosexual counselling that predated its introduction.

Intrauterine systems (IUS, formerly IUD/IUCD), such as the Mirena coil, which could be left in vivo for up to five years, were increasingly being used not just as a contraceptive device but also for the management of irregular menstrual bleeding, menorrhagia, and dysmenorrhoea. The NHS vigorously promoted long-acting reversible contraceptives (LARC) as both safer and more reliable than the combined contraceptive pill, and QOF rewarded their use. Female doctors and nurses found themselves taking on the bulk of any work relating to women's health.

Chaperones had to be trained and certified for the role!

---

[8] https://cks.nice.org.uk/topics/chronic-kidney-disease/management/management-of-chronic-kidney-disease/

6.8 METABOLIC/ENDOCRINE

The common endocrine diseases presenting in a GP surgery were diabetes mellitus, hypo and hyperthyroidism, gout, and osteomalacia (rickets).

6.8.1 1948–1975

Endemic in the post-war years of food rationing, children with rickets presented at GP surgeries with bowed legs and rosary ricket chests. Rickets had first been described by the English physician Daniel Whistler in 1645, and it was indefensible that it was still common three centuries later. Prevalence declined rapidly following the adoption of public health policy ensuring that every schoolchild was given a third of a pint of milk a day.

Gout, an even more venerable condition, was managed by colchicine, analgesia, ice, and elevation plus lugubrious advice to cut down on the port. Colchicine proved to be highly effective in managing gouty pain, as its use to the present day attests.

Complex endocrine diseases were managed almost exclusively by hospital specialists. The diagnosis of diabetes was based on clinical presentation, glycosuria, and raised blood glucose level. Acute hypoglycaemia was treated with intravenous glucose, a 50 ml vial that was an indispensable presence in any doctor's emergency bag.

Thyroid disease was diagnosed on clinical presentation and blood thyroxine/thyroid-stimulating hormone (TSH) levels.

Thyroxine was the first drug to be excluded from prescription charges. Other conditions in this historic group include.[9]

- Cancer (note that this includes treatment for the effects of cancer or treatment for the effects of current or previous cancer treatment)
- A permanent fistula requiring dressing
- Hypoadrenalism, such as Addison's disease
- Diabetes insipidus and other forms of hypopituitarism
- Diabetes mellitus except where treatment is by diet alone
- Hypoparathyroidism
- Myasthenia gravis
- Epilepsy requiring continuous anticonvulsive medication

6.8.2 1976–1999

Uncomplicated type 2 diabetes (T2DM) became a routine part of a GP's workload. Type 1 DM continued to be exclusively managed in secondary care. Monitoring no longer relied on blood glucose levels, a snapshot, following the introduction of glycated haemoglobin (HbA1c), which provided a video of glycaemic control over three months. Cheap finger-prick blood glucose machines replaced routine urine dipsticks as the method of choice for patients monitoring their glucose levels.

---

[9] www.nhsbsa.nhs.uk/exemption-certificates/medical-exemption-certificates

Practices introduced chronic disease management clinics for diabetes, run by practice nurses. Care in the community was increasingly managed by hospital-based specialist nurses.

Awareness of the long-term effects of steroid therapies, especially adrenal gland suppression and osteoporosis, led to a reduction of their use unless absolutely clinically indicated, as in the treatment of temporal arteritis and polymyalgia rheumatica. Long-term prescribing, even in such low doses as prescribed for hay fever or chronic urticaria, was strongly discouraged. Prophylactic co-prescribing of a bisphosphonate was recommended.

The cost of inhaled corticosteroids used in the treatment of asthma rocketed by over 500% as the propellant in metered-dose inhalers was switched to chlorofluorocarbon-free (CFC, hydrofluoroalkane), in accordance with the 1988 Montreal Protocol for reducing the hole in the ozone layer. The science behind the switch to CFC-free inhalers was questionable,[10] and patients found the new inhalers to be less responsive than those they replaced.

6.8.3 2000 Onwards

The parameters for diagnosis and control of diabetes mellitus were tightened: fasting blood glucose greater than 7.0 mmol/L and HbA1c below 48mmol/mol or 6.5%. The prevalence of T2DM in the community continued to rise inexorably and was blamed on poor lifestyle and obesity.

New classes of antidiabetic drugs were introduced, at first causing some confusion amongst clinicians who had become deskilled through lack of regular contact with their diabetic population.

More sophisticated insulin delivery and glucose monitoring devices were being prescribed by hospital specialist departments.

The improvements in diabetic care over the decades resulted in fewer hospital admissions for secondary complications of diabetes, such as renal failure and peripheral vascular disease. Meanwhile, emergency hospital admissions for hypoglycaemia and ketoacidosis continued to rise.[11]

6.9 HAEMATOLOGY

Common presentations were anaemia and lymphadenopathy. Both were usually due to a secondary cause, with the underlying aetiology demanding further investigation.

---

[10] Harrison E. Unlikely victims of banning CFCs—Asthma sufferers. Scientific American, 2008. Accessed 30 Apr 2019 from www.scientificamerican.com/article.cfm?id=unlikely-victims-of-banning-cfcs

[11] Fleetcroft R, Asaria M, Ali S, Cookson R. Outcomes and inequalities in diabetes from 2004/2005 to 2011/2012: English longitudinal study. Br J Gen Pract. 2017 Jan;67(654):e1–e9. doi: 10.3399/bjgp16X688381. Epub 2016 Dec 5. PMID: 27919938; PMCID: PMC5198605.

6.9.1 1948–1975

Iron deficiency, microcytic anaemia, in women was deemed due to excessive menstruation, until proven otherwise, and treated with iron supplements.

Vitamin B12 deficiency, pernicious, macrocytic anaemia was diagnosed on blood film and treated with monthly intramuscular vitamin B12 injections.

Lymphadenopathy was observed and referred for a hospital opinion if it persisted.

6.9.2 1976–1999

A broader haematology workup, including serum iron, ferritin, transferrin, vitamin B12, and folate, became available to GPs, but otherwise management remained unchanged.

The threshold for referral for any lymphadenopathy was lowered, especially for neck lumps.[12]

6.9.3 2000 Onwards

No change!

6.10 WOMEN'S HEALTH

Presentations relating specifically to women's health included contraception, fertility, cervical cytology, vaginal discharge, menstrual problems, menopause, and pelvic mass, often, happily, no more than an unexpected cyesis.

6.10.1 1948–1975

Before the 1960s and certainly in the early years following the introduction of oral contraception, family planning advice was given solely by specialised private services outside the NHS. Subsequently, the contraceptive pill had to be prescribed by a qualified medical practitioner. GPs were encouraged to provide family planning services funded separately through 'item of service' payments. A predominantly middle-aged, male GP population had the novel experience of seeing otherwise healthy, young, mini-skirted women seeking sexual freedom. It must have provided a pleasant change from their usual clientele! Oral contraception take-up was so rapid and dramatic, it soon became known as 'THE pill.'

The Abortion Act[13] was passed in 1967, allowing for the surgical termination of pregnancy up to 24 weeks' cyesis. Prior to the act, distraught women with an unwanted pregnancy had no option but to continue the pregnancy to term or resort to an illegal termination by an unqualified, back-street abortionist. The Act

---

[12] https://cks.nice.org.uk/neck-lump

[13] www.legislation.gov.uk/ukpga/1967/87/section/1

provided timely relief to the women and their doctors; the latter previously left to pick up the pieces when unlicenced procedures went wrong.

The terms of the Act were clearly defined, with the requirement that any woman seeking a termination of pregnancy must be seen by two registered medical practitioners, one of which was likely to be a GP. The doctors had to 'act in good faith' in referring the woman for termination. Some GPs with strong religious convictions refused to countenance any referral, and their beliefs often soured the relationships within the partnership. The debate on what was in the best interests of the mother and child remains unresolved to the present day.

Uncomplicated pregnancies were managed by the GP, with help from the midwife in the community.

6.10.2 1975–1999

Scare stories regarding 'the pill' waxed and waned. The association between larger doses of oestrogens and thromboembolic disease was confirmed and rectified by lowering the dose whilst maintaining efficacy. Similarly, progestogen levels were linked to raised blood pressure and the dose subsequently adjusted.

The provision of contraceptive services under the NHS was considered a public health responsibility, resulting in community family planning clinics running in parallel with the service provided in GP surgeries. This was not ideal; both services operated on strict patient confidentiality and, thus, did not communicate with each other. Thus, a woman could be taking a drug, the contraceptive pill, prone to adverse effects and drug interactions just like any other medication, and this would not be recorded in her medical records. The potential for a serious adverse event was high, but the anomaly was never rectified.

Pregnancy became the sole responsibility of the midwife.

Access to termination of pregnancy under the NHS remained limited. Local hospitals operated a strict quota on the number of terminations they would do in any month. GPs had to manage patient expectations, which was especially distressing for those young mothers who could not afford to pay for an abortion at a private clinic.

Infertility became an issue that could be treated. GPs undertook preliminary investigations covering male sperm analysis and menstrual temperature charts, before referring the couple for specialist care.

Cervical cytology screening was introduced for women aged 20–64 in 1988. Both doctors and nurses took routine cervical smears.

Menstrual problems, often related to benign fibroids, were managed by the Mirena coil, and referrals for hysterectomies declined.

6.10.3 2000 Onwards

Despite the widespread availability of free contraception in the UK, the incidence of abortion continued to rise from 8 per 1,000 women aged 15–44 in 1970, to peak at 18.2 in 2008.[14] Rates have since levelled off, partly due to the licensing in 2000, of mifepristone with misoprostol for medical termination of pregnancy up to nine weeks. Levonorgestrel, Levonelle, a palatable, safe, and effective post-coital contraception was initially only available on prescription but quickly moved to prescription-free purchase from chemists.

By 2010, any GP wishing to continue fitting an IUD had to have a basic qualification of Diploma of the Faculty of Family Planning, subsequently renamed Diploma of Family Sexual and Reproductive Health (DFSRH).[15] This requirement, coupled with medico-legal concerns regarding intimate gynaecological examinations, resulted in most male doctors discontinuing their interest in family planning, leaving their female colleagues to complain that they saw nothing but women in their clinics!

Practice nurses did all cervical screening. Male doctors shied away from any pelvic examination, partly in response to patient preference and partly due to medico-legal concerns.

Distressing symptoms arising from the menopause were managed with hormone replacement therapy (HRT) although not without controversy. The Million Women Study suggested a relationship between HRT and the risk of breast, endometrial, and ovarian cancer, creating huge anxiety in women who now had to balance benefit against risk. HRT use halved in the UK. By the 2010s, such concerns had been reversed.

6.11 DERMATOLOGY

The main dermatological conditions seen in general practice were eczema, psoriasis, acne, and fungal infections.

6.11.1 1948–1975

The mainstay of treatment for eczema, emollients, remained largely unchanged over decades, with each formulation coming in and out of fashion with time. As a rule, the greasier the application, ointment, cream, lotion, the more effective. A perennial issue in prescribing was GP reluctance to issue the large quantities required for an individual's needs.[16]

Formulations containing coal tar, ointment, and baths were used to manage psoriasis.

GPs tended to ignore acne. Advice ranged from 'cut down on sweets' to 'it's your hormones; you'll grow out of it.' Benzoyl peroxide cream (1930s) was rarely prescribed.

---

[14] www.statista.com/statistics/470890/legal-abortions-performed-in-england-and-wales/#:~:text=In%202000%20there%20were%20175%2C542,preformed%20in%20England%20and%20Wales

[15] www.fsrh.org/about-the-fsrh-diploma-and-nurse-diploma-dfsrh-and-ndfsrh/

[16] https://midessexccg.nhs.uk/medicines-optimisation/clinical-pathways-and-medication-guidelines/chapter-13-skin-3/2532-emollients-prescribing-guidelines-jan-2019/file

Antifungal compounds such as clotrimazole (1969) and miconazole (1971) provided effective treatment for minor fungal skin infections, such as tinea pedis, tinea cruris, and intertrigo.

All the above chemicals came in combination with steroids. The combination was popular with GPs, although dermatologists frowned on such practice.

Unsightly skin lumps, cysts, and moles were routinely excised in the surgery.

6.11.2 1976–1999

Little changed in the treatment of eczema, but newer, once-daily preparations were marketed for fungal infections and psoriasis. Severe, widespread, large plaque psoriasis had to be referred for specialist treatment of psoralen and ultra-violet A light therapy (PUVA).

Acne became recognised as a condition that could lead to facial scarring and mental health problems. Treatment became more aggressive with early introduction of oral antibiotics. Severe cases were referred to outpatient dermatology for isotretinoin, for hospital use only, due to potential serious side effects.

Unsightly skin lumps, cysts, and moles were still excised in the surgery but now attracted a minor surgery fee, £10 per procedure, under the provisions of the SFA.

6.11.3 2000 Onwards

No change generally, but new biologic and expensive immunotherapeutic agents were being licensed for the treatment of psoriasis, only available for hospital use.

Unsightly skin lumps, cysts, and moles were rarely excised in the surgery unless funded by Local Enhanced Services.

6.12 MUSCULOSKELETAL

Patients presented with acute muscular sprains and backache. Management of such conditions was based on ICE, ice, compression, and elevation for soft-tissue injuries, and analgesia, rest, and rehabilitation/exercise for back pain.

6.12.1 1948–1975

Back pain of any origin was treated passively by total rest for lengthy periods. Some GPs were adept at spinal manipulation, though clinical evidence of any benefit was scant.

Access to physiotherapy was non-existent.

6.12.2 1976–1999

General management remained unchanged, but access to NHS physiotherapy improved despite waiting times that could last months. Often the condition had resolved well before the patient was seen. Those who could afford to, paid for private physiotherapy. Patient advice leaflets on managing acute sprains and subsequent exercise regimes provided a temporary substitute for hands-on therapy. GPs could request a domiciliary visit by a hospital anaesthetist to perform a spinal nerve block for intractable back pain.

Swollen joints were aspirated and injected with steroids. The procedure attracted a £10 fee in the Statement of Fees and Allowances, following 1990 changes.

6.12.3 2000 Onwards

The emphasis on managing any pain shifted to active exercise after a minimal period of rest. Access to physiotherapy services improved, with many GP surgeries having a physiotherapy service on-site. Patients were allowed to self-refer to physiotherapy without having to see a GP first.

Domiciliary visits by a consultant anaesthetist became a rarity as hospitals introduced dedicated, multidisciplinary clinics for back pain.

Joint aspiration and injections became less popular, due to health, safety, and remuneration issues.

6.13 EAR, NOSE AND THROAT (ENT)

ENT conditions commonly presented in children and included tonsillitis, otitis media, otitis externa, and the various causes of rhinorrhea (foreign body, infection and allergy). Adults presented with hearing loss due to wax impaction and old age.

6.13.1 1948–1975

Any consultation where infection was suspected, regardless of viral or bacterial, resulted in the issuing of an antibiotic prescription.

Repeated episodes of tonsillitis, enlarged tonsils, and adenoids were referred to hospital and invariably resulted in tonsil and adenoidectomy.

Doctors removed ear wax using a dauntingly large, metal ear syringe.

6.13.2 1976–1999

Doubts were arising regarding the profligate use of antibiotics for mainly viral upper respiratory tract infections. Such doubts were not transferred to anxious parents who still expected a prescription for every cold.

Surgery for enlarged tonsils was rationed.

Nurses removed ear wax using electric irrigator machines.

6.13.3 2000 onwards

Relentless public health campaigns resulted in gradual parental acceptance that it was in their child's interest not to take an antibiotic for every cold. GPs spent more time explaining to parents why this was so.

Surgery for enlarged tonsils became a rarity.

Ear syringing was rarely performed in surgeries. Patients were encouraged to attend commercial providers.

6.14 AUTOIMMUNE AND INFLAMMATORY

The common rheumatology presentations were carpal tunnel syndrome, rheumatoid arthritis, seronegative inflammatory arthritis, giant cell arteritis, polymyalgia rheumatica, and lupus.

6.14.1 1948–1975

The diagnosis underlying any swollen, inflamed joint was clinical, supplemented by erythrocyte sedimentation rate (ESR).

Aspirin and other NSAIDs were the mainstay treatment for rheumatoid arthritis and seronegative inflammatory diseases. Disease-modifying agents of dubious provenance (gold and penicillamine) were prescribed and administered by GPs. The majority of cases were seen by hospital specialists, with ongoing management in the community.

6.14.2 1976–1999

Improved access to laboratory investigations (C-reactive protein (CRP), Rheumatoid Factor (RF), HLA B27) allowed for a more informed diagnosis.

Initial management was still undertaken in hospital, but ongoing management with newer chemical agents, such as COX-2 inhibitors and immunotherapies, azathioprine and methotrexate, were managed in primary care. The potential for adverse drug interactions had to be closely monitored.

Temporal arteritis and polymyalgia rheumatica were managed almost exclusively in primary care, with the diagnosis made on clinical presentation, supported by a significantly raised ESR and/or CRP. Treatment involved the immediate initiation of high dose (60 mg) prednisolone for the former, 40 mg for the latter.

Carpal tunnel syndrome was predominantly managed in primary care, by splinting and local steroid injection.

6.14.3 2000 Onwards

Care was transferred almost totally to specialist rheumatologists. Protocols were introduced for the rapid referral of suspected inflammatory joint disease. Novel biologic agents were highly effective, providing first-time genuine relief to patients suffering with these intractable conditions.

Guidance on the management of temporal arteritis, renamed giant cell arteritis, recommended emergency referral to a rheumatologist and ophthalmologist. If visual symptoms were present, then a same-day appointment with an ophthalmologist for temporal artery biopsy or ultrasound scan was mandatory.

In practice, this was not always possible, and high-dose steroids would be initiated, as before. In 40 years of practice, I never came across a single patient who had had a temporal artery biopsy.

6.15 ALLERGY

The common presentations were insect bites, urticaria, seasonal hay fever, and asthma.

6.15.1 1948–1975

The initial treatment for any allergic presentation was chlorpheniramine, rarely supplemented by steroids or adrenaline.

Prevention of symptoms became available through courses of desensitising injections against presumed, untested allergens. These could be undertaken in the GP surgery, often without access to resuscitation equipment!

6.15.2 1976–1999

More targeted therapies, such as topical (eyes, nose, skin) steroids and cromolyn sodium (Intal) provided some relief with few side effects.

Skin-prick allergen testing was offered to GPs by enterprising drug companies.

6.15.3 2000 Onwards

Drugs remained largely unchanged, but skin-prick testing was withdrawn, following safety fears.

Parents presented in increasing numbers with concerns over food, particularly peanut, allergies. GPs learned, and attempted to teach concerned parents, the difference between allergy and intolerance.

6.16 MENTAL HEALTH

The common mental health conditions included anxiety, depression, insomnia, the psychoses of schizophrenia and bipolar, and substance (drug and alcohol) abuse.

6.16.1 1948–1975

An accepted, binary division of mental health disorders prevailed. Diagnoses related to whether symptoms were exogenous or endogenous, the former classified as neurosis, the latter as psychosis.

In the early years of the NHS, the medical view towards mental health was one of acceptance tempered by a sense of despair. Treatment lay outside the remit of the average GP and in the hands of the specialist psychiatrist, often culminating in brutal therapies, such as ECT or lobotomy.

Following the introduction of the first oral antidepressant drugs, the mono-amine oxidase inhibitor in the 1950s, understandings changed, and specialist mental health services devolved the management of non-psychotic, still referred to as 'neurotic,' patients, to primary care.

Psychiatrists managed schizophrenia and manic depression, often involving lengthy inpatient care. Antipsychotics of the time, such as chlorpromazine (1950s), were effective but had profound side effects.

6.16.2 1976–1999

Depression was classified as being either endogenous, arising from within and due to a chemical imbalance within the brain, thus likely to benefit from a chemical intervention, or exogenous, a reaction to a life event and, thus, within the bounds of normal human emotional behaviour and, therefore, unlikely to be improved by a drug. To a degree, this simplistic classification, without the nomenclature, remains in place to this day, the former remaining within the purview of drug intervention, the latter more effectively managed by the talking therapies of counselling or cognitive behavioural therapy (CBT), carried out by counsellors, often untrained, based in GP surgeries.

Early treatment was advocated following the introduction of the 'safer' selective serotonin reuptake inhibitors (SSRIs). The attitude of 'try it and see' prevailed. The term Social Anxiety Disorder was coined; doctors viewed the condition as a cynical ploy by the pharmaceutical industry to create a disease for a drug, rather than the reverse.

Objective grading of the severity of mental health disorders was introduced in the 1990s, with a variety of scoring questionnaires, such as the Generalised Anxiety Disorder Assessment (GAD-7) and the Patient Health Questionnaire-9 (PHQ-9). The PHQ-9 had been developed by a pharmaceutical company (Pfizer) as a tool for drug clinical development.

Victorian mental hospitals were sold off and their occupants moved out into the community, managed by community mental health nurses/workers liaising with primary care. For many years thereafter, lonely, unkempt figures talking to themselves and clutching plastic bags of belongings stalked the town centres of Britain. It took some time for community care to be adequately funded.

GPs managed stable schizophrenia by using long-acting intramuscular phenothiazines.

Manic depression was relabelled bipolar disorder. Once stable, it too was managed by GPs using lithium carbonate (first used in 1948). Toxicity required regular testing of kidney and thyroid function.

6.16.3 2000 Onwards

The diagnosis and management of anxiety and depressive illness aspired to move away from chemical to behavioural therapies. Protocols for early referral for CBT were introduced but were not matched by the number of CBT counsellors. Online well-being tools were substituted to meet the demand. That some people may require lifelong medication for depression became established.

Drug classes for anxiety and depression were rationalised to three: SSRI, SNRI (serotonin and noradrenergic reuptake inhibitor; duloxetine if pain present, venlafaxine if not), and NaSSA (noradrenergic and specific serotonin antidepressant; mirtazapine if insomnia present).[17]

Newer antipsychotics, olanzapine and aripiprazole, were introduced but, as with all effective drugs, were duly found to have significant adverse effects, most notably weight gain and diabetes. Both required frequent biochemical monitoring.

The lexicon of mental health conditions expanded dramatically. Over 300 were listed in the 2019 edition of the International Classification of Disease (ICD-10),[18] a publication produced by the WHO and used by the NHS. These included examples such as nose-picking, sibling rivalry disorder, and sadomasochism. It became rare for anyone not to have had symptoms of a mental health disorder at some time in their life.

Community mental health services were repeatedly reconfigured, and GPs had trouble keeping up with the new structures and procedures for referral. Nevertheless, any service provided was well appreciated by local GPs if it removed some of the mental health burden from their surgeries. Patients could increasingly self-refer to counselling and drug and alcohol addiction services. Some GPs became 'local providers' of addiction services.

By the first decade of the 21st century, of the benzodiazepine class of drugs, only chlordiazepoxide (for short-course management of withdrawal symptoms in alcoholics), midazolam (for seizures), and the old warhorse, diazepam (mainly as a muscle relaxant), were still in widespread circulation. The hypnotic benzodiazepines were replaced by the nonbenzodiazepine 'Z-drugs' (zopiclone, zolpidem), marketed as being non-addictive. In due course, as their use became more widespread, they were found to have no advantages over their predecessors.[19] The dictum that 'where there is a need and a means to effectively meet that need, then dependence almost inevitably follows' remained extant.

6.17 PREVENTIVE MEDICINE

The benefits of disease prevention through immunisation had already been established, as were those of non-pharmacological interventions, nutrition, lifestyle,

[17] NICE Depression. Mar 2020. https://cks.nice.org.uk/depression#!scenarioRecommendation

[18] www.who.int/classifications/icd/en/bluebook.pdf

[19] Holbrook AM, Crowther R, Lotter A, Cheng C, King D. Meta-analysis of benzodiazepine use in the treatment of insomnia. CMAJ. 2000 Jan 25;162(2):225–33. PMID: 10674059; PMCID: PMC1232276.

and environment. Between 1980 and 2020, life expectancy in the UK[20] increased from 70 to 78 years for men and from 77 to 83 years for women. Within a single generation, individuals could expect to enjoy five more years of active life than their parents. Recognition of these factors gradually moved medical practice to placing increasing emphasis on the prevention of disease.

Primary care had neither the understanding nor the means to provide any alternative to therapeutic medicine in the first quarter-century following the creation of the NHS. Preventive interventions depended on the discipline of epidemiology, as the Oxford dictionary defines it, 'the branch of medicine which deals with the incidence, distribution, and possible control of diseases and other factors relating to health.'

The conundrum for those working in general practice was applying findings in the population to treatment of the individual. Understanding the statistical analysis of data was beyond the laity, and most doctors. Marginal improvements in morbidity and mortality were difficult to explain to a symptomless human. Preventive medicine became stigmatised as the medicalisation of the healthy.

The acceptance and publication of epidemiological studies from the 1960s onwards resulted in GPs increasingly including lifestyle advice in their consultations. Along with guidance on stopping smoking came advice on diet, reducing salt and saturated fats and increasing fibre, and regular exercise. These prompts tended to be patchy and unfocused. Many GPs remained unconvinced by the potential for words to replace drugs despite studies by one of their own, Dr Chris Steele, a GP in Manchester, who demonstrated that a significant number of smokers could be persuaded to give up the habit simply by asking them, at each consultation, whether they smoked. In short, a simple throwaway comment, provided that the words came out of a doctor's mouth, could have a profound effect on a person's lifestyle. Patients listened to doctors! That in itself must have come as a shocking revelation to most hardened, cynical GPs who had been the products of entirely science-based undergraduate medical education. It took many years for advice to replace the reflexive writing of a prescription. However, drugs provided the mainstay of disease prevention, their role demonstrated conclusively in the management of potential cardiovascular disease.

The case for treating symptomless hypertension had been made in the Framlingham Heart Study[21] from 1950 onwards, the findings of which were heavily promoted by pharmaceutical sales representatives. However, a British pioneer in the field of epidemiology, Sir James Mackenzie,[22] had pre-empted the findings from Framlingham in his own research 30 years earlier. Mackenzie, a medical

[20] Office for National Statistics. www.ons.gov.uk/peoplepopulationandcommunity/births deathsandmarriages/lifeexpectancies/bulletins/nationallifetablesunitedkingdom/2018to2020

[21] Dawber TR, Meadors GF, Moore FE Jr. Epidemiological approaches to heart disease: the Framingham Study. Am J Public Health Nations Health. 1951 Mar;41(3):279–81. doi: 10.2105/ajph.41.3.279. PMID: 14819398; PMCID: PMC1525365.

[22] https://academic.oup.com/ije/article/41/6/1525/749440; doi: 10.1093/ije/dys196

polymath, pioneered the use of the polygraph in diagnosing cardiac arrhythmia, founded the eponymous Institute of Clinical Research in St Andrews, and had a lasting influence on general practice through his encouragement of the local GP community keeping written records of their patients' long-term symptoms and illnesses, an innovation in the 1920s that could claim to make him the father of medical records.

The working hypothesis of the Framingham group was that hypertensive and arteriosclerotic cardiovascular disease did not have a single cause but was rather the culmination of multiple factors. Their published work in 1961 detailed a list of preconditions, hypertension, hyperlipidaemia, obesity, arrhythmia, and smoking (exercise was identified as decreasing risk) that became the 'cardiovascular risk factors,' the basis of all cardiovascular consultations. All these elements were subsequently refined into the Framingham cardiovascular risk score, the common tool for predicting cardiovascular morbidity in the NHS before the introduction of more UK-specific population algorithms, such as QRISK.[23]

GPs from 1970 onwards were bombarded by pharmaceutical sales teams with 'facts' coming out of the Framingham study, encouraging them to prescribe more antihypertensive drugs. The data was so compelling that GPs were made to feel incompetent if any patient on their list between the ages of 40 and 75 was not on such an agent. However, the salesmen were pushing on an open door. There is nothing that a doctor likes to see more than an abnormal number returning to normality following a therapeutic intervention. For hypertension, read diabetes, hyperlipidaemia, anaemia, asthma, or any number of markers, surrogate or otherwise, of disease. GPs adopted en masse the aggressive management of blood pressure, and over the years, the UK population benefitted by a steady decline in acute cardiovascular events and reduction in chronic morbidity and mortality from such events. Myocardial infarction and strokes, once common in primary care, are now a rarity. CVD mortality declined by 72% between 1979 and 2013.[24,25]

The other iconic study that became the staple of CV disease prevention in the mid-1990s was the Scandinavian Simvastatin Survival Study (4S).[26] One of the first 'megatrials,' the precursors of meta-analysis, 4S, along with the West of Scotland Coronary Prevention Study (WOSCOPS[27]), demonstrated the link between blood lipids and cardiovascular events that formed the basis for the universal use of statins.

[23] The QRISK 3 calculator. Accessed 1 May 2019 from https://qrisk.org/

[24] Bhatnagar P, et al. Trends in the epidemiology of cardiovascular disease in the UK. Heart. 2016;102(24). https://heart.bmj.com/content/102/24/1945.full

[25] https://heart.bmj.com/content/102/24/1945.full

[26] Randomised trial of cholesterol lowering in 4444 patients with coronary heart disease: the Scandinavian Simvastatin Survival Study (4S). Lancet. 1994 Nov 19;344(8934):1383–9. PMID: 7968073. https://pubmed.ncbi.nlm.nih.gov/7968073/

[27] West of Scotland coronary prevention study: identification of high-risk groups and comparison with other cardiovascular intervention trials. Lancet. 1996 Nov 16;348(9038): 1339–42. PMID: 8918276. https://pubmed.ncbi.nlm.nih.gov/8918276/

Framingham, 4S, and WOSCOPS were snowballs on a Swiss alp. The momentum for cardiovascular disease prevention gathered pace, and by the 21st century constituted a significant part of the workload in primary care.

GPs had become specialists in managing essential hypertension and dyslipidaemia, but the number of cardiologists in secondary care, rather than succumbing to redundancies, actually increased! They carved out a new role themselves. Exercise stress electrocardiograms became mandatory for the diagnosis of angina. Chest pain required percutaneous coronary artery angiography and perhaps subsequent coronary artery stenting. Percutaneous coronary intervention procedures per million population (UK) increased from 50 to 600 procedures a year.[28] Cardiac failure, a condition that GPs had previously and arguably quite adequately managed, was complicated by the mandatory requirement for echocardiography and newly identified diagnostic blood tests, all of which could only be done in hospital. Savings from preventive medicine were proving to be illusory.

Refinements in diagnostic investigations had further repercussions on GP confidence. Myocardial infarction, a diagnosis traditionally made on history, examination, ECG, and elevated non-specific cardiac enzyme levels, segued into a spectrum of presentations often with normal ECG and identifiable by highly specific blood troponin levels only available in hospitals. Previously clear waters had become turbid. Once hospitalised, a previously fit person would be discharged with a basket of drugs which, as of 2019, comprised aspirin, clopidogrel, bisoprolol, ramipril, atorvastatin, and eplerenone. It is quite humbling to experience the faith that patients have in their physicians, when one day they may be taking nothing, only to be taking a chemist's shelf of drugs the next.

The age of polypharmacy had begun.

People were living longer but they were not necessarily living healthier. Diseases of degeneration were still taking their toll. The UK population accumulated chronic diseases with age. Conditions were being recognised earlier, but effective management required drugs, and the more drugs used, the more opportunities presented themselves for drug interactions and adverse effects.

Medical student teaching had always placed 'iatrogenic,' from the Greek iatrós=doctor, genic=cause, or medically induced disease, at the top of any differential diagnosis list. A mandatory part of clerking patients included the list of medications that they were taking. The length of this list and its relevance increased with time, from almost nothing in the 1950s to upwards of a dozen drugs in, say, a patient with asthma and diabetes, in the 2000s. This explosion in polypharmacy, whilst arguably beneficial to the patient, created a heightened level of concern, even anxiety, in the physician. That drugs interact was not a novel concept. That drugs sometimes competitively use the same metabolic pathways in the human body was common knowledge. That the pharmacodynamics of a chemical compound at its site of action was fundamental to its licensing approval from the drug regulatory authorities was a legal requirement.

[28] www.nicor.org.uk/wp-content/uploads/2020/12/National-Audit-of-Percutaneous-Coronary-Intervention-2020-Summary-Report-FINAL.pdf

The competent physician took all these factors into account when prescribing any drug but needed a more accessible reference book than the *British Pharmacopoeia*, which, in all its majesty, weighed 3 kg in paper format, buckling the bookshelf of every GP's consulting room. The remedy was eventually supplied by the British National Formulary.[29]

Doctors were not alone in being bombarded by information on the drugs they prescribed. Patients, too, had their resources in the Patient Information Leaflet (PIL), an initiative of the European Commission and adopted by the UK MHRA in 2005.[30]

In an increasingly regulated pharmaceutical industry and a desire for a more informed society, the intention of the PIL was, in the Directive's own words:

> The provision of good quality patient information is intended to supplement and not replace the advice given to patients by health professionals. Every patient should be given a patient information leaflet with each medicine regardless of whether these are purchased over the counter, supplied on prescription or administered by a health professional.[31]

Whilst the principles behind the introduction of the PIL were laudable, in practice, the application strained the doctor-patient relationship at times. Patients often ignored the 'supplement and not replace' part of the above sentence.

Such a scenario was amusingly illustrated in a letter by Spanish doctors, the problems apply to healthcare systems worldwide, in the *Journal of Medical Ethics*,[32] on the outcome of a consultation where the patient's concerns over the side effects in the PIL outweighed those of their cigarette smoking.

The written advice the PIL provided often contradicted the doctor's verbal advice. Both participants in the consultation had unequal understandings of relative risk. The figures the PIL quoted could result in loss of confidence in the doctor's opinion, return appointments, non-compliance,[33] and even immediate disposal of the packet in the nearest bin. Thankfully, most patients never bothered to read it.

The PIL was not the first earnest policy to create problems with patient drug compliance. The child-resistant locking cap for pill bottles, which a Canadian

[29] www.bnf.org/about/

[30] Gov.UK. Medicines: packaging, labelling and patient information leaflets. 2016. Accessed 6 May 2019 from www.mhra.gov.uk/home/groups/pl-a/documents/publication/con2018041.pdf

[31] www.gov.uk/guidance/medicines-packaging-labelling-and-patient-information-leaflets

[32] Verdú F, Castelló A. Non-compliance: a side effect of drug information leaflets. J Med Ethics. 2004 Dec;30(6):608–9. doi: 10.1136/jme.2003.003806. PMID: 15574455; PMCID: PMC1733995.

[33] Cole A. Over 60s' use of prescription drugs has doubled in past decade in England. BMJ. 2008 Aug 1;337:a1132. doi: 10.1136/bmj.a1132. PMID: 18676445.

doctor, Henri Breault, invented in 1967, and the 'blister' packaging of tablets have created innumerable challenges for the elderly.[34] Such issues were long recognised in primary care and addressed through the introduction of pre-filled cards and dosette boxes, at the unquantifiable expense of the pharmacist's labour in filling them.

6.18 SUMMARY

The three arms of the NHS, public health, primary, and secondary care, have each had a beneficial impact on the health of the nation. The early decades of the NHS were remarkable for the virtual eradication of mortality from infectious diseases, driven by the introduction of mass vaccination and novel anti-infective agents. The terror experienced by every parent of an infant with fever, every child with watery diarrhoea, every adult with blood in their sputum, no longer needed to be realised. The serious residual defects arising from rheumatic fever, TB, and syphilis were consigned, as was the plague before them, to history. Novel compounds were being discovered and developed to combat conditions for which there had previously been no relief. The populace flocked to GPs for the cure to every ill.

Whereas the doctors of the 1940s had little to offer apart from healing hands and a handful of drugs, their 21st-century descendants had an abundance of technology and remedies. But the plethora of advances in therapeutic medicine had its own limitations, not the least being cost. Patented drugs and innovative technologies were often prohibitively expensive. In 1948, total government spending on healthcare for the UK population of 54 million was, allowing for inflation, £11.4 billion. Seventy years on, that had risen in England, for the same number of people, to £140 billion.[35]

A means had to be found to benefit the health of the nation without bankrupting it. One such way was reclaiming the adage 'prevention is better than a cure.' The healthcare and fiscal benefits of prevention had already been proved through the universal childhood vaccination programmes. Could this principle apply to the rest of the population?

The dawn of preventive medicine had arrived. Stop smoking. Limit alcohol. Eat a balanced diet. Exercise. Lose weight. Doctors began to offer, by rote, this basket of advice at every consultation. Health screening, weight, blood pressure, glycosuria, and lipidaemia became a part of routine practice. Any 'abnormalities' were rectified with chemotherapeutic agents. Doubts about such actions were allayed by research that seemed to point overwhelmingly to the benefits. The figures, particularly for cardiovascular disease, were irrefutable. From NICE to QOF, doctors felt negligent in their duty if they failed to prescribe. Responsibly, they tried to defray the costs by choosing generic, cheaper products, but this had minimal

---

[34] Swift CG. Prescribing in old age. Br Med J (Clin Res Ed). 1988 Mar 26;296(6626):913–5. doi: 10.1136/bmj.296.6626.913. PMID: 3129073; PMCID: PMC2546299.

[35] https://fullfact.org/health/spending-english-nhs/

impact on the overall primary care drug budget. The number of prescriptions ballooned. By 2019, primary care prescribing amounted to £8.6 billion.[36]

It has been difficult to evaluate the overall effect, medical, societal, and financial, of the shift in primary care towards preventive medicine. The debate continues regarding the medicalisation of the healthy and the morbidity arising from 'unnecessary' treatments.[37] Proponents would quote UK mortality data for cardiovascular disease, which had declined by 80% over the 70 years since 1948,[38] a period that has seen life expectancy rise from 65 to 80 years. Detractors would claim that such dramatic improvements were due to improvements in living standards and prosperity. Either way, people in the UK are living longer, healthier lives, and GPs can claim some credit for contributing to this joyous state through both the drugs and advice that they have dispensed over the decades.

[36] Prescribing costs in hospitals and the community 2018–2019. NHS Digital. https://digital.nhs.uk/data-and-information/publications/statistical/prescribing-costs-in-hospitals-and-the-community/2018-2019/results

[37] Fanu JL. Too Many Pills. How Too Much Medicine is Endangering Our Health and What We Can Do About It. Little Brown Books, 2018. ISBN: 9781408709771. https://www.hachette.co.uk/titles/james-le-fanu/too-many-pills/9781408709764/#:~:text=In%20Too%20Many%20Pills%2C%20doctor,memory%20and%20general%20decrepitude)%2C%20a

[38] Prevention is better than a cure. DHSS, Nov 2018. https://assets.publishing.service.gov.uk/government/uploads/system/uploads/attachment_data/file/753688/Prevention_is_better_than_cure_5-11.pdf

7

Drugs and Therapeutics

Doctors put drugs of which they know little into bodies of which they know less for diseases of which they know nothing at all.

(Voltaire)

7.1 INTRODUCTION

Do patients expect a pill for every ill? The historical jaundiced view of a general practitioner was that of a doctor with pen poised over the prescription pad as soon as the patient entered the consulting room. This unfounded caricature was based on the intimate bond a doctor has always had with the drug pharmacopoeia; a symbiotic relationship that has prevailed, from the use of digitalis by William Withering in the 18th century for the treatment of 'dropsy,' to zopiclone for insomnia three centuries later. Yet, despite the undeniable advances in drug discovery and development by the pharmaceutical industry over the past 50 years, the repertoire of drugs in use in primary care today has expanded little after the flurry of activity in the three decades following World War II. We are still using derivatives of digitalis for much the same purpose now as Withering did in Georgian times.

The GP of the 1940s had access to a limited drug armamentarium. The antibiotics streptomycin for treating tuberculosis; sulphonamides and penicillin for bacterial infections had only come into use in that decade and were still in short supply. Choices of analgesics were at the extreme ends of the spectrum for strength and side effects, aspirin, or morphine. Everything else was either a vitamin or a liquid of dubious provenance.

The research, and development, of a novel drug compound is both expensive (£800 million) and lengthy (up to ten years). Yet, the end-product is fundamental to how doctors do their job. The process is poorly understood and of little interest to most practising doctors, who have a somewhat snobbish and dismissive attitude towards the pharmaceutical industry and its scientists. Much to their chagrin, those scientists are likely to have a more profound impact on the welfare of the population than they do.

DOI: 10.1201/9781003256465-7

The rewards for bringing a successful compound to market are as eye-watering as the investment. Revenues for a 'blockbuster' drug can amount to well in excess of £1 billion a year for many years. The potential for such rewards drives innovation within the pharmaceutical industry, but it is the basic science and research that takes place within the universities that is increasingly providing the seed from which such drugs germinate.

What makes a drug a blockbuster? First, it must address a common, yet previously unmet clinical need. For example, the H_2 antagonists that effectively block gastric acid production were a step change in the treatments of dyspepsia and peptic ulcer, previous therapies for which comprised either barely effective simple alkalis or major surgery. Second, to be truly commercially successful, a drug must be aggressively marketed. Thus, ranitidine, a compound with no discernible advantage over the truly novel molecule cimetidine (the first drug developed through a rational approach to drug discovery, pioneered by Sir James Black and for which he received the Nobel Prize for Medicine in 1988), replaced it as the most widely prescribed antacid despite being brought to market five years after the former. Finally, the drug must be for a chronic disorder, such as hypertension, where its use is guaranteed for the lifetime of that condition.

A poignant description of a doctor's practice without drugs was written by Dr John S. Milne, a GP in East Lothian, Scotland, between 1946 and 1966. He recalled having access to around 30 drugs, including sulphonamide (antibiotic), mersalyl (diuretic), phenobarbitone (anticonvulsant), phenytoin (anticonvulsant), paraldehyde (anticonvulsant for use in status epilepticus), tincture of stramonium (for Parkinson's disease), potassium iodide (thyroid disease), soluble and protamine zinc insulins (diabetes), ephedrine (asthma), adrenaline (asthma), and aminophylline (asthma). Compare that to over 6,000 generic and branded products that are available to Milne's contemporary today. The BNF alone contains over 1,400 pages! Thankfully, doctors no longer have to remember each one. The presence of a well-thumbed BNF[1] or its commercial sibling, the Monthly Index of Medical Specialties (MIMS)[2] on every GP desk is as ubiquitous as that of a stethoscope or sphygmomanometer.

Despite the large numbers, the list of drug classes and individual drugs that have had a true impact on the practice of family medicine, and remain in daily use, is remarkably short. The following pages cover several that have been genuinely influential in bringing about the primary objective of any prescribed medicine, that is, to be effective in improving health whilst having a negligible risk of causing harm. The list, a personal one, covers those drugs that were truly innovative for their time, and which still provide the bulk of NHS prescriptions in primary care.

---

[1] A joint publication by the British Medical Association and the Royal Pharmaceutical Society. Distributed six-monthly. Free to all practising doctors. Available online.

[2] Published and distributed free to practising doctors every three months by Haymarket Medical Media. Available online.

7.2 CARDIOVASCULAR

Digoxin, Digitoxin, Digitalis—1785
Atrial Fibrillation, Heart Failure

Folklore for medical students, derived from the common foxglove plant and the cure for 'dropsy,'[3] for centuries, digitalis was the only drug that had a beneficial effect in managing cardiac failure and atrial fibrillation, having both a positive inotropic and negative chronotropic action on the heart. It had a small therapeutic window and required repeated but infrequent assay of blood levels. Still prescribed as an adjunct drug in managing refractory cardiac failure, it is now initiated by a cardiologist.

Methyldopa—1955
Hypertension

Methyldopa, an intriguing compound whose site of action is the central nervous system, but whose effect is on blood pressure, was first licensed for medical use in 1974. A moderately effective drug, it tended to cause fatigue and fell out of use once better-tolerated drugs were marketed. However, it inexplicably remains part of the triad of recommended drugs, the others being the equally ancient alpha/beta blocker, labetalol, and nifedipine, for the management of hypertension in pregnancy, a condition managed by specialist obstetricians.[4]

Hydrochlorothiazide—1958; Bendrofluazide—1959; Frusemide—1955
Hypertension, Heart Failure, Oedema

Hydrochlorothiazide was developed and marketed by Merck and CIBA and came into widespread use in 1958. Diuretics were the first drugs to have a beneficial effect in lowering blood pressure and promised to significantly reduce related morbidity and mortality. And they kept their promise! Within a decade, mortality from cardiovascular events, especially strokes, had been radically reduced.[5]

Diuretics dominated the pharmaceutical market in antihypertensive therapies for the following 15 years. Indeed, that they are still an integral part of the treatment of hypertension half a century later is testimony to the longevity of this class of drugs. Thiazide-like diuretics remain an integral part of the four-step 'ABCD' management algorithm recommended by NICE in 2019.[6]

---

[3] 13th-century term for oedema.

[4] https://cks.nice.org.uk/hypertension-in-pregnancy

[5] Pizzi RA. Developing diuretics. The Timeline, Modern Drug Discovery, Feb 2003. Accessed 30 Apr 2019 from http://pubs.acs.org/subscribe/archive/mdd/v06/i02/pdf/203timeline.pdf

[6] www.nice.org.uk/guidance/ng136/chapter/Recommendations#treating-and-monitoring-hypertension

Recognised adverse effects in their use included hypokalaemia and hyper-uricaemia (gout), both easily monitored once access to biochemical investigations became available to GPs. The prevalence of adverse effects was reduced when lower doses were found to be equally effective in reducing blood pressure.

A vitally important and dramatic use of diuretics, particularly such loop diuretics as furosemide, bumetanide, and ethacrynic acid, was in the rapid resolution of acute cardiac failure, where, within minutes, a single intravenous injection could raise a Lazarus from an ageing, prostrate, wheezing cadaver. Despite the somewhat laboured metaphor, the brand name for frusemide, Lasix, was based not on Lazarus but on the more prosaic 'lasts six hours.' Frusemide was the angel of redemption when the call came in the middle of the night to visit an elderly patient with 'a chest infection.'

As with many of the drugs in this account, dosages have decreased over the years as doctors have become more risk averse. IV injections of 80–160 mg were considered normal in the 1980s; today, 20–40 mg is used. Regardless of dose, the injectable formulation is now rarely used by GPs; patients with left ventricular failure tend to go directly to hospital via 999.

Spironolactone—1960
Oedema, Ascites, Hirsutism

Spironolactone is a potassium-sparing diuretic commonly prescribed by GPs as an adjunct to loop diuretics in the management of cardiac failure, oedema, and ascites. It has now been superseded for cardiac failure by eplerenone. Adverse effects include hyperkalaemia and, rather distressing for the patient, gynaecomastia. Both resolve on cessation of the drug, which is now more commonly initiated by a cardiologist.

Propranolol—1962, Atenolol 1969
Hypertension, Angina, Anxiety, Migraine, Headache

Sir James Black pioneered target-driven drug discovery with propranolol, the first of the β-adrenergic receptor blockers that would spawn so many others that the class became known as the 'me-too' drugs. There was even a generic called 'metoprolol'!

Launched in the late 1960s by ICI (subsequently Zeneca), propranolol revolutionised the treatment of angina before finding other uses in the treatment of such diverse conditions as hypertension, tachycardia, cardiac failure, anxiety, and migraine. It was not uncommon for doctors to self-prescribe propranolol to manage their own symptoms of anxiety when on call, a practice unlikely to occur today.

Refinements to the molecule resulted in atenolol, marketed in 1976. Atenolol had many advantages over its predecessor, once-daily dosage, cardio-selective, and fewer adverse effects, leading it to become the drug that single-handedly propelled ICI into the Financial Times 100 index.

Captopril—1976
Hypertension

In 1982, Squibb introduced captopril, the first ACE inhibitor, to the UK. GPs became as familiar with the renin-angiotensin pathway as they had previously been, as students, with the Krebs cycle. The lynchpin peptide that led to the identification of this compound had originally been isolated from the venom of the lancehead viper.

The ACE inhibitors were the first novel class of drugs developed for the management of hypertension since β-blockers 15 years earlier. They were a revelation and heavily marketed as effective, safe, and with few side effects. Anecdotal evidence suggested that many patients felt re-energised once they had been switched from a beta blocker to captopril.

GPs of the time were encouraged to listen for a renal artery bruit prior to initiating therapy since renal failure secondary to renal artery stenosis had been identified as a potentially serious adverse effect of the drug. The concern proved to be overstated, easily identified by measuring renal function, and generally reversible. The only drawback was the literally irritating cough that seemed to occur in around 5% of patients.

Captopril had the market to itself for some years, but competitor 'me-too' drugs inevitably followed, such as enalapril, lisinopril, and ramipril. These offered few advantages apart from once-daily dosing, compliance having always been an issue with thrice-daily captopril.

Like many previous drugs over time, since their initial introduction for the management of hypertension, other uses have been found for ACE inhibitors, not least in the counter-intuitive prevention of renal failure in patients with diabetes. There is now a good case for all patients with diabetes to be prescribed a low dose of ACE inhibitors, although even this, like most didactic statements in medicine, is debatable![7]

Angiotensin receptor blockers (ARBs) work further down the angiotensin-rennin pathway and have the advantage of not causing cough, although, unlike ACE inhibitors, they have not been shown to reduce cardiac mortality.

Nifedipine—1967, Amlodipine
Angina, Hypertension, Chilblains

Nifedipine was developed by Bayer and introduced to the UK market in the mid-1970s for the treatment of angina and hypertension. The drug had a cumbersome thrice-daily dosing regimen, leaving it wide open for replacement. This took a surprisingly long time to happen, until 1989, when once-daily amlodipine (Pfizer) came to market, with others including lacidipine, lercanidipine, and

---

[7] Suissa S, Hutchinson T, Brophy JM, Kezouh A. ACE-inhibitor use and the long-term risk of renal failure in diabetes. Kidney Int. 2006 Mar;69(5):913–9. doi: 10.1038/sj.ki.5000159. PMID: 16518351.

felodipine. Amlodipine came off patent in 2007, after which it pretty much had the market to itself.

As a group, side effects are few and minor, the most common being oedema, facial flushing, and headache.

Warfarin—1940s
Anticoagulant

Dicoumarols were first identified in the 1940s in decomposing sweet clover, following a serendipitous observation by a vet who noted cattle dying of a haemorrhagic illness after ingesting rotting silage. Coumarin was subsequently found in many sweet-smelling plants, such as liquorice and lavender. Warfarin, a more potent form of dicoumarol, was introduced as a rodenticide before finding a more humane use, in the 1950s, as an anticoagulant agent in man.[8]

Warfarin was never popular with physicians. It was old, clumsy, had a limited therapeutic window, a multitude of drug interactions, labour-intensive to manage and prone to potentially catastrophic adverse effects. Yet, with an ageing population and concomitant increase in the prevalence of atrial fibrillation, allied to meta-analyses that showed incontrovertible benefits in preventing thromboembolic effects, warfarin became the mainstay in preventing and treating such conditions. Unfortunately, the increase in use tended to be in the older population, the same group that had co-morbidities requiring polypharmacy.

The small therapeutic window required frequent monitoring of the international normalised ratio (INR). Many patients on anticoagulants were housebound, necessitating taking blood in their own homes and always in the morning; samples had to be analysed whilst fresh. Over the decades, INR monitoring switched back and forth between primary and secondary care. Regardless of where the test occurred, it was the GP who had to manage the emergency when the patient was in danger of bleeding through a substantially raised INR. Mistakes were not uncommon, some ending tragically.

Warfarin had one overriding advantage that inhibited the development of newer anticoagulants. It was, of course, laughably cheap.

Aspirin—1897
Analgesic Anti-Inflammatory Anticoagulant

Acetylsalicylic acid, aspirin, has been around since the dawn of man. Derived from the bark of the willow tree, Hippocrates used it to treat headache and fever in the 4th century BC. The active chemical, salicin, was isolated in 1829, purified to salicylic acid in 1838, recognised as a gastric irritant, buffered to the neutral acetylsalicylic acid in 1853, and finally marketed as aspirin by Bayer in 1899. Aspirin was originally used as an analgesic and anti-inflammatory drug, but research in

---

[8] Lim GB. Warfarin: from rat poison to clinical use. Nat Rev Cardiol, 14 Dec 2017. Accessed 8 Oct 2021 from www.nature.com/articles/nrcardio.2017.172.pdf

the 1980s found that it had an action on platelets in low dosage, 75–150 mg. It is now a bastion in primary and secondary care in the prevention of cardiovascular disease. Of historic note, the daily dose for managing rheumatoid arthritis in the 1970s was 7.2 grams.

NOAC/DOAC—2002
Novel or Direct Oral Anticoagulants

Most clinicians greeted the arrival of NOACs in 2008 with huge relief. This new class of antithrombin anticoagulants offered significant advantages over warfarin, with respect to effectiveness, compliance, monitoring, and safety. However, as always with the introduction of a novel class of drug, they were very expensive; the monthly prescription for a NOAC was around 50 times the price for warfarin. The excess cost to the NHS of switching every patient on warfarin (760,000) to a NOAC would have been in £700 million per annum.[9] This significantly impacted the initial uptake of these drugs. and it was not until relatively recently, as they came off patent and the price dropped, that their use has become widespread.

Simvastatin—1979
Hyperlipidaemia, Primary and Secondary Prevention CVD

Statins continued the paradigm of rational drug design through applied targeted biochemistry. Building on the correlation between raised blood cholesterol levels and ischaemic heart disease, the hypothesis that lowering blood lipids may benefit cardiovascular morbidity was posed, tested and proven . . . probably![10]

Early efforts at reducing blood lipid levels, such as sequestering agents, cholestyramine, and fibrates, were unpalatable, marginally effective, and had minimal impact on cardiovascular morbidity and mortality. The statins targeted the enzyme integral to the synthesis of cholesterol in the liver, and they were a therapeutic step change in lipid reduction.

By the late 1980s, Merck, the first company to develop a product (simvastatin) in this class of drugs, was spending huge sums on marketing. GPs were flooded with invitations to educational meetings where the local cardiologist would present data on the ubiquitous Scandinavian Simvastatin Survival Study (4S), with impressive graphs illustrating the direct correlation between lowered blood cholesterol levels and cardiac events. The data was compelling. Statins worked! However, despite the best endeavours of the pharmaceutical industry's marketing brains, the drug took some time to take off in the UK. Why? Cost, of course! As responsible public servants, GPs were and remain mindful of how they spend the

---

9 Gage BF. Cost of dabigatran for atrial fibrillation. BMJ. 2011 Oct 31;343:d6980. doi: 10.1136/bmj.d6980. PMID: 22042755; PMCID: PMC3281316.

10 Dr James Le Fanu. Much of this book is devoted to the prescribing of statins. There is no particular chapter specifically covering this. ASIN : B01MZF9Y46, *Too Many Pills: Too Much Medicine is Endangering our Health and What We Can Do About It.* Little Brown Book Group, 2018.

public's taxes. The concept of Quality Adjusted Life Years (QALY) and the field of health economics[11] took a long time gaining traction in primary care.

Not until simvastatin came off patent in the early 2000s, with the coinciding recommendation by the National Institute for Health and Care Excellence (NICE) for its widespread use in primary and secondary prevention of cardiovascular events,[12] that prescription numbers in the UK really exploded. By 2004, before generic switching, statins accounted for 9.1% of total NHS prescription costs of £8 billion. The numbers of people being treated continued to rise dramatically thereafter, but the overall cost dropped.[13] A decade later, simvastatin had become the most commonly prescribed drug in the UK with 34.4 million prescription items, amounting to only £46.5 million per annum.[14]

Statins heralded the shift from therapeutic to preventive medicine. Their prophylactic use not only dramatically reduced the blood levels of cholesterol and low-density lipids but that reduction resulted in demonstrable reductions in cardiovascular events, especially mortality.

Zocor, the brand name for simvastatin, had massive annual sales, but they were small change compared to Lipitor (atorvastatin), with annual global sales in excess of US$12 billion, again demonstrating the power of marketing. Lipitor had advantages over Zocor. It was a genuine once-a-day drug that did not have to be taken at night, with fewer drug interactions relating to metabolism through the cytochrome P450 pathway. However, its marketing was relentless. Sponsored medical meetings included a stall with a blood cholesterol analyser. Eager doctors queued to have their fingers pricked, staggering away minutes later, ashen-faced as they received their readings. Pharmaceutical companies marketing statins lent out such machines to GP surgeries, introducing the concept of 'point-of care' investigations in primary care.

In 2014, NICE advocated that anyone with a cardiovascular risk of more than 10% in ten years should be considered a candidate for taking a statin. This not only led to an increase in statin use but stoked the fires of debate around the morality of treating the otherwise well.

National tabloid newspapers, having developed an irrational hatred for this group of drugs, regularly mounted scare campaigns over their side effects. A previously healthy man need only be admitted to hospital with minor chest pain to be subsequently discharged virtually immobile on statins in industrial doses. Meeting the ever more stringent metrics of QOF left GPs inevitably over- rather than undertreating patients. Hospital biochemistry laboratories became

[11] MacKillop E, Sheard S. Quantifying life: understanding the history of Quality-Adjusted Life-Years (QALYs). Soc Sci Med. 2018 Aug;211:359–66.

[12] Raza et al. 92 Primary care prescriptions for statins in England 1998–2015. Heart (BMJ journals). 2017;103(Supplement 5). https://heart.bmj.com/content/103/Suppl_5/A67

[13] NICE technology appraisal 94 2009

[14] https://files.digital.nhs.uk/publicationimport/pub20xxx/pub20664/pres-disp-com-eng-2005-15-rep.pdf; www.ic.nhs.uk/news-and-events/press-office/newsreleases/drugs-to-treat-cardiovascular-disease-are-the-e

inundated by requests to measure lipids, resulting in unquantifiable costs.[15] Despite these concerns, statins remain the most widely prescribed drugs in the UK to this day.

7.3 RESPIRATORY

Isoprenaline—1947
Asthma, Heart Block

Isoprenaline was the first of the non-selective beta stimulants to be effective in managing acute asthma. It was also the first to be administered as an aerosol inhaler. However, its lack of selectivity could result in fatal tachycardia, and it was replaced by the much safer salbutamol in the 1960s.

I had a great affection for isoprenaline since I had severe childhood asthma as a child. Prior to its introduction, I can still recall frequent and seemingly endless nights with head bent over a bowl of steaming water, which was the only 'effective' treatment for bronchospasm up to that time. Isoprenaline cleared the wheeze in seconds.

Salbutamol—1966
Asthma, COPD

Salbutamol, a selective β-adrenergic agonist that Allen & Hanbury Ltd (now GSK) launched in 1969, remains the most widely used asthma drug to this day. It was a genuine lifesaver and almost unique in its action, providing instant and safe relief for a distressing symptom, bronchospasm. Perversely, despite its well-documented safety profile and efficacy, it was not licensed for use in the United States until 1982.

Salbutamol was available in several formulations: liquid, tablet, and nebuliser solutions, but primarily as an inhaler, both meter-dose and breath-actuated.

The main side effect of salbutamol, although not as severe as isoprenaline, remained tachycardia, but this did not lead to increased morbidity or, specifically, life-threatening arrhythmias. In short, it was magnificent! Yet, despite its increasing use in the community and theoretically improved management in primary care dedicated asthma clinics, hospital admissions and mortality remained inexplicably high.[16]

Ipratropium—1966
COPD/COAD. Asthma

---

[15] NICE. Lipid modification: cardiovascular risk assessment and the modification of blood lipids for the primary and secondary prevention of cardiovascular disease. Clinical Guideline CG67. 2008. Accessed 30 Apr 2019 from www.nice.org.uk/guidance/cg67

[16] Anderson HR, Gupta R, Strachan DP, Limb ES. 50 years of asthma: UK trends from 1955 to 2004. Thorax. 2007 Jan;62(1):85–90. doi: 10.1136/thx.2006.066407. PMID: 17189533; PMCID: PMC2111282.

Prior to the introduction of more recent muscarinic acetylcholine receptor blockers, such as tiotropium and ipratropium, Atrovent, as an inhaler, was the sole agent for reducing symptoms of chronic obstructive airways disease, or 'chronic bronchitis,' as it was known at that time. Ipratropium was moderately effective and had a good safety profile but was hindered by a short plasma half-life, requiring four-times-a-day dosing. It was eventually replaced by more convenient, long-acting muscarinic antagonists (LAMA), tiotropium (1989), glycopyrronium (2005), and umeclidinium (2013). LAMAs are an integral part of the GOLD (Global Initiative for Chronic Obstructive Lung Disease) guidance[17] on managing patients with COPD.

Aminophylline—1950s

This dramatic intravenous remedy for acute severe asthma served doctors well in the 1970s and 1980s, but it fell out of favour through its small therapeutic window and tendency to cause cardiac arrhythmia. Although it required slow injection over ten minutes, a luxury of time never afforded to a GP in an emergency setting, it rarely caused any problems in practice. Less effective oral formulations were used as an adjunct to salbutamol and inhaled steroids.

Pholcodine
Cough

Perhaps an unusual addition to any list of essential medications, pholcodine was the linctus of choice for any patient initially presenting with an acute cough of unknown aetiology. It was cheap, soothing, generally harmless, and, unlike codeine, non-addictive. It was a useful placebo, tidying patients over until symptoms had run their course. For all these reasons it is rarely prescribed nowadays.

7.4 GASTROINTESTINAL

Sodium Alginate (Gaviscon)
Dyspepsia

Sodium alginate was originally extracted from seaweed. Along with simple antacids, such as magnesium trisilicate, it was the mainstay of managing dyspepsia before the introduction of more targeted drugs. Gaviscon was aggressively marketed for heartburn, gastro-oesophageal reflux, with dubious claims of a dual action in acid suppression and coating the lower oesophagus, thus preventing mucosal irritation.

Prescribed simple antacids were largely made redundant following the introduction of the H_2 antagonists.

---

[17] https://goldcopd.org/wp-content/uploads/2018/11/GOLD-2019-POCKET-GUIDE-FINAL_WMS.pdf

Cimetidine—1976
Gastro-Oesophageal Reflux Disease, Peptic Ulcer

Introduced in 1976, cimetidine (Smith, Kline & French) became the first blockbuster drug to achieve sales of over US$1 billion per annum, only relinquishing that position ten years later to another H_2 antagonist, ranitidine (Glaxo Wellcome, 1981).

The introduction of the H_2 antagonists in primary care totally revolutionised the management of upper gastrointestinal conditions, such as dyspepsia, gastro-oesophageal reflux, and peptic ulcer. The drugs were a quantum leap in improved efficacy, tolerance, and compliance. Almost overnight, they consigned to the back shelf of the pharmacy the gallon flagons of Mist Mag Trisil/aluminium hydroxide and the ubiquitous Gaviscon. Among the GP community, their widespread use instantly reduced home visits and hospital referrals for such conditions.[18]

In fact, the downward trend in hospital admissions had preceded the widespread use of H_2 antagonists, probably due to improved living standards and smoking cessation; nevertheless, their introduction accelerated that trend.[19] A paradox subsequently developed. Emergency hospital admissions for upper-GI-related conditions began to rise! On closer scrutiny, this was found to be unrelated to the efficacy of H_2 antagonists but rather the increasing use of another novel group of drugs, the non-steroidal anti-inflammatory drugs, NSAIDs. In due course, the routine co-prescribing of H_2 antagonists or proton pump inhibitors with NSAIDs became standard practice.

Concerns, thankfully unfounded, were raised that unbridled suppression of gastric acid for lengthy periods could lead to stomach cancer. Although this debate is ongoing,[20,21,22] these fears have not led to any noticeable reduction in the prescribing of these compounds.

[18] Christensen A, Bousfield R, Christiansen J. Incidence of perforated and bleeding peptic ulcers before and after the introduction of H2-receptor antagonists. Ann Surg. 1988 Jan;207(1):4–6. doi: 10.1097/00000658-198801000-00002. PMID: 2892468; PMCID: PMC1493241.

[19] Higham J, Kang JY, Majeed A. Recent trends in admissions and mortality due to peptic ulcer in England: increasing frequency of haemorrhage among older subjects. Gut. 2002 Apr;50(4):460–4. doi: 10.1136/gut.50.4.460. Erratum in: Gut. 2003 Mar;52(3):458. PMID: 11889062; PMCID: PMC1773187.

[20] McColl KE. Acid inhibitory medication and risk of gastric and oesophageal cancer. Gut. 2006 Nov;55(11):1532–3. doi: 10.1136/gut.2006.103283. PMID: 17047103; PMCID: PMC1860103.

[21] García Rodríguez LA, Lagergren J, Lindblad M. Gastric acid suppression and risk of oesophageal and gastric adenocarcinoma: a nested case control study in the UK. Gut. 2006 Nov;55(11):1538–44. doi: 10.1136/gut.2005.086579. Epub 2006 Jun 19. PMID: 16785284; PMCID: PMC1860118.

[22] Cheung KS, Leung WK. Long-term use of proton-pump inhibitors and risk of gastric cancer: a review of the current evidence. Therap Adv Gastroenterol. 2019 Mar 11;12:1756284819834511. doi: 10.1177/1756284819834511. PMID: 30886648; PMCID: PMC6415482.

Omeprazole—1979
Gastro-Oesophageal Reflux Disease, Peptic Ulcer

Omeprazole (marketed in 1989 by Astra AB, now AstraZeneca) and the proton pump inhibitors, PPI, built on pre-existing target-driven drug innovation. Whilst undoubtedly more effective at suppressing gastric acid and arguably having a lower side-effect profile, their main benefit over the H_2 antagonists was compliance, a once-daily dosage. Despite this marginal benefit, omeprazole soon became the number one prescribed drug worldwide, a position it held for many years, establishing its parent company, Astra AB, as a global player.

An additional significant development in the eradication of peptic ulcer disease was the association of a previously anonymous bacterium, *Helicobacter pylori* and excess gastric acid secretion, first identified in Australia in 1982.

With a wonderful nod to the masochistic research methods of a bygone era, Dr Barry Marshall demonstrated the association between *H. pylori* and gastritis by downing a schooner full of the bacterial culture, immediately succumbing to excruciating gastric pain and vomiting. Subsequent gastroscopy confirmed his theory![23] Drs Barry Marshall and Robin Warren were awarded the 2005 Nobel Prize in Medicine and Physiology for their findings.

H. pylori became somewhat of a cause célèbre following the publication of Marshall and Warren's research. Even a reputable BBC current affairs programme, *Horizon*, devoted an hour of prime-time television to the subject. *H. pylori* identification and eradication became the primary objective in every GP consultation on upper gastrointestinal symptoms. Patients, driven by press coverage, flocked to see their GP.[24] For some years, anyone complaining of even the mildest postprandial dyspepsia was endoscoped, and GPs were trained to perform gastroscopies to meet the demand. The cycle of GP-led endoscopy clinics waxed and waned over the following decades, dependent on funding moving between primary and secondary care.

Combining proton pump inhibitors and antibiotics for the eradication of *H. pylori* became *de rigeur*, rapidly passing through several iterations impossible to remember without access to the latest BNF, making GPs routinely reach for the latest protocol whenever a patient burped.

Sulphasalazine—1950
Crohn's Disease
Sero-Negative Inflammatory Disease

---

[23] Charisius H. When scientists experiment on themselves: *H. pylori* and ulcers. Scientific American, 5 July 2014. https://blogs.scientificamerican.com/guest-blog/when-scientists-experiment-on-themselves-h-pylori-and-ulcers/

[24] Graham DY, Shiotani A. New concepts of resistance in the treatment of Helicobacter pylori infections. Nat Clin Pract Gastroenterol Hepatol. 2008 Jun;5(6):321–31. doi: 10.1038/ncpgasthep1138. Epub 2008 Apr 29. PMID: 18446147; PMCID: PMC2841357.

Sulfasalazine was a highly effective drug for the prophylactic, long-term management of Crohn's disease, for which there had previously been little relief apart from steroids.

7.5 UROGENITAL

Sildenafil—1996
Erectile Dysfunction

The discovery of Sildenafil (Viagra) was yet another story that has entered the annals of medical folklore. A serendipitous observation during clinical trials for a compound intended for cardiovascular conditions, Viagra, the 'little blue pill' became the first drug effective in treating an underreported, considered embarrassing, condition, erectile dysfunction. The drug had a rapid onset, was effective and safe but initially, perhaps prudishly, only available on a private prescription unless there were underlying medical conditions. NHS prescriptions were issued for a maximum four pills a month. Viagra was sanctioned for over-the-counter purchase in 2018.

Solifenacin—2004
Bladder Instability

Solifenacin, an antimuscarinic drug, was more effective, a once-daily, fewer-side-effects, and safer compound than tolterodine (1998), which it superseded in the treatment of overactive bladder/urge incontinence disorders. Solifenacin is now widely accepted as first-line treatment for these conditions.

Finasteride—1984
Benign Prostatic Hyperplasia Male Pattern Hair Loss

Finasteride, a 5α-reductase inhibitor antiandrogen, provided the GP with the only non-surgical treatment for benign prostatic hyperplasia and, thus, was invaluable in keeping frail, elderly men out of hospital.

7.6 ENDOCRINE AND METABOLIC

Insulin—1922
Diabetes Mellitus

The story of the discovery of insulin and its use in treating the previously fatal condition of diabetes mellitus forms yet another staple of pharmacology history for medical students.

The sourcing of the hormone moved from extraction from the pancreatic glands of cows and pigs to biosynthetic manufacture of human insulin (Eli Lilly 1982). Prescribing followed these developments, as did cost. In turn, GPs followed these trends but were ever mindful of both cost and bioequivalence. Dosing regimens also improved with combinations of long- and short-acting insulins.

Diabetes management, once under the sole guardianship of hospital endocrinologists, gradually devolved to their GP colleagues who, in turn, passed it over to their practice nurses. By the early millennium many GPs felt that they had become deskilled in this important, interesting, and common condition. A regrettable loss.

Metformin[25]—1957
Diabetes, Polycystic Ovarian Syndrome

Metformin, one of the biguanide class of chemical compounds, originated from the chance observation in the 17th century that extracts from the plant *Gallega officinalis*, or French lilac, had blood-glucose-lowering properties. Incremental research from the 1920s onwards finally resulted in the synthesis of metformin by Jean Sterne, a French physician and pharmacologist, who also coined the eventual trade name, 'Glucophage' or 'glucose eater,' in 1957. Since then, after lifestyle changes, it has become the first-line treatment for type 2 diabetes mellitus.

Metformin reduces insulin resistance by facilitating the cellular uptake of glucose. Unlike the other commonly used glycaemic drugs of the time, the sulfonylureas, it did not cause hypoglycaemia or weight gain. In fact, it had few adverse effects, the most common being diarrhoea. Metformin has since found other medical indications, its anti-androgenic properties leading to its unlicensed use in treating hirsutism and polycystic ovarian syndrome.

Chlorpropamide—1958
Diabetes

Chlorpropamide[26], a first-generation sulphonylurea, acts by stimulating pancreatic beta-cells to produce insulin. Therefore, by definition, it is ineffective when these cells are totally depleted, as in Type 1 Diabetes Mellitus (T1DM). It was an excellent drug at reducing blood glucose but had one major drawback, a long half-life that could, albeit infrequently, lead to profound hypoglycaemia and coma. It was a not uncommon cause, often overlooked by clinicians, of comatose patients being admitted to hospital. Chlorpropamide was the mainstay of treatment for Type 2 Diabetes Mellitus (T2DM) until the 1980s when second-generation sulphonylureas replaced it. Glibenclamide and gliclazide were no more potent but had a shorter half-life and, thus, were less likely to cause hypoglycaemia.

Following an increased interest in diabetes drug research at the turn of the 21st century, newer agents for managing T2DM, the glitazones, DPP4 inhibitors, and incretins were introduced. Apart from exenatide, 2005, they offered few benefits over the combination of sulphonylurea and biguanide that preceded them.

---

[25] www.jomrjournal.org/article.asp?issn=2347-9906;year=2014;volume=1;issue=2;spage=127;epage=130;aulast=Patade; doi: 10.4103/2347-9906.134435

[26] Quianzon CC, Cheikh IE. History of current non-insulin medications for diabetes mellitus. J Community Hosp Intern Med Perspect. 2012 Oct 15;2(3). doi: 10.3402/jchimp.v2i3.19081. PMID: 23882374; PMCID: PMC3714066.

Thyroxine—1914
Hypothyroidism

Thyroxine was isolated from the thyroid gland of a pig in 1914 and synthesised in 1927 by a team of British chemists. It is one of the top five most commonly prescribed drugs in the UK, unsurprisingly, since hypothyroidism has a prevalence of around 3% of the UK population. Blood levels needed to be monitored, less so once symptoms of hypothyroidism had stabilised, but annual checks became mandatory under the QOF.

Hydrocortisone
Prednisolone—1940s
Addison's Disease, Severe Allergy, Anaphylactic Shock, Inflammation

Prednisone was synthesised and brought to market in the late 1950s by Schering. The corticosteroids have been literal lifesavers, invaluable and used in a diverse range of conditions, from asthma to temporal arteritis, and in a variety of formulations, tablets, creams, injectables, eye drops, and inhalants.

They vary in potency from cortisone to dexamethasone. There is a sense that more recent generations of GPs are less familiar and confident regarding the relative potency and potential side effects, both short and long term, of this invaluable class of compounds and are thus misguidedly limiting their use.

Fludrocortisone—1953
Addison's Disease, Nocturnal Enuresis

Fludrocortisone, the first of the synthetic corticosteroids, was used as a hormone replacement for Addison's disease. Since its actions mimicked naturally occurring aldosterone, it could cause electrolyte imbalance and fluid retention resulting in oedema, cardiac failure, and cardiac arrhythmia. Urea and electrolytes required regular monitoring.

For many years, fludrocortisone was used in primary care as a last resort in treating children with nocturnal enuresis. The practice has largely been discontinued, due to concerns over safety.

Colchicine—1833
Hyperuricaemia, Gout

Famously derived from the autumn crocus and with a documented history going back to 1500 BC, colchicine entered modern usage for the management of acute gout in the 1950s but was only licensed in the United States in 2009!

Rare for any medication, it rapidly relieved symptoms. Dosage regimes vary. Historically, 500 mcg was given orally every 2–3 hours up to a maximum of six times a day or until the onset of diarrhoea, but the current NICE recommendation advises a more cautious approach!

Enovid—1951
Combined Oral Contraceptive, 1960

The first combined oral contraceptives were developed in the 1950s by Searle in the United States and introduced into the UK as an NHS-prescribed drug in 1961. Credit for promoting its use must go to an unlikely source, Enoch Powell, who was Minister for Health at that time.

7.7 DERMATOLOGY

Combination Emollients, Creams, and Ointments
Eczema, Psoriasis, Bacterial and Fungal Skin Infections

When I was a junior medical house officer, a wise consultant physician dismissed the whole specialty of dermatology by declaiming that one cream, Daktacort, a combination of emollient, antifungal, and steroid, cured all skin conditions[27]. I carried his advice throughout my career in general practice and rarely found it to be wanting.

Calcipotriol—1985
Psoriasis

Calcipotriol, a synthetic derivative of vitamin D, was the first topical treatment specifically targeted at plaque psoriasis. It provided a welcome alternative to the long-term use of topical steroids and coal tar, previously the only means for helping patients with this distressing skin condition. Combination therapy incorporating both calcipotriol and betamethasone provided even more rapid resolution of plaques.

7.8 NERVOUS SYSTEM

Phenobarbitone—1904
Epilepsy, Anxiety

The barbiturates were ubiquitous in the early decades of the NHS for managing anxiety, insomnia, and epilepsy. Their efficacy for these conditions led to long-term, chronic prescribing, resulting in drug addiction. In the 1980s, pragmatic GPs tried to replace their use with the 'safer' benzodiazepines, only to be stymied in their efforts when these too were found to be just as addictive.

---

[27] Nenoff P, Koch D, Krüger C, Drechsel C, Mayser P. New insights on the antibacterial efficacy of miconazole in vitro. Mycoses. 2017 Aug;60(8):552–7. doi: 10.1111/myc.12620. Epub 2017 Mar 30. PMID: 28370366.

Sodium Valproate—1962
Epilepsy

Sodium valproate, Epilim, along with carbamazepine, revolutionised the management of all forms of epilepsy, replacing the relatively toxic phenobarbitone and phenytoin that had previously been the mainstay of treatment for these conditions. Epilim became the first-line drug for absence and generalised seizures. Side effects were relatively minor, though reversible liver dysfunction could occur, easily monitored and resolving on discontinuation of the drug. More concerning was foetal valproate syndrome, neural tube defects, first identified in France in 1982. Unrelated to this association, folic acid was already being used as a vitamin supplement in women contemplating pregnancy. The dose was significantly increased for mothers who could not discontinue valproate during pregnancy. Nevertheless, extreme caution needed to be exercised leading to heightened anxiety in both the prospective parent and doctor, who was now more likely to be a specialist obstetrician.[28]

Carbamazepine—1963
Epilepsy, Neuropathic Pain

Carbamazepine, Tegretol, was mainly reserved for partial seizures, where it was highly effective with minimal adverse effects. It has since been found to be equally effective in managing neuropathic pain.

Noting its side effect of lowering libido, I once used it, off licence and many years ago, in a man who was sociopathically inclined towards sexual deviancy. It proved to be highly effective. I would not dream of taking such action today!

Levodopa[29]—1950s
Parkinson's Disease

A moving account of the impact of L-dopa in the management of the previously intractable Parkinson's disease cannot be better than in the 1968 book and subsequent film, *Awakenings*, by the neurologist Oliver Sacks.

Levodopa was commonly initiated in primary care; neurologists were few a scarce commodity in district hospitals until the 21st century. Thereafter, there was a shift towards early referral, diagnosis, and management in secondary care.

Sumatriptan—1991
Migraine

Perhaps a rather unusual choice to have in any list of drugs that changed general practice, the triptans, launched in the 1990s, were yet another example of a

---

[28] www.rcog.org.uk/globalassets/documents/guidelines/valproate-guidance-march-2019.pdf

[29] www.nature.com/articles/466S6a

novel chemical entity created to manage a common but previously unmet need, migraine. Sumatriptan was the first in the class of selective 5-hydroxytryptamine agonists, developed by Glaxo Wellcome and licensed in the UK in 1991. Its main drawback was that it was initially available only in an injectable form and, like all new drugs, was expensive.

Sumatriptan cleared migraine headaches faster than simple analgesics alone.[30] It gave GPs an alternative to the less effective therapies but also allowed them to avoid potentially toxic compounds, such as the ergot derivatives. All medical students from 1970 onwards had been taught about retroperitoneal fibrosis secondary to methysergide, an infinitesimally rare condition with a worldwide prevalence of less than 1 in 200,000. The profession was risk-averse long before NICE came to the fore. By 2008, annual global sales of triptans exceeded US$3 billion.[31]

7.9 MUSCULOSKELETAL AND RHEUMATOLOGY

Ibuprofen—1961
Pain, Anti-Inflammatory

Ibuprofen, developed by Boots in the UK in 1969, was the first of the non-steroidal, non-salicylate, anti-inflammatory analgesics, NSAIDs. It spawned an industry of similar 'me-too' products, each coming into and going out of fashion, largely depending on their marketing. Ibuprofen has stood the test of time, as has naproxen.

NSAIDs remain a significant contributor to hospital admissions for upper gastrointestinal haemorrhage. Most are now prescribed with concurrent proton pump inhibitors.

Paracetamol—1953
Analgesic

Paracetamol, acetaminophen, was discovered by Bayer in the 19th century and eventually marketed in 1953 under the brand name Panadol by Sterling Winthrop. Originally licensed in the UK as a prescription-only product, it moved to over-the-counter in the 1970s.

An NHS drive to reduce medicinal costs included encouraging patients to purchase paracetamol. As was the way with such policy initiatives, this advice was poorly received by patients, especially those on low income. Most doctors ignored the dictat and continued to prescribe paracetamol liquid for febrile infants.

---

[30] Humphrey PP. The discovery and development of the triptans, a major therapeutic breakthrough. Headache. 2008 May;48(5):685–7. doi: 10.1111/j.1526-4610.2008.01097.x. PMID: 18471110.

[31] Olesen J, Tfelt-Hansen P, Ashina M. Finding new drug targets for the treatment of migraine attacks. Cephalalgia. 2009 Sep;29(9):909–20. doi: 10.1111/j.1468-2982.2008. 01837.x. Epub 2009 Feb 25. PMID: 19250288.

Paracetamol overdose and the poor outcomes of acute, large dose inges-tion were recognised in the 1980s, following which the amount that could be issued on one prescription or sold at the chemist was restricted. This created problems for those patients taking the drug for chronic conditions, such as osteoarthritis. GPs are now encouraged to use their common sense in such situations.

Methotrexate—1947
Cancer, Inflammatory Diseases (Rheumatoid Arthritis, Crohn's Disease)

Methotrexate, developed as a chemotherapeutic/immunosuppressant agent for the treatment of some cancers, was found to have an additional beneficial effect in the management of inflammatory arthritis. A mainstay in these conditions since the 1990s, it is initiated by a hospital specialist rheumatologist leaving the GP to continue onward prescribing and monitoring.

Methotrexate is a relatively toxic compound with potentially fatal drug interac-tions. Its accidental prescribing alongside the common antibiotic, trimethoprim, remains a frequent item on significant-event audits. The incidence has not dimin-ished, despite sophisticated prescribing software, suggesting that human error can never be abolished in a pressurised working environment.

Sodium Aurothiomalate—1940s
Rheumatoid Arthritis

Gold injections, along with penicillamine, were the 'gold standard' of disease-modifying antirheumatic drugs in the post-war decades up to the 1990s. Administered by intramuscular injection every 3–6 months; sodium aurothio-malate was moderately effective in preventing disease progression. With a heavy metal, there was always a risk of renal damage, but thankfully, this was rare and did not prevent its use until hospital rheumatologists became more numerous. Both gold and penicillamine have since been replaced by tumour necrosis factor inhibitors (TNFI, 1989), the first of which, infliximab, Humira, went on to global blockbuster sales. Due to cost and parenteral administration, their use remains restricted to hospital specialist departments.

Pethidine—1939
Pain

Rarely used in its oral formulation, pethidine was a potent, relatively safe anal-gesic when administered IV or IM for the relief of severe pain, as in obstetrics labour, cholecystitis, ureteric colic, and back pain. It was omnipresent in 'the doc-tor's bag' for such emergencies and, as such, has fallen out of use as GP emergency callouts have diminished over the years.

Morphine—1804, Diamorphine (Especially in Combination with Cyclizine)
Pain

Diamorphine, more potent but with fewer side effects than morphine, as an intravenous or intramuscular preparation, was indispensable for managing the pain and distress of acute myocardial ischaemia, carcinogenic pain, or cardiac failure. Its use outside the out-of-hours services has become limited, and few doctors now routinely carry vials in their medical bag.

As with pethidine, it is a controlled drug requiring secure storage and a logbook of use. All prescriptions must be handwritten, documented, and accounted for in the records.

Naloxone—1961
Opiate Overdose

Naloxone, a literally lifesaving drug for both patient and doctor, was an essential item in any emergency bag for its instant and effective reversal of opioid sensitivity or overdose. It certainly saved my reputation on many an occasion.

Sadly, the son of Dr Fishman, the co-inventor, died of a heroin overdose in 2003.

7.10 MENTAL HEALTH

Diazepam—1963
Anxiety, Insomnia, Muscle Spasm, Epilepsy

Diazepam, marketed by Roche as Valium in 1963, was the second drug to be developed in the drug class of benzodiazepines, the other being chlordiazepoxide (brand name Librium, also by Roche). Its effectiveness in relieving anxiety symptoms quickly made it a blockbuster. For 13 years (1969–1982), it was the most widely prescribed drug in the United States.

Diazepam was a godsend to GPs. It provided a safe alternative to the barbiturates, widely prescribed at the time, in treating mild to severe general anxiety disorders and insomnia. It was the perfect drug for these conditions. It worked quickly. It had minimal, if any, side effects. It was safe in overdose. It was addictive. What? Shame about the last, really, but as its use increased, so the concerns regarding benzodiazepine addiction were confirmed. Nonetheless, it is a testimony to the market that it remained widely used long after dependence was demonstrated. In truth, despite no doubt desperate research to find an alternative, nothing has ever come close to managing anxiety symptoms since benzodiazepines fell out of favour.

An area where benzodiazepine use was never controversial was that of the treatment of status epilepticus. At last, doctors had a drug that could be easily administered, was safe, and provided instant and dramatic relief for a life-threatening event. Midazolam became a staple of the emergency bag, and status epilepticus became another condition that could be managed in the community.

Pharmaceutical companies viewing Roche's success vied with each other to produce variations on a theme, balancing anxiolytic effects against somnolence, onset against length of action. Eventually, diazepam spawned innumerable iterations of benzodiazepines, including nitrazepam and temazepam (both hypnotics), flurazepam, triazolam, alprazolam, chlordiazepoxide, clorazepate, diazepam, lorazepam, oxazepam, and midazolam. Clonazepam was mainly restricted to neurology and psychiatry, for use in epilepsy and psychosis, respectively.

Amitriptyline—1960
Depression, Insomnia, Neuropathic Pain

The tricyclic group of drugs, TCAs, first imipramine and then amitriptyline, were introduced to the market in the early 1960s and revolutionised the management of a previously widespread but poorly managed condition, depression. By 2017, 7.3 million people in England, 17% of the adult population, were receiving a prescription for an antidepressant,[32] at a cost to the NHS of around £260 million per annum.[33]

Given the large doses required to treat depression, 150–300 mg daily, the routine issue of monthly prescriptions and the drugs' predisposition towards cardiac arrhythmia led to a spate of overdoses and suicides, resulting in the tricyclics being replaced by the safer, but no more effective, SSRIs. However, amitriptyline, in low doses of 10–50 mg, had somewhat of a renaissance from the 1990s onwards, as an effective agent in the management of chronic headache and neuropathic pain.

Fluoxetine—1975
Depression

The SSRIs were first marketed in the United States in 1987, with fluoxetine (Prozac) rapidly achieving blockbuster sales. The SSRIs claimed to be both more effective and safer than the ageing TCAs, claims since widely disputed. Nevertheless, this class of drugs, including paroxetine, citalopram, and sertraline, are still featured in the top 20 most frequently dispensed drugs in England in 2019.[34] Prozac was so popular that it acquired its own cultural moniker, the 'little pink pill.'

7.11 INFECTION

Penicillin—1928
Respiratory Tract Infections

Although the term 'antibiosis' had first appeared in the 19th century, 'antibiotic'[35] only became common scientific currency after Selman Waksman, an

[32] Prescribed medicines review: summary. Public Health England, 10 Sep 2019. www. gov.uk/government/publications/prescribed-medicines-review-report/prescribed-medicines-review-summary

[33] www.theguardian.com/society/2017/jun/29/nhs-prescribed-record-number-of-antidepressants-last-year

[34] www.statista.com/statistics/378445/prescription-cost-analysis-top-twenty-chemicals-by-items-in-england/

[35] Hutchings MI, Truman AW, Wilkinson B. Antibiotics: past, present and future. Curr Opin Microbiol. 2019 Oct;51:72–80. doi: 10.1016/j.mib.2019.10.008. Epub 2019 Nov 13. PMID: 31733401.

American microbiologist, coined it in 1942. A similar delay took place in its application. Though discovered in 1928, penicillin did not come into use until 1942, and then was not widely available outside the armed forces until after 1945, the same year that its discoverers, Alexander Fleming, Ernst Chain, and Howard Florey, were jointly awarded the Nobel Prize for Medicine. It is a sobering thought that barely three generations have passed since the creation of this invaluable class of drugs that have gone on to save hundreds of millions of lives worldwide.

Amoxycillin—1972
Co-Amoxiclav
Respiratory Tract and Other Infections

Although preceded by benzylpenicillin, the combination of the penicillin nucleus with a beta-lactam ring by scientists at Beecham Laboratories (now GlaxoSmithKline) resulted in methicillin (1960), ampicillin (1961), and further iterations, including Augmentin, the combination of amoxicillin with clavulanic acid, generic co-amoxiclav (1981) that provided the flexibility of a wide-spectrum bacteriostatic antibiotic, administered orally with excellent bioavailability and safety profiles. Due to these properties, this class of antibiotics became widely used simply because they required little thought from the prescriber. Amoxicillin and co-amoxiclav became the drugs of choice in treating a wide range of conditions, including chest infection, earache, skin infection, cystitis, and to this day, amoxicillin still tops the list of prescribed antibiotics by number of prescriptions.[36] However, this widespread use has led to bacterial resistance. In response, dosage courses have evolved over the years from low dose/long time to high-dose/short-time regimens.

Other antibiotics, the macrolides and cephalosporins, became available and were used when resistance to or intolerance of the penicillins occurred.

Nitrofurantoin—1953
Urinary Tract Infections

Nitrofurantoin, a broad-spectrum antibiotic used almost exclusively for urinary tract infections, especially in pregnancy, is moderately free from side effects, apart from nausea. Despite being in common usage for over half a century, bacterial resistance remains remarkably low, 3%, according to NICE (2017).

---

36 Stewart C. Antibiotics prescribed in the UK in 2017. Statista, 8 July 2019. www.statista.com/statistics/1022598/antibiotics-prescribed-in-the-united-kingdom/

Metronidazole—1959
Anaerobic Infections

Metronidazole covered the anaerobic bacterial organisms resistant to the commonly used antibiotics. Its main indication was in the treatment of deep-seated areas of necrotic tissue, such as dental or pilonidal abscess. More directed indications included bacterial vaginosis. where it was effective against *Gardnerella vaginalis* and the eradication of *H. pylori* in upper GI disease.

Omission in informing the patient of its disulfiram-like properties was likely to result in an irate confrontation when prescribed to any oenophile.

Tetracycline—1948
Oxytetracycline
Respiratory Tract Infections, Acne

A commonly used bacteriostatic antibiotic with a wide spectrum of activity, the tetracyclines were for many years the first-line treatment of respiratory tract infections until more potent bactericidal compounds were discovered. Their primary use nowadays is in the management of acne.

Trimethoprim—1960
Urinary Tract Infections

The penicillins, or cephalosporins for those with penicillin sensitivity, were rarely used in urinary tract infections where trimethoprim reigned supreme for four decades, until the early 2010s. Originally combined with sulfamethoxazole, co-trimoxazole (brand name Septrin) was the antibiotic of choice, but its side effects, notably skin rashes, led to its replacement by trimethoprim alone. However, trimethoprim was a bacteriostatic agent, and by 2016, *E. coli* resistance to the drug had risen to 34% in England.[37] Nevertheless, it remains a first-line drug in the management of uncomplicated urinary tract infection.

Acyclovir—1977
Herpes Viral Infections

The acyclovir group of drugs is largely used in the treatment of herpes simplex and zoster infections. Oral acyclovir, with its five times daily dosing, has been largely replaced by famciclovir and valaciclovir, once the latter came off patent.

---

[37] English Surveillance Programme for Antimicrobial Utilisation and Resistance (ESPAUR) report 2016

7.12 ALLERGY

Adrenaline—1899
Cardiogenic Shock, Anaphylaxis

Adrenaline is primarily used by GPs in a self-administered, subcutaneous, injectable form for emergency use in severe anaphylaxis. Due to the relatively infrequent occurrence of such emergencies, vigilance is needed to ensure that the expiry date on the device has not been exceeded prior to plunging the needle into the patient's thigh. However, where needs must, doctors have been known to ignore this advice, with no adverse consequences.

Phenbenzamine, Chlorpheniramine—1948
Allergy

Antihistamines were first made available to patients around the same time as the NHS came into being. Phenbenzamine, the first compound in this group, was discovered by a Swiss-born Italian pharmacologist, Daniel Bovet, who won the Nobel Prize for Physiology and Medicine in 1957.

Chlorphenamine was introduced soon afterwards, and it is humbling to note that it is still in worldwide use 60 years later. The newer antihistamines have provided no additional advantage from the originals, apart from once-daily dosing regimens and a relative lack of sedation. They are certainly no more potent or effective.

The first of the 'non-sedating' antihistamines, terfenadine, was not introduced until 1985. Terfenadine (Triludan) a prodrug, was metabolised to its active chemical, fexofenadine by the liver, through the ubiquitous cytochrome P450 pathway. As such, it reacted with a variety of drugs using the same metabolic pathway. This would not have been a problem had terfenadine not been cardiotoxic and arrhythmogenic in higher blood concentrations. Though patient deaths were rare, the anxiety created in physicians was not, and terfenadine was discontinued in 1997, once fexofenadine had been isolated. In turn, fexofenadine (Telfast) became a blockbuster with global sales in excess of £1.8 billion. Both drugs had come from the same pharmaceutical company, Hoechst Marion Roussel. Readers can draw their own conclusions.

Other new antihistamines included loratadine (Clarityn), which, in generic form after 2002 and available without a prescription, contributed over 36% of the sales revenue of its parent company Schering-Plough.

It is hard to imagine a doctor's bag without an antihistamine amongst its contents.

7.12.1 Commonly Prescribed Drugs

The NHS Prescriptions Services, a division of the NHS Business Services Authority (NHS BSA), monitors the number and cost of all medications prescribed in the UK.

The list of the top 20 drugs prescribed in England should come as no surprise to any practicing GP. Many are as ancient as the doctor writing the prescription. All have certain features in common. They are cheap, generic, and used for common chronic medical conditions.

The top 20 chemical drugs dispensed in England 2019, by items, included:[38]

1.	Atorvastatin	Hyperlipidaemia. Primary and secondary prevention of cardiovascular disease
2.	L-thyroxine	Hypothyroidism
3.	Omeprazole	Dyspepsia. Gastro-oesophageal reflux. Peptic ulcer.
4.	Amlodipine	Hypertension. Angina
5.	Ramipril	Hypertension. Cardiac failure. Secondary prevention renal disease in diabetes
6.	Lansoprazole	Dyspepsia. Gastro-oesophageal reflux, Peptic ulcer
7.	Bisoprolol	Hypertension, Ischaemic heart disease, Cardiac arrhythmia
8.	Cholecalciferol	Vitamin D deficiency
9.	Metformin	Diabetes mellitus, Polycystic ovarian syndrome
10.	Aspirin	Primary and secondary prevention ischaemic heart disease
11.	Simvastatin	Hyperlipidaemia. Primary and secondary prevention of cardiovascular disease
12.	Salbutamol	Asthma
13.	Paracetamol	Mild pain
14.	Sertraline	Anxiety. Depression
15.	Co-codamol	Moderate pain
16.	Citalopram	Anxiety. Depression
17.	Amitriptyline	Chronic headache. Migraine. Neuropathic pain
18.	Furosemide	Cardiac failure. Odema
19.	Beclometasone	Asthma. COPD
20.	Losartan	Hypertension. Cardiac failure, Secondary prevention renal disease in diabetes

None of these drugs was registered as a new chemical entity in the past 25 years. To some degree, this reflects the pharmaceutical industry's move away from inexpensive, small chemical compounds for common use to expensive, targeted biologics for relatively rarer conditions, such as cancer. The paucity of new drugs available to primary care is partly the reason why drug reps rarely visit GP surgeries compared to their heyday in the 1980s.

---

[38] www.statista.com/statistics/378445/prescription-cost-analysis-top-twenty-chemicals-by-items-in-england/

In 2003, the *BMJ* published a paper that first coined the term 'polypill,'[39] a single pill that combined a low dose of aspirin, statin, and antihypertensives, all agents still well represented in the list of commonly prescribed drugs above. The author made a compelling case that 80% of cardiovascular disease would be prevented if the UK adult population took the daily pill; a cost-effective, cheap, and safe strategy for the health of the nation. The conclusions of the article were so compelling that the *Lancet* was still promoting the benefits, never implemented, some 18 years later![40]

7.12.2 Emergency Drugs

Whilst the overall number of drugs available for GPs to prescribe remained high, those for use in emergencies were, for practical reasons, limited. The carriage of these drugs plus any additional equipment that might be required, such as stethoscope, sphygmomanometer, thermometer, syringes, took place in the doctor's bag, a case that has evolved from the weather-worn, creased, leather Gladstone of the 1950s to bespoke, sleek, metal briefcase, and finally the wheeled, cantilevered, plumber's mate version of today.

Publications by the Drug and Therapeutics Bulletin and Care Quality Commission 2017[41] provided recommendations for drugs for emergency use in the community. As with the container in which they were carried, these too evolved.

Drugs GPs were expected to carry in 1950 and 2010.

DRUG	Indication	1950	2020
Adrenaline injection	Anaphylaxis	Yes	Yes
Aminophylline injection	Asthma	Yes	No
Aspirin—low dose	Acute coronary syndromes	No	Yes
Atropine injection	Bradycardia	No	Yes
Benzylpenicillin injection/ cefotaxime injection	Bacterial meningitis	Yes	Yes
Chloramphenicol injection	Bacterial meningitis	No	Yes
Chlorpheniramine injection	Anaphylaxis	No	Yes
Cyclizine/prochlorperazine/ metoclopramide injection	Nausea and vomiting	No	Yes
Dexamethasone	Croup	No	Yes

[39] Wald NJ, Law MR. A strategy to reduce cardiovascular disease by more than 80%. BMJ. 2003 Jun 28;326(7404):1419. doi: 10.1136/bmj.326.7404.1419. Erratum in: BMJ. 2003 Sep 13;327(7415):586. Erratum in: BMJ. 2006 Sep;60(9):823. PMID: 12829553; PMCID: PMC162259.

[40] Mant J, McManus R. Polypills with or without aspirin for primary prevention of cardiovascular disease. Lancet. 2021 Sep 25;398(10306):1106–7. doi: 10.1016/S0140-6736(21)01913-9. Epub 2021 Aug 29. PMID: 34469762.

[41] www.cqc.org.uk/guidance-providers/gps/nigels-surgery-9-emergency-medicines-gp-practices

DRUG	Indication	1950	2020
Diamorphine/morphine injection	Severe pain relief MI/LVF	No	Yes
Diazepam injection	Status epilepticus	No	No
Diclofenac injection	Analgesia	No	Yes
Furosemide injection/tablets	LVF	No	Yes
Glucagon injection	Hypoglycaemia	No	Yes
Glucose injection or oral solution	Hypoglycaemia	No	Yes
Glyceryl trinitrate spray	Angina	No	Yes
Haloperidol/chlorpromazine injection	Acute psychosis	Yes	No
Midazolam (buccal)	Epileptic fit	No	Yes
Naloxone injection	Opioid overdose	No	Yes
Paracetamol/ibuprofen	Mild/moderate analgesia	No	No
Prednisolone soluble tablets/ Hydrocortisone injection	Asthma	No	Maybe
Procyclidine injection	Adverse effects of antipsychotics	No	No
Salbutamol inhaler (+ spacer device)/nebuliser solution	Asthma, Anaphylaxis	No	Yes
Syntometrine injection	Post-partum haemorrhage	Yes	No

Since 2004, GPs are rarely called out to emergencies. The maintenance of a doctor's bag with a comprehensive list of medications that needed regular updating for time expiry has largely been made redundant. It was simply too wasteful.

7.12.3 Drug Formularies

The exponential growth in the number of chemotherapeutic agents required a single source reference easily accessible to clinicians, the BNF.

The BNF evolved from the National War Formulary (NWF), created in 1939, containing 380 preparations.[42] The drug names in the NWF were in Latin, the doses in minims and grains. Its contents included an exotic assortment of tonics, cough mixtures, and aperients; *Mistura Ammonii Chloridi et Morphini* and *Mistura Cascarae et Nucis Vomicae*. There were three enemas, including the rather disconcerting *Enema Fellis Bovini* (bovine bile enema). Amid all these panaceas were three recognised chemotherapeutic agents: sulfanilamide, sulfathiazole, and sulfapyridine.

Following the end of the war, the British Pharmaceutical Society and British Medical Association felt that despite its archaic collection of chemicals, the concept of a standardised formulary was not only sound but worth preserving. The collaboration led to the publication of the first *BNF* in 1949. From 1949 to 1976, updated editions were published every three years. By 1963, English had at last replaced Latin,

---

42 www.bmj.com/content/bmj/306/6884/1051.full.pdf

and metric measurements were introduced. New sections on antibiotics and cortico-steroids were written. And yet, it was still only being updated every three years, at a time when new classes of drugs were coming on the market almost monthly. Thus, the pharmaceutical industry decided to take matters into its own hands and began its own publication in the early 1970s, the MIMS, present on every GP's desk ever since.

At first, the BNF could not keep pace with this brash upstart. A survey at the time showed that only 20% of young doctors were using it, the rest preferring the smaller, more up to date and legible MIMS. A revamp of the BNF was ordered in 1981, coupled with an undertaking to deliver it free to every doctor in the UK. It has been updated six-monthly ever since. Each update involved 3,000–4,000 changes. By 2020, the BNF had grown to over 1,000 pages. The BNF for children, BNFC, was introduced in 2005. Both editions of the BNF were available in a wide variety of digital formats, as of 2010.

Running in parallel with the BNF and with the purpose of limiting both the unmanageable number of available drugs and their cost, practices developed their own, abridged drug formularies. Individual doctors were left free to prescribe any drug, provided the cost was reimbursable from the Drug Tariff. In due course, this principle was facilitated by the introduction and development of clinical IT systems, where the default on the prescription screen would automatically be a generic drug from the practice formulary.

Generic prescribing had always been encouraged as a means of bringing down the overall NHS drug budget, although the pharmaceutical industry had stymied this laudable practice at times by overcharging for generic formulations.[43]

GP performance and productivity came under closer scrutiny following the GMS contract of 2004. The PCT introduced and managed the concept of an 'indicative' drug budget based on historical prescribing data. A practice was given a notional annual drug budget and instructed not to exceed it. In practice, the innumerable challenges in meeting the budget included hyperinflationary drug pricing and increasing volumes of prescribed medications in preventive medicine. Some doctors viewed underspending as synonymous with undertreating. Following 2013, CCGs adopted a stricter policy, publishing their own locality-based drug formularies, with roving pharmacists ensuring that practices adhered to their contents. The CCG published and circulated charts comparing a practice's prescribing costs with other practices, a nudge to shame extravagant prescribers to reduce their costs. The initiative had mixed success. A practitioner could still prescribe any drug, but the CCG had the statutory right, rarely used, to refuse reimbursement of cost.

7.12.4 The Drug Tariff

The Oxford English Dictionary defines a tariff as 'a list of the fixed charges made by a business.' The Drug Tariff[44] outlined the price of medicines and appliances the NHS paid to the contractor, the doctor, for services provided.

---

[43] Walley T, Burrill P. Generic prescribing: time to regulate the market? Price rises are a blow to nascent primary care groups. BMJ. 2000 Jan 15;320(7228):131–2. doi: 10.1136/bmj.320.7228.131. PMID: 10634713; PMCID: PMC1128727.

[44] www.drugtariff.nhsbsa.nhs.uk/#/00446515-DC_2/DC00446511/Home

The Pharmaceutical Directorate of the NHSBSA published the Drug Tariff monthly for the DH and supplied it to pharmacies and doctors' surgeries. It defined the rules for dispensing, the value of the fees and allowance, the drug and appliance prices, and what was and was not allowable. It was a legal document; unsurprisingly, rather large and unwieldy, albeit divided into logical, clinical sections.

The sum of the basic price of the drug, discount scale, VAT allowance, dispensing fees and out-of-pocket expenses determined reimbursement for a prescribed drug or appliance. The calculations were time-consuming and complex, and few non-dispensing practices bothered to do them, instead relying on the NHSBSA to arrive at an honest sum. However, dispensing practices could not afford to be so relaxed. There were around 1,250 dispensing out of around 9,000 GP practices in the UK in 2019. These were mostly rural and covered around 8.7 million patients and 7% of all prescribed items.

Doctors could dispense from either an on-site dispensary or a standalone pharmacy. More rigorous regulations covered the latter than the former. Creating an on-site commercial pharmacy was time-consuming, expensive, and potentially controversial.[45] The practice had to provide evidence to the CCG, supporting the claim that a proportion of its patient population resided more than 1.0 miles from the nearest high street chemist. Patients within that radius retained the right to have their prescription dispensed at the surgery or any pharmacy. Few chose to do go elsewhere, since the convenience of a one-stop shop, consultation and medication, outweighed choice. The on-site pharmacy had to be registered as a business independent of the GP partnership. Any conflict of interest had to be avoided.[46] A qualified pharmacist had to be in charge. Rent had to be paid to the practice if the pharmacy was sited in the practice building. All business accounts had to be separate from those of the practice.

Above all else, as healthcare professionals, pharmacists and doctors were expected to put the interests of patients before their commercial interests.[47]

7.12.5 The Blacklist

The explosion in the number of pharmaceutical compounds and their presence in an enlarged pharmacopoeia containing rigorously researched drugs that were safe and effective led to a re-evaluation of the many medicines included prior to the dawn of highly regulated drug research and development.

---

[45] The Pharmaceutical Journal, 6 June 2015, Vol 294, No 7865, online. doi: 10.1211/PJ.2015.20068279

[46] https://pcpa.org.uk/assets/documents/Guide-for-GPs-considering-employing-pharmacist.pdf

[47] Goldacre B, Reynolds C, Powell-Smith A, Walker AJ, Yates TA, Croker R, Smeeth L. Do doctors in dispensing practices with a financial conflict of interest prescribe more expensive drugs? A cross-sectional analysis of English primary care prescribing data. BMJ Open. 2019 Feb 5;9(2):e026886. doi: 10.1136/bmjopen-2018-026886. PMID: 30813120; PMCID: PMC6377511.

In the 1980s, with minimal consultation with the profession, the DH removed many 'medicines' from the list that could be prescribed on an FP10. This naturally led to knee-jerk howls of indignation and railing from doctors, directed at government interference. It was all a matter of principle. There was little dispute over the more outrageous remedies in the existing tariff, such as Nurse Sykes Bronchial Balsam or Dr. De Jongh's Cod Liver Oil with Malt Extract & Vitamins Fortified Syrup or even Father Pierre's Monastery Herbs. Nevertheless, the profession felt that this was yet another assault on their independence by the men from the Treasury. The invective raged for some time before doctors admitted that the blacklist had had zero impact on their day-to-day practice. The great majority of blacklisted items were branded names for which alternative generic products were both available and cheaper, for example, Panadol and paracetamol. Justifying freedom to prescribe quack medicines was difficult, against the DH's calculations of annual savings of £75 million from this measure. On closer scrutiny, the list was fair and generally reflected contemporary thought and usage.

Reflecting on the uproar regarding the blacklist only reinforces the maxim of knowing when to pick your fights. The profession's childish outcry at its introduction only succeeded in reinforcing the jaundiced view civil servants held of the profession.

7.12.6 The Cost of Drugs

The NHS had a long history of targeting prescribing costs in primary care, a subject first discussed by the Central Health Services Council, set up in 1948 to advise the Ministry of Health. However, no action was taken until 1988, when the Prescription Prescribing Authority (PPA) began producing regular, personalised Prescribing Analysis and Cost and Prescribing Analysis Reports (PACT),[48] which were distributed to individual GPs. An electronic version replaced the original hard copy in 1995. The PPA extracted and analysed data from the millions of FP10 prescriptions that NHS doctors and dentists had generated. In 1995, GPs in the UK issued 550 million prescriptions, at a total cost of £4.7 billion. By 2016, those figures had doubled, to 1.1 billion and £8.3 billion, respectively.[49]

At a local level, the data guided policy on drug formularies, clinical governance, and budget-setting. The overall intention was commendable as a soft attempt to nudge all doctors towards national standards of 'excellence' in prescribing. Quantifying whether PACT succeeded in this aim was difficult. Initially, the document, in its distinctive glossy envelope, was eagerly received and the contents pored over. However, over time, the novelty wore off, and thereafter, the

---

[48] Majeed A, Evans N, Head P. What can PACT tell us about prescribing in general practice? BMJ. 1997 Dec 6;315(7121):1515–9. doi: 10.1136/bmj.315.7121.1515. PMID: 9420496; PMCID: PMC2127947.

[49] The rising cost of medicines to the NHS Kings Fund. Apr 2018. www.kingsfund.org.uk/sites/default/files/2018-04/Rising-cost-of-medicines.pdf

unopened envelope was directly consigned to the bin. Anecdotal testimony suggests that few doctors continued to access the online replacement.

In any perpetually relabelled administration such as the NHS, neither the term PPA nor PACT remained undisturbed for long. By 2006, the former had become NHS Prescription Services (NHSPS), the latter the Prescribing Analysis Report (PAR).

NHS Prescription Services (NHSPS) was a division of the NHS Business Services Authority (NHSBSA). Its duties mirrored those the redundant PPA had previously undertaken, including calculating and reimbursing the costs of drugs and appliances dispensed on NHS prescriptions. To give some idea of their workload, they handled over 4 million individual prescription items every working day of the year. The number of prescriptions increased year on year, driven by an expanding population, especially the elderly with multiple co-morbidities and complex medical needs, a peripatetic medical workforce, nurse prescribing, a risk-averse culture, and preventive medicine. The last had a particularly profound impact on prescription numbers, if not necessarily cost, as the prescribing of statins demonstrated. Annual UK prescriptions for all statins soared from 295,000 items in 1981 to 52 million in 2008 and 71 million in 2018, at which time over 7 million people were taking the drugs.[50,51]

7.13 SUMMARY

Where there's a will there is a way; where there's a pill there's dismay. Man has always sought ways of alleviating physical and mental distress with the solution invariably supplied by chemicals, drugs. Modern medicine is predicated on a supply of medicines and patients have become attuned to expecting a cure for every ailment, regardless of how trivial. Yet increasingly medicines are prescribed for asymptomatic conditions, hypertension, hyperlipidaemia, Type 2 DM and patients have had to adjusted to being medicated on need rather than want.

Doctors, and their patients, have been in thrall to the benefits of drugs since the time of Asclepius in classical Greece. That feeling prevailed in the half-century following the foundation of the NHS when a succession of new drugs, especially antibiotics, finally provided relief from the infections that had previously ravaged societies. The public expected a prescription for antibiotics at the first symptom of a cough or high temperature; doctors were only too willing to oblige. Knowledge of the clinical presentations of viral and bacterial infections was in its infancy. Symptoms overlapped and outcomes were unpredictable. What harm could there be in prescribing an antibiotic; just in case? The prescription was a

[50] Trusler D. Statin prescriptions in UK now total a million each week. BMJ. 2011 Jul 14;343:d4350. doi: 10.1136/bmj.d4350. PMID: 21757438. www.bmj.com/content/343/bmj.d4350.full

[51] www.bhf.org.uk/for-professionals/healthcare-professionals/blog/statins-10-facts-you-might-not-know

panacea for both patient and their physician. The public became accustomed to expecting a prescription at the end of every medical consultation.

The cosy scenario changed with the advancement of scientific knowledge and in particular, two factors, antibiotic resistance and preventive medicine. The former vexed the doctor more than the patient. Medicine is a science discipline informed by rigorous research. GPs are just as mindful of developments in medicine as their hospital colleagues. Their message on treatment became more complicated as they attempted to differentiate between viral and bacterial illness before resorting to drugs. Patients were not attuned to the doctors reasoning for the delay. Consultations could become heated. Doctors ruminated on cases where patients had been admitted to hospital and been told that their GP had been negligent in for not prescribing an antibiotic earlier. Eventually, the downward trajectory of antibiotic prescribing stalled.[52]

Meanwhile that for preventive medicines has accelerated but not without producing its own issues. Cardiovascular disease prevention, epitomised by the introduction of the statins in the 1990s, heralded a move for primary care into public health. Whilst the population of the UK had seen the benefits of vaccination programmes in substantially eliminating childhood diseases, they were less convinced of the need for medication in a healthy adult. Once more their family doctor was called upon to communicate a subtle message, based on science, to a sceptical audience. Consultation times lengthened. Workload increased as asymptomatic individuals were recalled for repeat appointments to review their condition and medication. More surgery time was needed to monitor an erstwhile healthy population. The result? Fewer appointments for acute illnesses. Whilst the benefits to the population were proven, those for the individual were more nuanced.

To some degree, the choice of whether or not to treat has been removed from the front-line physician. The management of many conditions, acute and chronic, have become guideline and protocol-driven. It remains only for the doctor to convince the patient that whatever course of action taken has been done so in their best interests. There is a sense within the profession that with the passage of time, patients have become less convinced that this is so.

52 Pouwels KB, Dolk FCK, Smith DRM, Robotham JV, Smieszek T. Actual versus 'ideal' antibiotic prescribing for common conditions in English primary care. J Antimicrob Chemother. 2018 Feb 1;73(suppl_2):19–26. doi: 10.1093/jac/dkx502. PMID: 29490060; PMCID: PMC5890776.

8

Education and Training

The life so short, the craft so long to learn.

(Hippocrates)

8.1 INTRODUCTION

Here is a fact that may astonish any recently qualified GP: prior to 1981, doctors did not need any specialist training to enter general practice as a GP principal. In other words, any 'unqualified' GP in post prior to that date could still be legally practising 30 to 40 years later, despite never having trained for that role in the first place. To reassure those of a more nervous disposition reading this, no research has shown that this cohort of doctors has harmed the population any more than those who followed it. So, purely as a hypothesis, has mandatory training for the role made any difference to a doctor operating as a GP or, more vitally, to their patients?

Historically, general practice as a career choice tended to be one of default rather than aspiration. Becoming a hospital specialist was far more arduous; roles were few, the training lengthy, gruelling, and incompatible with family or social life. The peripatetic existence of a training specialist prevented any laying down of roots until trainees were well into their 30s. The specialist examinations were exceedingly difficult and expensive, first-time pass rates low, and career progression not guaranteed. All these hurdles would be on top of the five to six years of undergraduate training followed by two mandatory foundation years of high-octane hospital jobs. In short, there were and still are many sound reasons for not choosing a hospital career. The alternative, general practice, was far more appealing. Prior to 1981, a doctor could become a fully registered GP principal, independent and on a high income, immediately upon completion of one year of junior house jobs. Despite the attractions of doing so, most medical students of the time remained wedded to a hospital career, and it is remarkable that little has changed in their view to the present day. Yet, despite their initial preferences, many graduate doctors end up having general practice thrust upon them. The author became a GP after becoming exhausted, embittered, and thoroughly sick of studying for and failing exams to become a physician. He was not alone.

DOI: 10.1201/9781003256465-8

Against this background of medical student apathy towards a career in general practice, the RCGP strove to enhance the reputation of general practice by introducing postgraduate training, on a par with that for physicians, in the 1960s before becoming compulsory in 1981.

Since then, whether by coincidence or design, attitudes among medical students have changed. In 2013, the British Medical Association undertook a survey of medical students to gauge their views on career choice.[1]

For the question, 'Are you considering a career in general practice?' half of those polled answered positively and with a maturity that belied their age. In addition, the qualitative element of the survey provided heartening reading to their colleagues in practice. Examples included:

- 'In the past GPs have been undervalued by the medical profession as a whole. I believe a career in general practice can be exciting, varied, challenging, and rewarding.'
- 'With an ageing population and a high burden of chronic disease and mental health problems, we need to shift towards a more generalist, community-focused healthcare model, which means that we need to give general practice the recognition it deserves.'
- 'General practice has for too long been seen as the soft option when compared to hospital medicine.'
- 'The reality is that with our generation's push for more care in the community, becoming a GP is an exciting prospect with a wealth of opportunities for innovation.'
- 'I've been put off a lot when, at the start of every teaching session with a new doctor, they usually ask "So what specialties do you want to do?" then say "Well, half of you are going to be GPs anyway." This really bugs me as it's as though they are saying general practice is just a job pool where most will end up regardless of whether they want to, or whether they would be any good.'
- 'I think many students wrongly believe that GPs have an easy job.'
  Personally, I believe they have the most difficult job along with emergency department doctors, absolutely anything can walk through the door.'

These perceptive comments highlight certain preconceptions within the undergraduate medical curriculum that have remained constant over centuries. Specifically, hospital specialists still deliver much of the clinical content in hospitals. Thus, it is no surprise that the teaching favours those specialties. Yet, despite noting (then ignoring) such bias, it remained resistant to change until 2002, when the creation of a raft of new medical schools brought in a more enlightened, holistic, problem-based syllabus, at the heart of which was greater primary care input via GP practice-based placements.

---

[1] British Medical Association Survey—18 July 2013. *Students decide: is your future in general practice?* Available from: http://bma.org.uk/news-views-analysis/ news/2013/july/students-decide-is-your-future-in-generalpractice

The foundations of medical knowledge lie in the sciences of anatomy, physiology, and pharmacology, subjects best taught in the lecture theatre or within a clinical setting, a hospital where access to complex cases can be optimised. The academic lecturers are hospital-based, so, understandably, medical students would only consider a career in an environment familiar to them. Despite the comment made above that 'absolutely anything can walk through the door' in general practice, the paradox remains that most students still look on primary care as being predictable and boring, with GPs having none of the lustre that sparkles off their hospital counterparts.

The same BMA survey that asked the students if they thought that GPs had an image problem confirmed this point as well. Two-thirds of those polled agreed.

Again, the comments showed that those surveyed had wisdom beyond their years:

- 'There seems to be a common view that becoming a GP and not a hospital doctor is a cop out.'
- 'From what I've encountered, it seems GPs are stigmatised because they're not "specialised." But while a consultant may only be up to date in his or her relevant field, a GP must have knowledge of all areas of medicine, this is a specialty in itself.'
- 'Although many GPs are very popular among their patients, hospital doctors often seem to view them as lazy and overpaid. I think this is partly because hospital doctors only notice bad practice by GPs and are not so aware of the large volume of patients whose GP cares for them and never refers them to secondary care.'
- 'My experience suggests that there is a large stigma associated with practising GPs and those who aspire to be one are seen as failed hospital doctors. This is a shame as the discipline of general and community practice is an area of expertise itself, requiring specific training and a natural flair.' Mea culpa!

This survey took place in 2013. To put that into historical perspective, it was 60 years after the creation of the College of General Practitioners and 40 years after it gained its royal charter, with the avowed intent of elevating general practice to the professional status that physicians, surgeons, and gynaecologists enjoyed. Their endeavours have yet to bear fruit.

However, all is not lost. More medical students than ever are choosing a career in general practice, and there is even a suggestion that such thoughts gain traction as they progress through their undergraduate training. A survey of Scottish medical students, published in 2014, showed that the percentage choosing general practice as one of three top preferred options increased from 45% to 55% as they progressed through the course.[2] The study was not broken down by gender, but

2 Cleland JA, Johnston PW, Anthony M, Khan N, Scott NW. A survey of factors influencing career preference in new-entrant and exiting medical students from four UK medical schools. BMC Med Educ. 2014 Jul 23;14:151. doi: 10.1186/1472-6920-14-151. PMID: 25056270; PMCID: PMC4131477.

anecdotal evidence suggested that general practice had a greater appeal to female medical students.

8.2 GP DEMOGRAPHICS

A Kings Fund report of medical workforce trends published in 2011[3] enumerated the increase in the number of students entering medical school, the proportion of female students, and the changing demographics of general practitioners. The figures included:

- First-year medical student places increased from 2,000 in 1960 to 7,889 in 2010, 400% over 50 years. In the following decade, the figure increased further to 8,730.
- Female medical students made up more than half of all medical students in 2010, and 59% by 2017.

Meanwhile, data published by the GMC[4] (2016) on the demographic make-up of the GP workforce (England and Scotland) of 54,000, revealed:

- Gender   Male 46%; Female 54%
- Ethnicity (where recorded)   White 68%; BME 32%
- Age   Under 50 years 60%; Over 50 years 40%
- Country of origin   UK 78%; Overseas 22%

The trend has been towards an increasingly younger, gender and culturally diverse workforce. The workforce is getting younger, partly due to the increased output from medical schools but also to GPs retiring early, following changes in pension provisions, enacted in the 2010s, that punitively taxed excessive earnings.

General practice has become a more attractive option for female medical students looking for flexible part-time work, compatible with raising a family. The proportion of doctors from a Black, Asian, and other ethnic (BME) backgrounds, at around one-third of the workforce, has remained remarkably constant over the decades, but the country of primary medical degree has changed as more, particularly second- and third-generation British BAME students chose medicine as a career option. The mix of nationalities working in the NHS has varied over time. Initially, doctors from the Commonwealth predominated, but of late, with the freedom of movement that EU membership allowed, the UK has proved to be an attractive destination for doctors from both Western and Eastern Europe. Their numbers are likely to fall following the UK exit from the EU in 2020.

---

[3] Medical Workforce King's Fund, 2011. www.kingsfund.org.uk/projects/time-think-differently/trends-workforce-medical

[4] www.gmc-uk.org/-/media/documents/what-our-data-tells-us-about-gps_pdf-74830685.pdf

But perhaps the premise for the debate on whether general practice is a positive career choice is specious. Teenagers drawn to a career in medicine arrive from a variety of socioeconomic backgrounds and with characters and abilities developed in infinite ways. Other chapters have noted that those entering a career in medicine after World War II were almost exclusively white, middle-class males from families with a medical heritage, many of whom were expected to enter medicine much as their historic relatives had entered the military or the clergy. The egalitarian society of the present offers greater opportunities for all school leavers to consider medicine as a realistic career option. Diversity in the GP workforce enriches the patient experience of primary care.

However, the entry costs for a career in medicine remain prohibitive, especially for those applicants from a disadvantaged background. Support for further education through state-paid tuition fees and means-tested maintenance grants, in place from 1962, was abolished in the 1990s, replaced by university tuition fees to be repaid over the working life of the graduate. Thus, a medical student could be faced with a bill in excess of £50,000 on graduating. Regrettably, such eye-watering sums of money might deter teenagers with lower socioeconomic backgrounds from considering a career in medicine. The healthcare of the population of the UK, apart from Scotland where tuition fees remain free, is poorer for their exclusion.

An often-overlooked means of attaining a university education was through sponsorship by the armed forces, requiring a short-term commission to remain in the armed services for a minimum of five years after graduation. The postgraduate training of military doctors was and remains closely entwined with the NHS. That is particularly so for GP vocational training.

The history of GP vocational training in the armed forces started in 1973, when the Armed Services General Practice Approval Board was established, chaired by Pat Byrne and with members from both military and civilian backgrounds. The board appointed GP trainers and selected civilian training practices in the UK but also on military bases worldwide, including Germany, Cyprus, Gibraltar, and Hong Kong. Military trainees spent 18 months in practice instead of the 12 of their civilian peers, during which they became firmly embedded in the practice team. The trainees also benefitted from generous funding through non-NHS sources. The hospital training was supernumerary to the hospital service posts, placing less pressure on the trainee and allowing more time for learning.

Once qualified, the clinical experience of a military GP could be patchy. Doctors were posted abroad with their regiments. The demography of the patient population was skewed towards the young and fit. Exposure to complex, multifactorial, co-morbidity chronic diseases of the elderly, the bread and butter of civilian practice, was negligible. Still, the road from military to civilian practice always remained open, provided that a certificate of completion in specialist training had been achieved, and ex-military GPs were as welcome in primary care as their forebears had been after World War II.

A final route to a career in medicine in the UK was through training in the European Union, previously the European Economic Community (EEC). In the early 1980s, the UK was one of only a handful of European countries that had established mandatory postgraduate training for general practice, in line with the 1975 EEC Doctors' Directive. For the Directive to be relevant, other countries had to be persuaded to follow suit. Given the variations in the style of general practice between member states, this was no easy matter. Eventually, after prolonged negotiations, EU member countries agreed that by the mid-1990s, all qualified GPs would have had to complete a minimum period of specialist postgraduate training before being allowed to operate independently in any jurisdiction.[5] Despite these strictures, the training and experience of doctors working in health systems across Europe differed greatly from those in the UK. European doctors required a sometimes-lengthy period of adjustment when joining the NHS. Whereas medical knowledge was easily transferrable across borders, soft skills, such as language, in particular the local vernacular, and customs, so vital in understanding the local culture, could be problematic. EU doctors found that they experienced the same initial antipathy from the British population as had greeted the arrival of Asian doctors in the 1950s and 1960s but, like them, quickly became an established part of the community.

8.3 GP STATUS

Despite countless initiatives over the decades to elevate GP status vis a vis their specialist peers, public and professional opinions have remained stubbornly fixed.

In 2016, Health Education England and the Medical Schools Council supported a task force headed by Dr Valerie Wass, Emeritus Professor of Medical Education at Keele University, to look into the negative perception of general practice among medical students and possible remedies. The Wass Report made several recommendations, including increasing the proportion of the syllabus based on and in general practice, less negative stereotyping of general practice by hospital consultants, and embedding GPs within the career advisory service.[6] Sadly, a survey of the 36 medical schools done four years after the publication of the Wass Report suggested that, if anything, the situation had regressed further, with GP input remaining static or falling![7,8]

The way society at large sees GPs also reflects the way they see themselves. Patients view the status of hospital consultants as higher than that of GPs.

[5] Framework for Professional and Administrative Development of General Practice/ Family Medicine in Europe. WHO. EUR/ICP/DLVR 04 01 01. https://apps.who.int/iris/ handle/10665/108066

[6] Wass V, Gregory S. Not 'just a GP': a call for action. BJGP. 2017;67(657):148–9. doi: 10.3399/bjgp17X689953

[7] Barber S, Brettell R, Perera-Salazar R, Greenhalgh T, Harrington R. UK medical students' attitudes towards their future careers and general practice: a cross-sectional survey and qualitative analysis of an Oxford cohort. BMC Med Educ. 2018 Jul 4;18(1):160. doi: 10.1186/s12909-018-1197-z. PMID: 29973203; PMCID: PMC6030758.

[8] Lawson E. The Wass Report: moving forward 3 years on. doi: 10.3399/bjgp20X708953

Arguably, this may be largely due to access to healthcare services. GPs are always available, local, and can (theoretically, at least) be seen at short notice and at any time. Conversely, hospital specialists can only be seen with a referral and a prearranged appointment, at a remote site and only after a long wait. Rarity enhances the value of a product. Partly to address the balance in public opinion, the RCGP proposed a specialist qualification for primary care doctors. Did they succeed in this aim? The MRCGP became the single-entry point to a career in general practice in 2007. There is little to suggest that society's views have changed since then. The matter of status vexed the public less than it did the profession.

The mandatory requirement of MRCGP had a long gestation period. In the 1970s, the RCGP sought to raise the status of GPs by focusing on improving standards in practice and introducing mandatory training and career progression, akin to that in place for the established specialties. Much has been written about the motives of the RCGP in seeking such training. Whilst accepting the College's expressed desire to enhance the profile of general practice as a career option for all doctors, some commentators, perhaps cynically, also mused over whether the proposed changes had more to do with enhancing the College's own status. They noted that up to that time, during negotiations with the government, the RCGP, very much the junior lightweight among the senior, long-established colleges, had been slighted in matters of strategy.

Whatever the RCGP's motives, individual doctors working in general practice had always been aware of disparities in the competencies of their colleagues. Some were uncomfortable with the fact that without any further training, a newly minted doctor could set up their plate on a wall and practice as a GP principal, without any further assessment of their capabilities until retirement decades later. The NHS charter of 1948, which even went so far as to recommend a trainee practitioner scheme, originally contained the need for continuing professional development and training. Piloted on a patchy basis across the UK from the 1960s, such schemes became more widespread a decade later.[9]

The GMC further promoted the central tenet that only a lifetime of continued learning could sustain a career in any branch of medicine. In 1967, it published *Recommendation as to Basic Medical Education*,[10] at the heart of which was the principle that completion of medical undergraduate training should be considered a steppingstone towards medical education attainment, not an endpoint. The political weight that the GMC report provided, alongside the granting of a royal charter to the College of General Practitioners, renewed the momentum for a postgraduate training curriculum for general practice. Ultimately, that heralded the birth of general practice vocational training, completion of which became the sole entry point to independent practice as a GP principal.

---

[9] Horder JP, Swift G. The history of vocational training for general practice. J R Coll Gen Pract. 1979 Jan;29(198):24–32. PMID: 399785; PMCID: PMC2158966.

[10] Medical Education 1979;13:239–241.

8.4 GP VOCATIONAL TRAINING

The Nuffield Foundation in the 1950s and the University of London a decade later sponsored early VTS. The first structured GPVTS programmes in Wessex and Inverness included two years in hospital, comprising one year in any specialty but a mandatory six months in obstetrics and gynaecology (O&G) and a further year in general practice. In recognition of general practice as community-based, all training posts had to be undertaken in one geographic locality. All the hospital posts were supernumerary to the service posts of a similar level. In retrospect, the programme structure proved remarkably robust and remained largely unchanged to the present day.

In 1964, the innovation of a weekly, half-day release course was introduced in Canterbury, for doctors in their GP training year. The syllabus on these days was intended to cover elements of medical education relevant to general practice but unlikely to have been covered in any other postgraduate setting. Such topics included practice organisation, administration, and finance; social medicine; ethics; medico-legal; psychological and psychosomatic medicine; and the 'Cinderella' specialties: dermatology, ophthalmology, and ENT.

The year 1964 also witnessed the creation of the RCGP vocational training working party, comprising the renowned GP intellectuals of the time, John Horder, Patrick Byrne, Paul Freeling, Conrad Harris, Donald Irvine, and Marshall Marinker, to further develop ideas and lobby government for the introduction of mandatory postgraduate specialist training for GPs. The group set about defining the role of the GP and the knowledge, skills, and attributes needed to be one. Their deliberations were published under the title *The Future General Practitioner*, and this book, now out of print, provided the template (not universally accepted at the time) for the implementation of vocational training schemes across the UK.[11]

Meantime, recognition of general practice as an academic discipline came with the 1963 appointment of Richard Scott to the chair of general practice in Edinburgh, a world first. England followed suit somewhat belatedly, appointing Pat Byrne to the chair in Manchester a decade later. Both Richard Scott and Pat Byrne deserve further mention for their pioneering work in establishing general practice as an independent discipline within medicine.

Richard Scott (1914–1983) graduated with a medical degree from the University of Edinburgh in 1936 and went on to serve in the Royal Army Medical Corps for the entirety of World War II, demobilised with the rank of lieutenant colonel. He returned to Edinburgh to pursue a career in public health and general practice, uniquely combining both disciplines on-site at the university. In 1963, the General Practice Teaching Unit became the Department of General Practice, the world's first such independent department, and Scott was appointed to the chair. A feature of doctor's lives at that time, he retired from medicine in 1979, dying just four years later.

---

[11] Correspondence. https://bjgp.org/content/25/152/208

Patrick Byrne (1913–1980) was the son of a butcher; his academic ability gained him scholarships not only to his local grammar school in Liverpool but subsequently to Liverpool University to study medicine. Upon graduating in 1936, he worked as a GP principal in Westmorland for 42 years before retiring and, sadly, dying only two years later. He was one of a group of cerebral GPs scattered around the UK who, despite being geographically separate, collaborated in developing the nascent ideas that eventually led to the creation of the RCGP, with Byrne as its president from 1973 to 1976. His seminal treatise on the subtleties underpinning the doctor-patient relationship, *Doctors Talking to Patients*,[12] written with Barrie Long and published in 1976, would become obligatory reading for any practising doctor wishing to expand his or her interests into medical education.

Debate within medical academia continued in the early 1970s over the length and content of GP training. At that time, the consensus favoured a five-year rotation of three years in hospital posts and two years in general practice. However, this ambition was quickly abandoned, primarily on the grounds of cost. Likewise, the hope that doctors on the GPVTS would be supernumerary senior house officers (SHOs) whilst in hospital was quietly shelved, with these positions becoming service roles as for others in training.

In 1968, a Royal Commission looking into medical education published the Todd Report.[13] Informed by the GMC's own publication of the previous year and compelling presentations from the now 'Royal' College of General Practitioners, the authors' recommendations prioritised the recognition of general practice as a separate discipline within medicine, requiring its own specialist postgraduate training. These recommendations were finally enacted eight years later in 1976, when parliament approved the National Health Service (Vocational Training) Act, making vocational training compulsory for any doctor seeking to become a principal in general practice. General practice had come of age.

This was a huge boost to the prestige of the RCGP, which had pushed for such recognition against the antipathy and sometimes openly hostile opposition of the other royal colleges, the BMA, and, surprisingly, many GPs. However, it was a just reward for all the stubborn endeavours and hard labour of its executive committees over the years.

By 1982, no doctor could become a GP principal without having passed through a GPVTS. A Certificate of Satisfactory Completion of Training (CSCT), basically a certificate of attendance, was awarded on completion of the three-year course. The CSCT was tacitly accepted as defining the doctor's basic (some suggested minimal) level of competency that allowed them to practice medicine independently and safely in the community.

The CSCT was neither a final assessment nor an examination. Thus, the scheme was an educationist's dystopia, where everyone passed, provided that they attended the various elements of the training scheme. Clinical tutors signed attendance forms, the GP tutor confirmed their provenance, and the Joint

---

12 Byrne P, Long B. *Doctors Talking to Patients*. London: HMSO, 1976.
13 Report of the Royal Commission on Medical Education, 1968. H.M.S.O.

Committee on Postgraduate Training for General Practice (JCPTGP) issued the CSCT. From 1989 to 1992, only 0.26%, 16 out of 6200 GP trainees, failed to obtain their CSCT.[14]

The flaws in this system were self-evident, with no set curriculum, no core subjects, no assessments, and no quality control. There was no integration or communication between the various placements, especially those in primary and secondary care. Many of the tutors, undoubtedly excellent in their service roles, were themselves uneducated in education theory.

The quality of teaching varied. The hospital posts were training in name only, with hospital managers and consultants alike ignoring any supernumerary element. Concerns also began to arise regarding the competency of doctors coming off vocational training schemes. Those that went on to take the MRCGP examination failed at a worryingly high rate. Doubts in the process were partially alleviated in 1997 when the more rigorous certificate of *competence* in training replaced the certificate of *completion* of training. A summative assessment at the end of the three years tested competence in six elements: factual knowledge, problem-solving, practical work, clinical knowledge, consultation skills, and trainer's report.

Over the following years, the RCGP vigorously promoted the case for a gold-standard endpoint assessment, the MRCGP exam. Bolstering the RCGP argument were figures for medical litigation, complaints to the GMC, and erasure from the GMC Register, all of which showed higher numbers for doctors without the MRCGP.

The merits of summative (with or without MRCGP) and formative assessments were also troubling rank-and-file GP trainers across the UK. Many felt put in an invidious position, judging rather than supporting their postgraduate students, a concern mirrored two decades later over the role of GP appraisal and revalidation. Eventually, a consensus emerged. The GMC stated in 1996 that in time it would be usual for new principals to hold the MRCGP, but it should not be mandatory for entry to NHS general practice. The statement went some way towards defusing the anxieties of doctors in training, wary that failure in a difficult exam might result in premature termination of their career. Their fears were further allayed when the RCGP agreed to merge some elements of summative assessment, such as a video consultation, with the MRCGP exam, thus dispensing with the need for duplication. Despite the softening in its position, the College remained steadfast in its prime objective of making the MRCGP qualification a marker of excellence rather than of minimum competence in general practice training.

By the end of the 20th century, it was becoming increasingly apparent that the MRCGP exam would be the mandatory exam at entry into a lifelong career as a GP. Summative assessment alone as an endpoint remained a flawed concept. But what would happen to trainees who failed? Would they undergo further training and assessment? If so, for how long, and how would this be funded? The answer to

[14] Murray S. Summative assessment: a historical perspective. Br J Gen Pract. 2008 Dec;58(557):894–5. doi: 10.3399/bjgp08X376357. PMID: 19068175; PMCID: PMC2593553.

the last question was, 'with difficulty!'[15] Any troubling questions were postponed for future policy makers' attention.

As it was, trainees were independently accelerating the move towards the MRCGP, by voluntarily taking the exam in increasing numbers. The overlap between sections of the summative assessment and MRCGP drove the logic for doing so. A little extra effort resulted in a lot of extra letters after one's name. Despite wide acceptance of the MRCGP examination becoming the endpoint of GP vocational training, at the 11th hour, professional educators suddenly began questioning the robustness of the exam for that purpose. The Committee of General Practice Education Directors, COGPED, had arrived! A committee of eminent medical educationists, the Postgraduate Medical Education and Training Board (PMETB), was set up to advise, encourage, and maintain a consistent approach to general practice training across the UK[16]; it was only one of many medical education acronyms in the latter half of the 20th century.

The structure of governance overseeing GP training in the UK was complex, convoluted, and had more letters than the Royal Mail! Whilst the RCGP had an overview of standards in general practice, several other professional bodies dealt with the development, authorisation, and accreditation of educational programmes. The road to becoming a qualified doctor began on entry to medical school.

8.5 UNDERGRADUATE MEDICAL EDUCATION

Medical schools had never rested comfortably within the established structure for undergraduate education in the arts or sciences. They were only formally recognised as centres of further education following the passage of the Medical Act 1858, which sought to put the previously poorly regulated medical profession on a more publicly accountable footing. For the following century, the 12 medical schools in London and the 13 in the rest of the UK operated largely independently from their affiliate universities. In due course and following several governmental reviews on medical manpower and an increase in the number of funded places, additional medical schools were established; by the 21st century, the total had increased to 37.

The London medical schools, attached to their local hospital, predated (often by centuries) the establishment of the University of London in 1836. Subsequently, although the University of London oversaw the curriculum and awarded the final degree, the majority of learning occurred in lecture theatres and the wards of the hospitals whose names appeared on those degree certificates. Even historic centres of excellence, Oxford and Cambridge, could only teach the basic sciences; London medical schools subsequently provided any clinical experience.

[15] Carnall D. Summative assessment in general practice. BMJ. 1996 Sep 14;313(7058):638–9. doi: 10.1136/bmj.313.7058.638. PMID: 8811746; PMCID: PMC2352003.

[16] Murray S. Summative assessment: a historical perspective. Br J Gen Pract. 2008 Dec;58(557):894–5. doi: 10.3399/bjgp08X376357. PMID: 19068175; PMCID: PMC2593553.

The curriculum had no general practice component; thus, perhaps it is not surprising that in the milieu of specialist hospital practice, most students were encouraged to and did look on a hospital career as the likely outcome of their years of study.

The complex relationship of the hospital and its medical school in the Victorian era was summarised by Henry Charles Burdett:[17]

> Not only are the hospitals placed at the disposal of the authorities of the medical school for the clinical instruction of their pupils, but the two institutions are very largely manned by the same individuals, an appointment on the staff of the hospital very often carrying with it, by custom if not by by-law, some definite status in the medical school, and similarly the junior appointments in the medical school being very sure stepping stones to the medical and surgical staff of the hospital. The control and management of the medical school is often vested in the governing body of the hospital, and in nearly all cases in this country the financial relations between the hospital and the school are very close. The hospital is called upon to provide the proper facilities for the carrying on of the clinical teaching within its walls, involving the provision of larger outpatient rooms, operating theatre, lecture rooms and laboratory; and the other school buildings—theatre, classrooms, library, museum, laboratories etc., are either provided by the hospital authorities or built with money advanced to the school by the hospital.[18]

The arrangement Burdett described remained largely unchanged until the 1970s. The creation of new medical schools in Nottingham, Leicester, and Southampton, followed by the amalgamation of the London medical schools in the late 1980s, caused much outcry at the time The newer medical schools were closely integrated into their parent university. Their medical curriculum introduced innovative teaching theory, including problem-based learning, practice-based teaching, and professional actors roleplaying patients. Medical students were introduced to patients in their first term and found the holistic approach to teaching medicine far more interesting than the traditional lectures on such topics as the Krebs cycle.

The medical degree course typically lasted five years, six if an intercalated degree was included. The newer medical schools also introduced four-year-degree courses for mature students with a previous scientific degree.

The syllabus of the traditional course, still in place in some universities to this day, consisted of two years spent entirely in lecture halls, studying anatomy, physiology, pharmacology, and biochemistry, followed by three years of mixed teaching of the major specialties on the wards. By the 1980s, most medical schools had

---

[17] Henry Charles Burdett (1847–1920). Hospital administrator of Seamen's Hospital Society and notable philanthropist.

[18] Rivett G (undated). The development of the London hospital system. Accessed 7 Oct 2021 from www.nhshistory.net/hospitals_and_medical_education.htm

introduced a general practice element to the curriculum, initially a short elective based in a GP practice. By 2019, general practice contributed around 20% of the syllabus. Communication and consultation skills training became increasingly prominent during the 21st century.

The Responsible Officer for delivering the undergraduate curriculum was the Dean of Medicine, a university appointee. Lecturers appointed by the university and clinical lecturers both undertook teaching with joint appointments by the universities and the NHS and attached to NHS teaching hospitals.

A delightful summary of undergraduate medical education before 1948, written by Prof Steve Field, is worth a read.[19]

Medical students qualified with a degree of Bachelor of Medicine, Bachelor of Surgery—MBBS, MB BChir (Cantab), or MBChB, depending on the institution. A legacy of the Victorian era, 'Conjoint,' Licentiate of the Royal College of Physicians (LRCP) and Master of the Royal College of Surgeons (MRCS), available only to London, Oxford, and Cambridge graduates provided an alternative route to entry to a career in general practice. Conjoint degrees were gradually discontinued in the post-war years, though doctors holding only this qualification were still practising into the 1990s.

On graduating with a basic medical degree, the newly qualified doctor was expected to continue advancing knowledge and skills through a lifetime of learning and continuing professional development, a term not yet coined at that time. But were they going on to be trained or educated? The terms were interchangeable, the difference best explained in an article by Dr John Lister, published in the *Postgraduate Medical Journal* in 1994[20] where he summarised training as the acquisition of specific skills aimed at achieving technical competence whereas education has a broader concept encompassing critical thinking and problem-solving.

As well as creating a register of medical practitioners, The Medical Act 1858 also proposed suitably training for those practitioners. The act led to the creation of the General Council of Medical Education and Registration (GCMER) retitled the GMC in 1951. The GCMER set about standardising the quality of medical education across all medical schools in the UK, dictating that a basic degree and registration without further training did not qualify a doctor for a lifetime's practice in all areas of clinical medicine. However, compulsory preregistration hospital training was not introduced until 1953.

8.6 SUPERVISION AND QUALITY

No specific academic body oversaw all postgraduate medical education until 1967 when the Central Committee on Postgraduate Medical Education (CCPME) was

---

[19] Field S. The story of general practice postgraduate training and education. In: *A Celebration of General Practice*. pp. 117–30. London: RCGP, 2003.

[20] Lister J. The history of postgraduate medicine education. Postgrad Med J. 1994 Oct;70(828):728–31. doi: 10.1136/pgmj.70.828.728. PMID: 7831169; PMCID: PMC2397773.

created. This rapidly morphed into the Central Council for Postgraduate Medical Education (so, another CCPME), with the newly minted council comprising members whom the Secretary of State for Health appointed from the royal colleges, universities, profession, and NHS. The CCPME advised the government on all matters relating to postgraduate medical education and training.

The Council for Postgraduate Medical Education in England and Wales (CPME) (Scotland and Northern Ireland had significantly different bodies) sat below the CCPME and acted as a bridge between the NHS as resource provider, and the academic bodies developing the curricula. The CPME liaised with the regional academic deaneries on all matters pertaining to postgraduate medical education but had no authority to enforce or sanction any region that failed to comply with its recommendations. These additional powers arrived with the Standing Committee on Postgraduate Medical Education (SCoPME), which replaced the CPME in 1988[21] and answered solely to the Secretary of State.

Further devolution of postgraduate medical education took place with the establishment of regional Postgraduate Medical Education Committees (PGMEC) with a postgraduate dean as their executive officer. A subcommittee of the PGMEC was tasked with developing GP vocational training and raising standards in training practices. The membership of the general practice subcommittee was drawn largely from the Local Medical Committees and RCGP. The lower rungs of the training ladder were occupied by GPVTS course organisers, GP trainers, and training practices.

General practice training needed to be quantified and quality assured. The curriculum was generally ill-understood by trainers, and the quality of teaching and assessment varied widely across the country. The triple tenets of training; objectives, methods, and assessment, were hazy to most trainers, who had come to the role without any previous experience of education theory. Fierce disagreements continued within the profession as to how to proceed in producing the ideal GP. The RCGP, led by Denis Pereira Gray and Donald Irvine, strongly promoted an academic route but the BMA resisted. As the doctors' advocate, the BMA bridled at the setting of the bar at a height that would exclude a great number of doctors from choosing a career in practice. These differences were finally resolved through the establishment in 1981 of yet another committee, the JCPTGP. To ensure equal representation of all views within the profession, membership of the JCPTGP was drawn from the RCGP, representing academia, the General Practitioners Committee of the BMA, representing rank-and-file doctors. They even rotated the chair! A grant from the Department of Health and RCGP provided funding.

The JCPTGP became the competent authority that issued the final certificate of completion of training, CCT, without which a doctor could not practice as a GP principal. To this day, the CCT, now focused on competence rather than completion, remains the sole endpoint of GP training; however, since 2007, it can be issued upon attainment of success in the MRCGP examination.

---

[21] Lister J. The history of postgraduate medicine education. Postgrad Med J. 1994 Oct;70(828):728–31. doi: 10.1136/pgmj.70.828.728. PMID: 7831169; PMCID: PMC2397773.

These changes owed their existence almost entirely to the fortitude and vision of two elder statesmen of general practice, Denis Pereira Gray and Donald Irvine.

Sir Denis Pereira Gray had followed both his father and grandfather into the family GP practice in the West Country, establishing in Exeter the first post-graduate university department of general practice in Europe. Subsequently, his significant roles during a lengthy career included the presidency or chairmanship of the GMC, RCGP, JCPTGP, Academy of the Medical Royal Colleges of Great Britain and Ireland, and the GMC Standards Committee, which developed the first draft of *Good Medical Practice*. He was knighted for services to medicine, the citation highlighting his work on the witheringly dry subject of quality assurance in the setting of standards for medical competency.

Sir Donald Irvine also followed his father into practice but at the opposite end of the country, in Northumberland, where he was a GP, Regional Advisor for General Practice at the University of Newcastle upon Tyne, President of the RCGP, and the first GP elected President of the GMC. Like Pereira Gray, he was an early leader in the drive to improve quality in medical education and training; unlike Pereira Gray, his career, especially at the GMC, was dogged by controversies. He was unlucky to have been in post when the triple fallout from the Harold Shipman case, the Bristol heart surgery disaster and the subsequent hysteria over self-regulation and revalidation of doctors left him stuck between the rock of government and the hard place of rank-and-file doctors. Ultimately, these overwhelming burdens gave him little option but to resign from the presidency of the GMC in 2001, a sad end to a glittering career.

The JCPTGP provided a step change in the development of postgraduate GP education. The whole process was put on a more professional footing.

The 1997 NHS Vocational Training for General Medical Practice regulations and their 1998 equivalent regulations in Scotland and Northern Ireland gave the JCPTGP the responsibility for approving all training posts for GP training, in both hospitals and training practices across the UK. The JCPTGP became the designated body responsible for assessing the training and experience of all prospective GPs, confirmed in 1994 as the competent authority under European Council Directive 93/16/EEC.

The JCPTGP oversaw postgraduate training through a programme of tri-annual inspections of each region of the UK, conducted by three experienced GPs drawn from regional and associate advisors. The visits focused on the quality of the systems underpinning the educational content and process in each deanery, rather than on individual GP training. However, its powers were hamstrung by having little influence over the hospital component of GP training, though theoretically it could veto their use should they be found wanting. This power was seldom exercised since it would annul all GP training within that deanery. This unfortunate anomaly was rectified in the Vocational Training Regulations amendments of 1998, which allowed derecognition of individual posts in hospital without mutually assured destruction (MAD), the term used by the JCPTGP. The same amendment introduced summative assessment as the endpoint of GP training, despite fierce opposition from the General Practitioners Committee and, once published, the trainees themselves.

A plaintive letter to the *BMJ* highlighted a common concern of trainees at this time:[22]

Editor—My colleagues and I are among the first group of general practice registrars who have to pass the new compulsory summative assessment.

Although we are all enthusiastic about general practice and understand that assessment is needed to produce well trained general practitioners of suitable competence, the current situation seems somewhat unacceptable. Most of us aim to take the MRCGP examination in our final six months of training in general practice. The additional compulsory requirement to complete a summative assessment at the same time has unnecessarily increased our workload, especially as there is considerable overlap between the two examinations: the summative assessment seems to be a common denominator in both. The production of video work for the doctor-patient consultations requires typed assessment of each consultation. Unfortunately, summative assessment requires a different format for typed work from that required for the MRCGP examination. If done properly, the work is likely to take many weeks. This not only means that less time can be spent revising for the MRCGP examination but, more importantly, the enjoyment of general practice training is lost and vital follow up of patients is sacrificed. Implications may go further. I am sure the current situation is not attractive to junior doctors undecided on their future career.

The current situation needs to be revised. At least, if video work is good enough to pass the MRCGP examination it ought to be of sufficient standard to satisfy summative assessment and avoid the need to produce separate work.

The author's plea, initially at least, fell on deaf ears.

But what was the career path for the newly graduated doctor? Having obtained an MBBS or equivalent, all recently qualified doctors had to spend a prescribed period in hospital roles before being granted a licence to practice, essentially to prescribe medications and sign death certificates, and be registered as an independent medical practitioner with the GMC. Prior to 2005, the doctor spent the year working in a supervised position as a junior house officer (JHO), split between general medicine and surgery, although the option, not widely publicised, also offered six months in general practice. After 2005, the period of hospital training was extended to two 'foundation' years, but

---

[22] Cunliffe TP. Summative assessment compounds workload for MRCGP examination. BMJ. 1997 Oct 11;315(7113):950. doi: 10.1136/bmj.315.7113.950. PMID: 9361558; PMCID: PMC2127620.

registration with the GMC still took place on completion of the first of those years. Included in the six four-month rotations were mandatory placements in medicine, surgery, and for the first time, general practice, with the remainder in specialties of the training doctor's choice. JHO became FY1 and FY2 (Foundation Year Doctor 1 and 2).

Hospital training posts were initially intended to be supernumerary to service jobs, but by the 1970s, the boundaries had blurred to such an extent that the service provider, the NHS, absorbed the funding for these posts in their entirety.

All doctors in training, from Junior House Officer (FY1) through to Senior Register, had to be approved and, theoretically, supervised whilst in post by the royal colleges. Initially, these were the Royal College of Physicians and the Royal College of Surgeons, but in the 1970s, the Royal College of General Practitioners was finally included.

The training in the early years in hospital was essentially an apprenticeship. Junior doctors were expected to learn through experience on the job, with supervision patchy at best and varying widely from unit to unit and hospital to hospital. The guiding phrase in acquiring any skill was 'see one, do one, teach one'! Doctors certainly had ample opportunity to acquire experience; the working week was often well over 100 hours in 1:2 or 1:3 on-call rosters.

During the JHO year, doctors could independently apply for and expect to get a place on a GP vocational training scheme (GPVTS) of their choice. The standard GPVTS would be two years in six-month hospital rotations, followed by a year based in a local training practice. The hospital posts on the scheme continued to be service posts underwritten by the royal colleges, with the regional deanery approving the GP training practice.

Regrettably, especially in the early years, the principle of the GP trainee as a supernumerary apprentice tended to be blurred in many practices, though not to the same degree as their counterparts in hospital. GP trainees came into a practice as licensed doctors; thus, they were expected to operate as a GP principal, albeit with access to supervision and support if required. The trainee undertook consultations in booked surgeries, home visits, and out-of-hours. In truth, they became a source of cheap labour for many practices. However, they were allowed a ring-fenced half or full day a week for formal teaching with other trainees, usually in the local postgraduate education centre.

Having performed teaching duties informally before 1972, GP trainers did so after that date under the auspices of the regional deanery. Previous education theory and practice was not a prerequisite for such appointments, nor was RCGP membership, though it was encouraged.

Recruitment to GPVT schemes fell off in the late 1980s for lack of applicants. Some schemes had to fold. Schemes recruited doctors from Western Europe to remain viable. Ironically, European doctors were less familiar with our healthcare education and systems than their counterparts from the Commonwealth, but EU freedom of movement and migration law counted against the latter. Many continental trainees stayed to become GP principals.

8.7 THE CONSULTATION

A focus on the patient consultation became a prime differentiator between the training in general practice and hospital.

Medical students are taught to diagnose and manage disease using the basic template of history, examination, and investigation, but analysis of the consultation required a more thoughtful understanding of why the patient attended and what the consultation had achieved. It was precisely this precept that led to a closer study of the subject by the notable pioneers in the field. Their individual conclusions followed the same path; the consultation process could be broken down into well-defined elements. Adherence to the process ensured that nothing would be overlooked; that patient expectations were fully met. But was it unrealistic to expect such outcomes in the limited time available, especially as extraneous factors began to increasingly intrude on that time? Target setting, QOF, and the need to demonstrate efficiencies for political and financial reasons all posed distractions and challenges to the primary purpose of the consultation. Such intrusions could confuse the interaction and lead to a breakdown in communication and trust. Ignoring them, or at least striking a balance between the doctor's agenda and the patient's, was far more likely to lead to a harmonious relationship. Such wisdom only came with experience.

Consultation analysis became a routine part of the post and undergraduate medical curriculum, afforded time and resources equivalent to the teaching of anatomy, physiology, and pharmacology.

Analysis required observation obtainable through real or simulated (using actors) consultations. Conspicuous observation of the consultation was more likely to affect what went on within the consultation, although it was surprising how rapidly patients adapted to this 'fly-on-the-wall' scenario when exposed to it.

Subsequent discussion and analysis usually took place with reference to the various consultation and feedback models in vogue at the time.[23] Commonality between models revolved around the benefits accruing from the participation of all involved within the consultation, that is, the observed/observer/patient, rather than by abstract, academic or theoretical analysis alone.

Many of the publications on consultation analysis were very much of their time, but a brief review of notable contributions to the literature included:

1957: Michael Balint, *The Doctor, His Patient & the Illness*[24]

Michael Balint and his wife, Enid, both psychoanalysts and refugees from Hungary, worked with GPs in London in the 1950s and 1960s. The book was the

---

[23] Consultation models Pawlikowska, Leach, Lavallee, Charlton, Piercy Bradford VTS. www.bradfordvts.co.uk/wp-content/onlineresources/communication-skills/consultation-models/consultation%20models%20chapter.pdf

[24] Balint M. *The Doctor, His Patient and the Illness*. Edinburgh: Churchill Livingstone, 1957. Updated in 1964. ISBN-10: 0443064601. ISBN-13: 978-0443064609

result of a research project involving 14 GPs and a psychiatrist at the Tavistock Clinic in London. Meetings, 'Balint Groups,' of GPs took place, during which psychological aspects of their consultations were encouraged. The majority of GPs, who ascribed an almost cult-like status to the movement, viewed such groups with some scepticism at the time.

Balint described the most frequently used drug in general practice as the doctor himself ('the drug doctor'). Balint described the act of listening, rather than hearing, as an acquired skill and held that 'asking questions only gets you answers.'

Balint's seminal finding was the importance of 'attentive' listening. He was the first to suggest that the quality of the brief GP consultation, rather than the time itself, was the most important contribution to a satisfactory outcome. Patients liked to feel that the doctor was genuinely engaged and focused on their problem rather than operating on the doctor's own agenda. Many GPs would claim that this was difficult to achieve in the multitasking setting of a Monday morning surgery.

1964 Eric Berne, Games People Play[25]

Eric Berne was an American psychologist whose book, Games People Play, became a huge international bestseller with over five million copies sold. He introduced the term 'transactional analysis,' where each party enters any social engagement with the predetermined aim of obtaining gains or advantages from the other participant. He described the scenario as akin to a game involving rituals, pastimes, intimacy, and activity, during which the contestants alternated through three ego states: parent, adult, and child.

1972: John Horder et al., The Future General Practitioner

The Future General Practitioner originated from discussions within the RCGP on the definition of general practice and the ways of addressing the patient's physical, psychological, and social conditions.

The book was the first to set out the differing requirements of the consultation between primary and secondary care.

1976: Byrne and Long, Doctors Talking to Patients[26]

Pat Byrne and Barrie Long were the first to adopt one of the basics of informed research, namely, that meaningful statistical analysis needed big data. They listened to over 2,500 tape-recorded consultations from over 100 doctors in the UK and New Zealand. The study is now considered overly doctor-centric, as the title

[25] Berne E. Games People Play: The Psychology of Human Relationships. London: Penguin, 1964.

[26] Byrne PS, Long BEL. Doctors Talking to Patients. London: Royal College of General Practitioners, 1984.

implied. However, their study identified the influence of the personalities of the doctor and patient on the style of the consultation, on a spectrum from doctor-dominated, with minimal input from the patient, to a virtual monologue by the patient where the doctor remained a passive listener.

The consultation had six stages:

- The doctor establishes a relationship with the patient
- The doctor attempts to discover the reason why the patient attended. This might not be as transparent as it first seems. What is the patient's agenda? What are his or her fears and concerns?
- History-taking and possibly examination
- The doctor, in partnership with the patient, considers the condition
- Treatment or further investigations are discussed and set in place
- The consultation is terminated

Doctors using open, rather than closed questions tended to see their patients less frequently.

Byrne and Long's research was the first to break down the consultation into bite-size chunks, the forerunner of the ubiquitous Calgary-Cambridge model that Silverman suggested in 2005, widely used throughout medical teaching today.

1979: N C Stott and R H Davies, *The Exceptional Potential in Each Primary Care Consultation*[27]

Both Stott and Davies were Senior Lecturers in the Department of General Practice at the Welsh National School of Medicine. Their paper described four areas that must be systematically explored in each patient consultation:

- Management of the patient's presenting problem
- Modification of help-seeking behaviours
- Management of continuing problems
- Opportunistic health promotion

The paper's central thesis was the use of the consultation to educate and empower patients to manage their own symptoms and effect lifestyle changes to improve their overall health and prevent disease. Anecdotal evidence would suggest that this has been impossible to achieve despite 40 years of trying.

1984: David Pendleton et al., *The Consultation: An Approach to Learning and Teaching*

Pendleton, a social psychologist at the University of Oxford, together with three local GPs (Schofield, Havelock, and Tate), sets out seven tasks, arising from

[27] Stott NC, Davis RH. The exceptional potential in each primary care consultation. J R Coll Gen Pract. 1979 Apr;29(201):201–5. PMID: 448665; PMCID: PMC2159027.

patients' needs and with their cooperation, that needed to be addressed in a consultation. These included:

- Defining the reason for attendance
- Considering other problems
- Collaborating with the patient in prioritising and actioning each problem
- Achieving a shared understanding of the problem
- Enabling the patient to share responsibility in managing the problem
- Managing time and resources appropriately
- Establishing and maintaining a relationship whereby the patient is happy to present any other problems; the 'hidden agenda'

The paper built on previous work on the subject by being the first to adopt video technology as a tool for allowing objective evidence of the consultation to be used for subsequent discussions. The authors were the first to coin the triplet of patients presenting with an agenda encompassing ICE, which remains the foundation of all consultations to this day.

In addition, Pendleton formulated a set of rules governing the constructive ways of giving participants feedback on the consultation. The principle of structured feedback remains an essential element of all observed medical education.

Pendleton's rules on constructive feedback:

- Check the learner wants and is ready for feedback
- Let the learner give comments/background to the material that is being assessed
- Invite the learner to state what was done well
- Invite the observer(s) to state what was done well
- Let the learner state what could be improved
- Let the observer(s) state how it could be improved
- Make an action plan for improvement

1987: Roger Neighbour, *The Inner Consultation*

Roger Neighbour was a Hertfordshire GP whose career culminated in his election as President of the RCGP in 2003. His textbook, *The Inner Consultation*, has been aptly described as a medical classic. In it, he defined an intuitive five-stage model of consultation:[28]

- Connecting with the patient and developing rapport and empathy
- Summarising with the patient his or her reasons for attending; their feelings, concerns, and expectations
- 'Handing over' or sharing with the patient an agreed-upon management plan that hands back control to the patient

---

[28] Neighbour R. *The Inner Consultation: How to Develop an Effective and Intuitive Consulting Style*. 2nd edn. Abingdon: Radcliffe, 2004.

- 'Safety-netting' or making contingency plans, in case the clinician is wrong or something unexpected happens
- 'Housekeeping' or taking measures to ensure the clinician stays in good shape for the next patient

These suggestions removed the doctor from the previous role of manager of the patient's condition and suggested that better outcomes would result by including the patient, as an equal partner, in the decision making process.

1994: Peter Tate, *The Doctor's Communication Handbook*

Peter Tate developed some of the themes from the cooperative work he had undertaken with David Pendleton.[29] A doyen of the RCGP, he was responsible for the introduction of the video module to the MRCGP examinations in 1996.

In the text, he reaffirms that patients often did not feel fully engaged in the consultation and that this could be simply remedied by eliciting their ICE.

1996 Kurtz, Silverman, and Draper, *Calgary-Cambridge Observation Guide to the 'Medical Interview'*

Drs Suzanne Kurtz, Professor of Emerita, University of Calgary; Jonathan Silverman, Associate Clinical Dean and Director of Communication Studies, University of Cambridge; and Juliet Draper, GP and Research Fellow at the University of Cambridge; collaborated on devising the Calgary-Cambridge method of teaching and analysing consultation skills, now the basis of the communication curriculum in most UK undergraduate and postgraduate departments.[30,31] Their model derived from Pendleton's and was an evidence-based approach to the integration of the 'tasks' of the consultation and improving skills for effective communication. Once again, the emphasis was on collaboration.

The consultation was divided into:

- Initiating the session (rapport, reasons for consulting, establishing shared agenda)
- Gathering information (patient's story, open and closed questions, identifying verbal and non-verbal cues)
- Building the relationship (developing rapport, recording notes, accepting patient's views/feelings, demonstrating empathy and support), see ICE

---

[29] Tate P. *The Doctor's Communication Handbook*. Oxford: Radcliffe Medical, 1994.

[30] Calgary-Cambridge guide to the medical interview—communication process. Accessed 4 Oct 2018 from www.gp-training.net/training/communication_skills/calgary/guide.htm

[31] Kurtz S, Silverman J, Benson J, Draper J. Marrying content and process in clinical method teaching: enhancing the Calgary-Cambridge guides. Acad Med. 2003 Aug;78(8):802–9. doi: 10.1097/00001888-200308000-00011. PMID: 12915371.

- Explaining and planning (giving digestible information and explanations)
- Closing the session (summarising and clarifying the agreed-upon plan)

2002: John Launer, *Narrative-Based Practice in Health and Social Care*

John Launer, a London GP and Honorary Senior Lecturer in Primary Care, University of London, wrote his PhD thesis on the subject of a 'narrative-based' model of the consultation. His dissertation was interesting in that it offered a return to a more intuitive model where the consultation was managed like a general conversation. The salient points were:

- Circular questioning or picking up patients' words help to form open questions and assist patients in focusing on their answers
- Active listening was vital for an effective interaction (for example, avoiding note-taking during the consultation, a perennial complaint from patients, especially after the introduction of desktop computers)
- Exploring the context of the problem could often identify a non-medical cause, such as social, family, or work issues
- The conclusion should be a common narrative that encompasses the patient's concerns
- Other forms of information, for example, pictures and diagrams, help to assist the patient in understanding problems

2002: Lewis Walker, *Consulting with Neurolinguistic Programming*

Lewis Walker, a GP in Buckie, Scotland, suggested that neurolinguistic programming techniques or the use of 'body language' could improve communication with patients; only 10% of a message could be conveyed by words alone, with the remainder communicated by subtle variations in speech tone and body posture. To many GPs, this was overcomplicating what occurred naturally using 'social skills.' Nevertheless, Walker's text provided a useful guide to those lacking such insight and was particularly relevant in the sympathetic management of patients presenting with mental health problems.

2005, Jonathan Silverman et al., *Agenda-Led, Outcomes-Based Analysis (ALOBA)*

Subsequent generations of teachers thought Pendleton's rules on constructive feedback were too didactic and overly biased towards the teacher's rather than the pupil's agenda. Silverman and colleagues sought to rectify such bias through an Agenda-Led, Outcomes-Based Analysis (ALOBA) model. The process commences with the teacher eliciting learners'/students' agendas, the problems they experienced, outcomes they are trying to achieve, and what help they would like to achieve them. The student should initially be encouraged to consider how any problem could be resolved before including the teacher/group in the feedback. Feedback should be descriptive, formative, balanced, objective, and never judgemental.

Fundamental to all advice on feedback was the principle that people learned best in a 'safe' environment, free of negative criticism. This novel concept was totally at odds with the destructive model that had preceded it for much of the history of medical teaching, as illustrated by the *Doctor* books and films of Richard Gordon, in particular, the character of the irascible Sir Lancelot Spratt! ALOBA was based on the following stages:

- Start with the trainee's agenda
- Look at the outcomes the interview is trying to achieve
- Encourage self-assessment and self-problem-solving first
- Involve the whole group in problem-solving
- Use descriptive feedback
- Balance feedback (what worked and what could be done differently)
- Suggest alternatives
- Rehearse suggestions through role-play
- Be supportive
- Keep the interview a valuable tool for the whole group
- Introduce concepts, principles, and research evidence as opportunities arise
- At the end, structure and summarise what has been learned

2020 James Sherifi, *A Non-Academic Consultation Model*

An attempt at summarising all the above noteworthy consultation models has led me to formulate my personal humble contribution to managing the consultation process. The model is based on eight stages:

- *Ambience*
  - Your consulting room is clean and tidy. You are a professional offering a service
  - Photos of your family allow the patient to see that you are human and likely to have life experiences outside of the surgery
  - A framed degree certificate on the wall reinforces your credentials as a professional doctor
  - Dress code—smart or casual but freshly laundered. If you cycle to work, leave the Lycra in the bike shed
- *Welcoming*
  - Simple social etiquette. Stand to greet the patient as they enter. Introduction by name; not given name but title and surname; they are expecting to see a doctor, not their neighbour at the supermarket
  - Complete the notes for the last patient before the arrival of the next
  - Check the records before the patient enters to be able to offer full and undivided attention. It may be mundane to you, but to the patient, this is likely to be the most important event in their immediate calendar
- *Questioning*
  - 'How are you? What can I do for you today?' are good ways to open the dialogue

- Initially, questions should be open, giving the patient the opportunity to expand. Allow time, 'the golden minute,' without interruption, for them to explain why they are seeing you
- Avoid closed, limiting, or leading questions until you inevitably have to step in, to manage agenda and time
- Try not to interrupt unless for clarification, though some people need reining in. Listen and maintain a flow. Sometimes patients say something that needs further enquiry, but it is generally unproductive breaking their stream of consciousness
- Any additional concerns that arise should be revisited later in the consultation, but this is easily forgotten. A useful tip is to jot a note, an aide memoir, as you go along
- *Listening*
  - Appear attentive and maintain eye contact as much as possible. Vary your posture naturally in response to the narrative and their non-verbal cues and body language
  - It may or may not be appropriate to make notes as the patient speaks. Be tuned to the patient's alertness. Do not fall into the trap of, 'the doctor was more interested in that screen than in me'
- *Responding*
  - This is a dialogue. To succeed, it needs two people to engage
  - Clarify points raised. Summarise repeatedly. Reflect statements and feelings. Ascertain knowledge and understanding. Be tuned in to changing mood; possibly defusing anger before it establishes a hold
  - Empathy is vital. It may be all the therapy needed[32]
- *Explaining*
  - Use language that the patient will understand
  - Give important information first
  - Repeat important points and ascertain that the patient understands
  - Provide written information or visual aids to reinforce understanding and advice
- *Closure*
  - 'Have we covered everything you wished to see me for?'
  - Safety-netting. Always append a self-preservation clause. Give clear instructions as to actions to be taken by the patient should the situation change or worsen
  - Stand and usher the patient to the door
  - Reflect on what has taken place in the consultation. What do I expect to happen if I am right? How will I know if I am wrong? What would I do then?
  - Make contemporaneous, accurate, and suitably detailed notes

Follow the above rules and you will make a fine doctor, my friend.

---

[32] Bub B. The patient's lament: hidden key to effective communication: how to recognise and transform. Med Humanit. 2004 Dec;30(2):63–9. doi: 10.1136/jmh.2004.000164. PMID: 23671291.

8.8 MEDICAL TRAINING, 2000 ONWARDS

Postgraduate medical training underwent a seismic upheaval following the publication of Modernising Medical Careers (MMC)[33] in 2003; a policy statement to 'improve patient care by improving medical education with a transparent and efficient career path for doctors.'[34] The proposal sought to align the early years of specialist hospital and GP training in the UK with the European Union, including implementation of the European Working Times Directive, which would substantially reduce the average working week for a junior hospital doctor from 80+ to a maximum of 48 hours.

By 2005, the JCPTGP and the Specialist Training Authority covering hospital specialist training, both being the competent authorities for assuring medical training under the European medical directives, had been unified under the banner of the PMETB. The JCPTGP had done a good job during its ten-year existence and many educationists mourned its demise.[35]

The PMETB, with an acronym no more memorable than those that preceded it, never quite gained the respect of the royal colleges that its predecessors garnered. Thus, it came as no surprise when it was duly absorbed into the GMC.

During its brief existence, the PTEMB set about modifying, rearranging, and overhauling the training curriculum. Clinical competency was the new buzz phrase. It had been noted with some concern that doctors were gaining specialist certificates but lacked simple skills in practice, such as the taking of a blood pressure or a cervical smear. There were gaps in the training and assessment of clinical skills, which needed to be addressed. Unusually, before concluding its report, the PMETB sought out the views of the stakeholders, the trainees, educators, assessors, and laity.

The trainees wanted a robust assessment package worthy of effort, an educationally focused, effectively delivered trainer's report, fair, reliable and relevant examinations, fewer summative hurdles and future developments mindful of costs.

The educators wanted more time to teach, less assessment, a single route process, formative approaches, flexible career progression, avoidance of multiple workplace assessments and opportunities for remedial support for any struggling trainees.

The assessors wanted assessments that drove the education agenda, content reflective of real practice, continuing high standards for assessor selection and training, maintenance of a national panel of assessors, and fairness and equal opportunities for trainees and assessors.

The lay representatives wanted appropriate, reliable standards for completion of training, assurance that registrars were safe for independent practice, lay involvement in standard-setting, and clinical skill tests.

---

[33] https://publications.parliament.uk/pa/cm200708/cmselect/cmhealth/25/25i.pdf

[34] www.mmc.nhs.uk/default.aspx?page=310

[35] Keighley B. The JCPTGP; the passing of an era. BJGP. 2005;55(521):970–1.

The PMETB responded to these suggestions by proposing that the assessment for GP registrars needed streamlining, and a single route to certification of competence in training (CCT) and RCGP membership should be developed, that is, no duplication of exams. In addition, more focus on formative workplace assessment, exams that tested both applied knowledge and clinical skills, completion of assessments that informed both CCT and College membership, and a two-phase licensing test.

Despite the recommendations, dual (some might say confused) entry to a career in general practice remained in place. Any prospective GP still had to complete the assessment of specialist training (formerly, the summative assessment), in addition to passing the revised MRCGP examination. However, the summative assessment was revised to include two formal elements:

1. The Applied Knowledge Test (AKT), a multiple-choice questionnaire with the focus on applied knowledge relevant to primary care, as defined in the RCGP curriculum, and on critical appraisal of the evidence base that informs current UK practice, i.e. good clinical practice
2. The Clinical Skills Assessment (CSA), an objectively structured clinical exam (OSCE), with 14 stations simulating experiences in a primary care environment

These tests could be sat at any time during the three years of training, but logically would offer the best chance of success if taken in the final year.

The standards set for these tests would be reviewed regularly, under the scrutiny of both the PMETB and RCGP, to ensure that the exit from vocational training assured the public that GP registrars were safe and 'fit for purpose,' to practice independently.

Thus, after much agonising and years of lobbying within the profession, the adoption of the MRCGP exam as the entry qualification into general practice alongside elements of the summative assessment for the CCT became mandatory in August 2007. The debate surrounding this conclusion had been conducted not only between traditionalists and modernisers but even within the RCGP itself, with several academic members expressing concern that the stature of the examination and thus RCGP membership might be diluted by an exam with an almost 100% pass rate. However, the group mainly affected by these changes, the trainees, largely welcomed the prospect that a little extra work over and above that required for summative assessment would, at the very least, add a few extra letters after their name, elevate them to the same status as their hospital specialist colleagues, and, if they chose, be the last exam they would ever have to take in their professional lives!

As of 2010, the GMC became the responsible body for policing standards for the entirety of postgraduate medical education in the UK,[36] including the approval

---

[36] Promoting excellence: standards for medical education and training. GMC. www.gmc-uk.org/-/media/documents/Promoting_excellence_standards_for_medical_educa-tion_and_training_0715.pdf_61939165.pdf

of GP trainers, curricula and assessment systems, training posts, GPVTS programmes, and foundation programmes (FY1 and FY2).

Within a year, the GMC produced its first report on the state of medical education in the UK, pithily titled *The State of Medical Education and Practice in the UK!*[37]

The executive summary acknowledged that an unacceptable variation in the standards of medical practice remained (the report covered all specialties, not just primary care) and highlighted concerns regarding clinical investigations, treatments, and communication with patients. The report identified that a small (0.03%) but worrying number of doctors were falling seriously short of the standards expected of them. One in 3,000, 73 from the total of 240,000 GMC registered doctors, had been struck off in that year. The report set a marker that the GMC would tolerate nothing but perfection.

The report went on to state, in somewhat damning terms, the pre-GMC administration that had overseen medical education:

Medical education and training need to be more responsive to changes in healthcare needs, the organisation and delivery of care, and the shifting expectations of patients.

There is a tension between service delivery and protected time for education and training and this has been exacerbated by the Working Time Directive.

Trainee doctors need high-quality supervision and positive role models with strong leadership skills. Yet there is variation in trainees' experiences of supervision.

To rectify these issues, the report recommended a wider, more flexible approach to training, to be delivered by higher-quality educators. UK GP vocational training schemes were put under the spotlight with more frequent inspections, review of reports and action plans, a national training survey, and exam data collected by individual trainees. These initiatives proved effective. *The State of Medical Education and Practice in the UK* report for 2019 proved to be more comfortable reading for all involved in postgraduate medical education; 82% of trainees rated the quality of their experience as good or excellent whilst 92% of trainers rather enjoyed their role as a trainer![38]

The vocational training of doctors to become GPs was of little interest to those front-line doctors not in a training practice. Nevertheless, the quality of UK-trained VTS GPs was guaranteed and VTS alumni were keenly sought for vacant partnerships. That need alone ensured that all practising GPs retained more than a passing interest in the training of the GPs of the future.

Having remained unchanged for the first half of the NHS's lifetime, the entry to becoming a GP had progressed through four incrementally difficult iterations; basic medical degree, formative assessment with trainer's report, summative

[37] www.gmc-uk.org/-/media/documents/somep—report-about-the-state-of-medical-education-and-practice-in-the-uk-73730345.pdf

[38] www.gmc-uk.org/-/media/documents/somep-2019-full-report_pdf-81131156.pdf

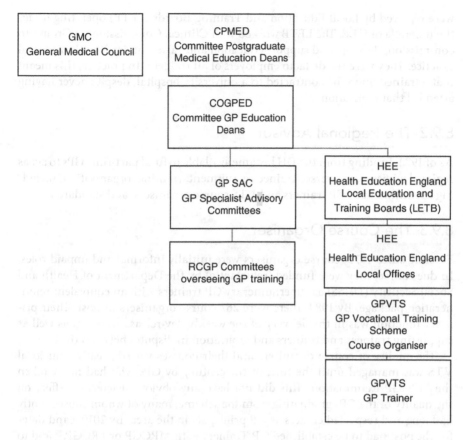

Figure 8.1 The administrative structure overseeing GP training, 2013.

assessment, and MRCGP. General practice was no longer the easy opt-out for the failed physician but had finally become a specialty in its own right. Whether that increased the status of GPs with their specialist colleagues or, indeed, the public, remained a matter of opinion.

8.9 THE ADMINISTRATION OF GP VOCATIONAL TRAINING

The administrative structure responsible for the local delivery of the GP vocational training schemes was headed by the regional dean and delivered at the grassroots by the GP trainer.

8.9.1 The Dean

Although the strategy for medical education emanated from the national designated authorities, the implementation at the local level began with the regional dean, an academic post based in a centre of higher education. In 2013, deaneries were replaced by Local Education and Training Boards (LETB) operating under the umbrella of HEE. The LETB worked with Clinical Commissioning Groups to commission, develop, and support education and raise standards within general practice. They were the de facto employers of all trainees. In practice, this meant that a trainee might be contracted to a university hospital, despite never having attended that institution.

8.9.2 The Regional Advisor

As of 1972, funding from the DH became available to fund part-time GPs to act as regional advisors, to oversee trainee recruitment, training, organisation, including appointment of GP trainers and VTS course organisers, and standards.

8.9.3 The Course Organiser

Existing since 1972, course organisers were initially informal and unpaid roles. In due course, they were funded (reluctantly) by the Department of Health and Social Security (DHSS) as supernumerary GP trainers with an equivalent remuneration package. By 1984, there were 267 course organisers in post. Their primary function was in the delivery of the weekly day-release training, as well as supporting trainees and trainers and arbitration in disputes between the two.

The quality of course organisers and their courses varied greatly. Our local VTS was managed until the turn of the century by GPs who had never taken the MRCGP examination. This did not have any obvious deleterious effect on the quality of the GPs graduating from the scheme; many of whom subsequently had long and respected careers as GP principals in the area. By 2010, candidates for the post had to be established GP Trainers with MRCGP or FRCGP,[39] and to have completed a Postgraduate Certificate in Medical Education,[40] followed by a formal practice inspection by the local GP training programme director.

8.9.4 The GP Trainer

Prior to 1973, the Local Medical Committee (LMC), an arm of the BMA, appointed GP trainers. The regional Postgraduate Medical Education Committee now makes appointments, usually following an interview with the subcommittee for PMEC GP. The role appealed to those doctors with a general interest in education but also a selfish desire to ensure that their protegees would be competent enough to treat them when, with age, they, in turn, became patients! Despite the role requiring the incumbent to have MRCGP, this was never rigorously enforced.

Over time, as for the course organiser, the training and qualifications for a GP trainer became more daunting. The professionalisation of the role was beautifully

---

[39] Fellow of the Royal College of General Practitioner.
[40] BMJ. 2008;337. doi: 10.1136/bmj.a880 (Published 30 July 2008). Cite this as: BMJ. 2008;337:cf_zaca_educationdip

illustrated in the lengthy job description within the Essential Handbook for GP Training & Education, first published in 2012.[41] GP training had travelled far from a time when the only attribute needed to become a trainer was the insight to recognise when it was your round at the pub!

Until relatively recently, all of these roles (apart from dean) were open to any established GP principal, yet few chose to apply, citing the burden of daily work and diffidence when facing the education establishment. The acronyms that had bedevilled the administration of medical education meant nothing to them, as indeed to many of those delivering that education. Those that did apply to become GP trainers did so for reasons of personal development, adding variety to their own working lives, altruism in wanting to enhance the learning experience of the young, and, rarely, income. The barriers to entry have increased in recent years, demanding an ever-stronger commitment from those wishing to enjoy a supplementary career in medical education. Those barriers have put off many experienced doctors with much to offer in educating the doctors of tomorrow, to the detriment of all, including patients.

8.10 CONTINUING PROFESSIONAL DEVELOPMENT

8.10.1 Training the Trainers

In parallel with the organisational developments in vocational training in the 1970s, thought was given as to how regional advisors, course organisers, and trainers could develop and advance their teaching, in line with contemporary education theory.

In 1965, the RCGP published The *Future General Practitioner—Learning and Teaching*,[42] a seminal work describing the process of education. Sir Denis Hill stated the guiding principles of the book:

> The family physician's role is a difficult one. If it is to be sustained and developed, the general practitioner must become the most educated, the most comprehensively educated, of all the doctors in the health service.[43]

The authors defined the content of vocational training as falling into five domains: health and diseases, human development, human behaviour, medicine and society, and the practice. The contents and conclusions of the report were both original and prescient; original in that they did not focus exclusively on

---

[41] Mehay R. *Essential Handbook for GP Training & Education*. CRC Press, 2012. https://www.taylorfrancis.com/books/edit/10.1201/9781846197918/essential-handbook-gp-training-education-ramesh-mehay

[42] Royal College of General Practitioners. The future general practitioner—learning and teaching. BMJ. J R Coll Gen Pract. 1972 Sep;22(122):581–2. PMCID: PMC2156233

[43] https://bjgp.org/content/bjgp/22/122/629.full.pdf

disease; prescient in including human development, behaviour, and environment. The pre-eminence of anatomy, physiology, and pharmacology, the 'physical' diseases, in traditional teaching never provided the holistic view required for care in the community. *The Future General Practitioner* addressed that omission whilst also defining the ethos, attributes, activities, and aspirations of family medicine and its practitioners. It is as relevant today as it was 50 years ago, although, as would be expected of any historical text with 'future' in the title, some of the concepts and wording now seem a little outdated.

Educating the educators proceeded apace. In 1973, the RCGP, with financial support from the Nuffield Provincial Hospitals Trust, established the first of three courses designed primarily for course organisers and regional advisors. The inaugural tutor, Paul Freeling, from the Department of General Practice at St. George's Hospital Medical School, combined educational theory with a novelty at the time, small-group learning.[44]

In 1976, Freeman and Byrne, from the Manchester University Department of General Practice, published their work on rating scales for use in the assessment of trainees.[45]

In 1977, Pereira Gray published a paper on vocational training, in which he explained educational theory and set out objectives, methods, and assessments piloted at the Exeter University Department of General Practice.[46]

The 1980s saw a plethora of activity in the field of medical education resulting with worthy contributions from Byrne and Long in *Doctors Talking to Patients*;[47] N. C. Stott and R. H. Davies in *The Exceptional Potential in Each Primary Care Consultation*; David Pendleton in *The Consultation—An Approach to Learning and Teaching*;[48] and Roger Neighbour in *The Inner Consultation*. All became essential reading for any aspiring GP.

The national funding of medical education and GP training was as complex as its organisation.

There are currently four streams of funding under the overall umbrella of medical and professional education and training, (MPET), overseen since 2012 by Health Education England (HEE).

- Non-medical education and training: For paramedics, nurses, physiotherapists, radiologists, psychologists, and physician associates
- Service Increment for Teaching (SIFT): Covers the costs of tutors (usually clinical tutors in hospitals and general practice) and facilities required for teaching
- Dental SIFT, SIFT but for dental training

[44] White P, Freeling P. Randomised controlled trial of small group education on the outcome of chronic asthma in general practice. JRCGP. 1989 June;39(322):182–6.

[45] Freeman J, Byrne PS. *The Assessment of Postgraduate Training in General Practice*. Guildford: Society for Research into Higher Education, University of Surrey, 1976.

[46] Pereira Gray DJ. A system of training for general practice. RCGP. 1978 Sep;28(192):441–2.

[47] Byrne PS, Long BEL. *Doctors Talking to Patients*. RCGP, 1984. Royal College of General Practitioners ISBN-10: 0850840929 ISBN-13: 978-0850840926

[48] Pendleton D, et al. *The Consultation—An Approach to Learning and Teaching*. Oxford: Oxford University Press, 1984.

- Medical and Dental Education Levy (MADEL): Covering the salaries for those doctors and dentists in training, replacing the previous funding for general practice training through the GMS Statement of Fees and Allowances. The element of MADEL covering general practice funds the three-year GP VTS, including 100% of the trainee salary, and GP premium plus associated employer national insurance and pension contributions. The trainer grant amounted to £8,350 in 2020[49]

For the year 2020/2021, HEE had an annual budget of £4.2 billion.

Accountability for these significant sums of money has not always been transparent. A BMA publication (2007), *Medical Service Increment for Teaching (SIFT) Funding*,[50] reported that half the trusts that responded to its survey could not account for SIFT expenditure over the previous five years! As an idea of the variation of sums involved, teaching hospitals were receiving between £35,000 and £100,000 per year for each student under their wing.

SIFT was first introduced in 1976 to cover the additional service costs the NHS incurred in providing hospital facilities for the clinical teaching of medical students. GP practices were only included following the publication of the Winyard Report (1995), at a woeful rate of £12 per half-day teaching session per student.[51] SIFT was replaced by a more responsive, tariff-based system, the Department of Health and Social Care (DHSCC) Education and Training Tariff in 2013.

Doctors do not stop learning after qualifying for their chosen medical specialty. The RCGP promoted a lifetime of learning at its inception in 1952, and other august bodies, such as the GMC and royal colleges have reinforced the principle throughout the decades. A structure for organising and overseeing postgraduate education was accelerated following the publication of the Royal Commission on Medical Education, the 400-page Todd Report, in 1968, although GPs had always recognised that you never stopped learning through experience.[52]

From the 1960s, all hospitals had postgraduate medical centres, and GPs regularly attended the educational meetings that took place there. The popularity of these meetings progressively dropped as GP practices grew in size and initiated their own in-house educational meetings. Most surgeries had a library, of sorts, containing at least the free weekly medical journals as well as the *BMJ*. In due

---

[49] NHS Education Funding Guide. NHS HEE. 2020. https://www.hee.nhs.uk/our-work/education-funding-reform/nhs-education-funding-guide

[50] Bevan G. The medical service increment for teaching (SIFT): a £400m anachronism for the English NHS? BMJ. 1999 Oct 2;319(7214):908–11. doi: 10.1136/bmj.319.7214.908. PMID: 10506054; PMCID: PMC1116729.

[51] Rosenthal J, McKinley RK, Smyth C, Campbell JL. The real costs of teaching medical students in general practice: a cost-collection survey of teaching practices across England. Br J Gen Pract. 2019 Dec 26;70(690):e71–e77. doi: 10.3399/bjgp19X706553. PMID: 31636129; PMCID: PMC6805166.

[52] Royal Commission on Medical Education. *Report of the Royal Commission on Medical Education, 1965–8*. London: HMSO, 1965–8.

course, the Internet also encouraged contemporaneous, 'trigger point' learning. This too fell prey to the march of acronyms, becoming PUNs/DENs (Patients Unmet Needs/Doctors' Educational Needs), the eponymous book first published by Richard Eves in 2003.

The GP contract of 1990 encouraged GPs to engage in maintaining their knowledge by attaching a monetary incentive, the postgraduate education allowance (PGEA) to learning. To qualify for PGEA, the Regional Advisor in general practice had to approve meetings. A somewhat arbitrary minimum of 30 hours a year of learning was set. Failure to achieve the mandated hours resulted in the withholding of up to £2,000, roughly 6% of target net remuneration of a GP principal at that time.

As generalists, GPs were only too aware that their knowledge on all medical matters was likely to be wanting. Continuous, reflective learning was a natural part of the job. The introduction of annual GP appraisals in 2002 changed that perception. Whilst everyday learning continued as before, providing onerous, written evidence that it was so was regarded as a bureaucratic affront by many front-line GPs. That sentiment has remained unchanged to the present day.

8.11 THE MRCGP EXAMINATION

Passing the MRCGP examination became the sole route of entry to the GMC register of general practitioners, as of 2007. A doctor could not practice as a GP without a GMC licence.

The MRCGP examination was originally introduced in 1965 as a requirement solely for membership of the Royal College of General Practitioners. Membership was optional, and GPs chose to take the exam partly to challenge themselves and to gain a qualification for entry into other fields of medicine, such as academia. Initially few, annual applications for the exam increased steadily, 2,000 in 1986, 3,500 by 2015. Of the total applicants in 2015, 80.3% were UK graduates, 3.9% from EEA, and 15.8% categorised as 'Rest of the World.' Pass rates were UK 83%, EEA 59%, and RoW 50%.[53]

The structure of the exam evolved over the years. The original format[54] contained two parts; part 1, a written exam including a multiple-choice questionnaire, a modified essay testing problem-solving and management skills, including attitudes, and a traditional essay. Part 2, an oral exam, covered case records examiners provided, testing problem-solving and patient management, and a review of a logbook of 50 cases that the candidate provided.

Educationists always considered the old MRCGP exam flawed because it did not include an assessment of how the doctor operated within a general practice setting. The logbook of consultations had only acted as a surrogate test for these competencies, and the preferred option, video consultations, was considered too

[53] MRCGP Statistics 2015–16. Annual Report. www.rcgp.org.uk/-/media/Files/GP-training-and-exams/Annual-reports/MRCGP-Statistics-2015-16-Final-Draft-Feb-17.ashx?la=en

[54] Byrne PS. Report of a conference on examination for MRCGP. J R Coll Gen Pract. 1970;19:240–1. https://bjgp.org/content/bjgp/19/93/240.full.pdf

cumbersome. The exam also had to comply with GMC standards on validity, reliability, feasibility, cost-effectiveness, opportunities for feedback, and impact on learning, in addition to following best practice in assessment, quality assurance, and standard-setting. Few parts of the exam adhered to these aims. Thus, the exam was revised to cover a broader spectrum of work relevant to general practice, with the new format introduced in 2000.

The revised 'n,' for 'new,' MRCGP, had three components covering the spectrum of knowledge, skills, behaviours, and attitudes, as defined by the GP Specialty Training Curriculum, and rigorously validated prior to the introduction of the exam.

These were grouped under the headings:

- Applied Knowledge Test (AKT)
- Clinical Skills Assessment (CSA)
- Workplace-Based Assessment (WPBA)

8.11.1 Applied Knowledge Test[55]

As the name suggested, the AKT was intended to test problem-solving cognition rather than the acquisition of theory. The format of the examination included:

- Multiple-choice questions, computer-based; 200 questions to be answered over 3 hours and 10 minutes (the 10 minutes was added after a review in 2014, suggesting that non-UK graduates may be disadvantaged by language, needing more time to understand the content of the question. The same review allowed a calculator to be brought into the exam room!)
- 80% of the total questions covered clinical medicine; 10% critical appraisal and evidence-based medicine; and 10% health informatics and administrative issues

The cost of taking the AKT was £459 in 2020. This was a tax-allowable expense that could be partially reclaimed from Her Majesty's Revenue and Customs (HMRC).

8.11.2 Clinical Skills Assessment[56]

The CSA tested a doctor's ability to operate in a holistic manner, gather information, understand disease processes and make evidence-based decisions that could

[55] Royal College of General Practitioners. The Applied Knowledge Test content guide, Aug 2014. Accessed 18 Sep 2018 from www.rcgp.org.uk/gp-training-and-exams/mrcgp-exams-overview/~/media/D96EB4E0188E4355BCC9221B55859B08.ashx

[56] Royal College of General Practitioners. MRCGP Clinical Skills Assessment (CSA). 2018. Accessed 18 Sep 2018 from www.rcgp.org.uk/gp-training-and-exams/mrcgp-exams-overview/mrcgp-clinical-skills-assessment-csa.aspx

be communicated effectively to patients and colleagues. In summary, it sought to emulate the various elements of a typical clinical consultation. The assessment was based on the OSCE comprising 13 stations, each containing a specific clinical scenario likely to occur in general practice.

The content for each station covered elements from the GP training curriculum, including:

- Management of common medical conditions in primary care
- Problem-solving skills: gathering and using data for clinical judgement, choice of physical examination, investigations and their interpretation, and demonstration of a structured and flexible approach to decision-making
- Comprehensive approach: demonstration of proficiency in the management of co-morbidity and risk
- Person-centred care: communication with patients and the use of recognised consultation techniques to promote a shared approach to managing problems, including safety-netting
- Attitudinal aspects: practising ethically with respect to the accepted professional codes of conduct
- Clinical practical skills: demonstrating proficiency in performing physical examinations and using diagnostic and therapeutic instruments
- Paediatric care

The cost of taking the CSA was £1,352 in 2020.

8.11.3 Workplace-Based Assessment[57]

The WPBA evaluated the trainee's progress in areas of professional practice best tested in the workplace. It was a contemporaneous assessment of the trainee's performance. Events were documented in a logbook over the three years in specialist training. Evidence of reflective learning focusing on capability and, most importantly, patient safety, had to be visible. The assessment was undertaken by the GP trainer who was expected to verify that the trainee was fit to progress towards completion of training and ultimately fitness to practice as a GP. This was no easy task since interrogation of the logbook had to cover the wide range of activities[58] in general practice, including:

- *Fitness to practise.* The doctor's awareness of when his/her own performance, conduct, or health, or that of others, might put patients at risk, and taking action to protect patients
- *Maintaining an ethical approach.* Practising ethically, with integrity and respect for diversity. This includes the ethical principles of medical practice, autonomy, beneficence, non-maleficence, and justice

---

[57] www.rcgp.org.uk/training-exams/training/mrcgp-workplace-based-assessment-wpba.aspx
[58] www.rcgp.org.uk/-/media/Files/GP-training-and-exams/WPBA/WPBA-capabilities-with-IPUs-detailed-descriptors.ashx?la=en

- *Communication and consultation skills.* Communication with patients, and the use of recognised consultation techniques, e.g. Calgary-Cambridge[59]
- *Data gathering and interpretation.* For clinical judgement, choice of physical examination and investigations and their interpretation
- *Clinical examination and procedural skills.* Competent physical examination of the patient with accurate interpretation of physical signs and the safe practice of procedural skills
- *Making a diagnosis/decision.* A conscious, structured approach to decision-making
- *Clinical management.* Recognition and management of common medical conditions in primary care
- *Managing medical complexity.* Aspects of care beyond managing straightforward problems, including management of co-morbidity, uncertainty, risk, and focusing on health rather than just illness
- *Working with colleagues and in teams.* Working effectively with other professionals to ensure good patient care, including sharing information with colleagues
- *Maintaining performance, learning, and teaching.* Maintaining performance and effective continuing professional development (CPD) for oneself and others
- *Organisation, management, and leadership.* Understanding the use of computer systems to augment the GP consultation and primary care at individual and systems levels, the management of change, and the development of organisational and clinical leadership skills
- *Practising holistically, promoting health, and safeguarding.* Operating in physical, psychological, socioeconomic, and cultural dimensions, taking account of feelings as well as thoughts. Mandatory training in the safeguarding of children
- *Community orientation.* Management of the health and social care of the practice population and local community

These tasks and evidence required would have taxed most experienced GPs! Nevertheless, the GP trainer had to review progress in the above descriptors every six months, using the Educational Supervisors Review, ESR,[60] to highlight those areas that needed further work and those that had been satisfactorily completed.

There were no fees levied for the WPBA.

Successful attainment of the MRCGP exam included the first year's membership in the College. Thereafter, membership was optional. The membership fee in 2020 for a fully qualified GP earning more than £46,350 per annum was £519.

---

[59] What are consultation models for? Claire Denness. doi: 10.1177/1755738013475436
[60] www.rcgp.org.uk/training-exams/training/mrcgp-workplace-based-assessment-wpba/esr-for-workplace-based-assessment.aspx

The RCGP produced an annual report containing extensive data and insights on those taking the MRCGP exam,[61] such as the dominance of UK graduates, women, and military doctors successfully passing the exam.

A mini-industry of commercial courses has developed to bolster the chances of candidates achieving a successful outcome. They vary in price but, as a rule, were worth the expense.

8.12 MEMBERSHIP BY ASSESSMENT OF PERFORMANCE (MAP)

MAP[62] was introduced in 2000 as an alternative route to attaining MRCGP for those established general practitioners who had not bothered with the MRCGP in the past. There was little reason, apart from academic fulfilment, for doctors choosing to challenge themselves in this way since the work involved in providing the portfolio of evidence was time-consuming. Nevertheless, the promotion, with its 95% pass rate, proved to be popular, and by 2017, over 1,350 doctors had used this route to membership.

MAP had two parts, a portfolio documenting evidence in a logbook covering much the same descriptors as the WPBA and an oral assessment using a similar OSCE format to the CSA. Part of the reason underlying the high pass rate for the exam was the College's willingness to facilitate the process by allowing multiple submissions until a successful conclusion was reached. Some cynics claimed that this was to boost their memberships and coffers! They could have been right. The fees in 2020 were £100 for each of the 13 domains, £250 for the evaluation panel. Despite the cost, GPs gaining MRCGP through MAP had a warm feeling of gratification, some using the qualification to further a career in academia or medical research.

MAP was discontinued in 2021, replaced by the awarding of MRCGP to any GP who had successfully been revalidated to practice following five annual appraisals. At a stroke, all GPs now had the qualification!

8.13 CONTINUING PROFESSIONAL DEVELOPMENT

Heartening as it was to see grizzled old GPs submitting themselves to taking any exam, the MRCGP examination was never intended to be the endpoint of GP learning. The rough diamond needed further shaping and polishing. The lapidarist would take the form of continuing professional development and its able assistant, reflective learning.

Historically, GPs could devote as little or as much time as they wished to acquiring knowledge within their chosen field. Like contented catfish in a swamp, their views were somewhat murky. Many felt that general practice was an ideal environment for

---

[61] RCGP. MRCGP annual reports and research. 2018. Accessed 4 Oct 2018 from www.rcgp.org.uk/training-exams/mrcgp-exams-overview/mrcgp-annual-reports.aspx

[62] www.rcgp.org.uk/training-exams/practice/membership-by-assessment-of-performance-map-the-route-to-rcgp-membership-for-established-gps.aspxwityh

experiential learning, where day-to-day medical encounters were layered upon one another to provide an incremental gain in overall knowledge, skills, performance, and confidence. As such, they eschewed the need for any formal education.

Most GPs grazed the weekly periodicals such as *Pulse*, *GP*, and *Doctor* and occasionally dipped their intellectual toes into more scholarly journals such as the *BMJ* or *BJGP*. They attended 'educational' meetings and symposia organised by the pharmaceutical industry, the latter often held in high-end restaurants or abroad, with all expenses paid. All was not unbridled hedonism; the industry also sponsored medical meetings in local postgraduate centres that tended to be more responsive to locality needs and fostered closer cooperation between primary and secondary care. Indeed, the drug industry at that time was the foremost sponsor of postgraduate medical education. The topics covered at these meetings were often repetitive, responding to whatever class of drugs was in fashion at the time. Of course, many GPs, unbidden, sought an independent path to continued professional learning. Over time, some of these went on to set up the RCGP and its educational publication, the *British Journal of General Practice*.

To encourage doctors to maintain their knowledge, the DH introduced the Postgraduate Education Allowance (PGEA) in the GP contract of 1990. The PGEA was highly prescriptive regarding the areas in which GPs needed educating. These were grouped under three domains: health promotion and illness prevention, disease management, and service management. Recycled money already paid to GPs was used to reimburse them for attending. The full allowance could only be claimed for attendance at a minimum 25 days of accredited postgraduate education spread over five years.

As with many DH initiatives, GPs soon learned to game the system. Pharmaceutical companies continued providing sponsorship for courses that they devised for their marketing needs. The criteria for accreditation were minimal, described in a letter to the *BMJ* as having a 'never mind the quality, just feel the width' philosophy.[63] In response, the education establishment seized the responsibility for course accreditation, which now had be approved by a Director for Postgraduate Medical Education, Regional Advisor, and GP tutor. By the early millennium, industry sponsorship, once a raging river, through a combination of rigorous self-regulation and GP apathy, had dried to a trickle.

The introduction of GP revalidation finally put the stake through the heart of GP indolence by making CPD an integral and mandatory part of appraisal, revalidation, and ultimately relicensing. GPs were required to provide evidence, with reflection, of learning, of 250 hours over five years. Reflection spawned an industry of its own. A scribbled note was replaced by the 'reflective template,'[64] a bureaucratic, cumbersome beast that negated all the learning on which it was applied.

---

[63] Bahrami J. Postgraduate education for general practitioners. Centrally funded scheme would not necessarily be better. BMJ. 1997 Dec 6;315(7121):1543. PMID: 9420516; PMCID: PMC2127940.

[64] www.aomrc.org.uk/wp-content/uploads/2016/06/Reflective_template_for_revalidation_0312-2.pdf

Title and description of activity or event

- Dates of activities or events.
- Which category of activity does this match?
- General information about your practice.
- Keeping up to date.
- Review of your practice, for example, quality improvement, significant event.
- Feedback on your practice, for example, patient/carer/colleague feedback, complaints, compliments.

What have you learned?

- Describe how this activity contributed to the development of your knowledge, skills or professional behaviours.
- You may wish to link this learning to one or more of the GMC *Good Medical Practice* domains to demonstrate compliance with their principles and values.
- Knowledge, skills and performance.
- Safety and quality.
- Communication, partnership and teamwork.
- Maintaining trust.

How has this influenced your practice?

- How have your knowledge skills and professional behaviours changed?
- Have you identified any skills and knowledge gaps relating to your professional practice?
- What changes to your professional behaviour were identified as desirable?
- How will this activity or event lead to improvements in patient care or safety?
- How will your current practice change as a result?
- What aspects of your current practice were reinforced?
- What changes in your team/department/organisation's working were identified as necessary?

Looking forward, what are your next steps?

- Outline any further learning or development needs identified (individual team/organisation, as needed).
- If further learning and development needs have been identified, how do you intend to address these?
- Set SMART objectives for these (Specific, Measurable, Achievable, Relevant and Time-bound).
- If changes in professional practice (individual or team/department) have been identified as necessary, how do you intend to address these?

Figure 8.2 Generic reflective template, 2008.

The formal reflective template was excessively time-consuming with little practical utility. It was also pointless since doctors opted for a file and forget philosophy. By 2017, such elaborate record-keeping was finally recognised as a disincentive to further learning. The generic template[65] was whittled down to:

Learning objectives
- Were my objectives met?
- What I learned
- Was this the most effective way to learn this for me?
- How could it have been improved?
- How does this fit in with what I already know?
  - How might I use this?
  - Record change in practice related to a specific, anonymised, patient
- Areas needing further study/follow-up
- Was information disseminated to colleagues?
- Time taken
- Reflection time

This was hardly better, and many appraisers chose to ignore it altogether, reverting to trusting the word of the appraisee on such matters.

The original PGEA payments were subsumed into the overall practice budget in the GMS contract of 2004, thus removing any direct financial incentive to encourage continuing education. Since learning has been rolled up into the revalidation and relicensing process, GPs now do so for purely altruistic motives, giving no thought to the threat of having their licence to practice and, thus, their livelihood removed for non-compliance. Such coercive considerations could be argued to be marginally less ethically dubious than those of financial gain.

Older GPs continued to baulk at the idea of recorded learning. Acceptance was higher in the younger generation of doctors that had passed through their medical education imbued with the ethos of written reflective learning. Both cohorts were united in recognising that the vast majority of their learning took place in their primary service activity, the consultation.

8.14 SUMMARY

For half of the current lifetime of the NHS, any medical graduate could become a GP without further formal training. Theoretically, a registered doctor could enter general practice at the age of 24 years and practice for the next 50 years without ever setting eyes on another medical text. General practice had long been considered an apprenticeship, a role where one learned on the job and where knowledge was honed by the thousands of consultations that took place each year. The opportunity to learn was inherent in the very fabric of the job. There are no data to suggest that such experiential learning harmed patients or that doctors of the time were any less able than those that followed them.

---

[65] www.gpappraisals.uk/reflection.html

Despite the ease of entry to the profession, there was little resistance from incumbents to the introduction of formal postgraduate training to qualify for independent practice as a GP. At the very least, such training provided the young with the basic tools to practice and the time to mature in age, experience, and insight as they sought to better navigate the multifarious nature of the role. Vocational training schemes were introduced in the 1960s; the format, two years in hospital and one year in general practice, remained largely unchanged to the present day. The schemes were initially voluntary, formative in nature before becoming more widespread, and eventually, in 1980, summative and mandatory for licensing as a GP. The endpoint of training moved from a certificate of completion, a roll call of attendance, to competence, a formal assessment of learning and skills. Eventually, after years of lobbying by the Royal College of General Practitioners, the MRCGP exam was adopted.

Did the MRCGP make for a better general practitioner? The answer is hard to come by since all GPs adhere to the GMC's guidance, Good Medical Practice, on 'what it means to be a good doctor.'[66] There have been no quantifiable studies to suggest that doctors with MRCGP, now the vast majority in primary care, outperform those without. The same can also be said for the views of their customers, patients, who neither know nor care whether their family physician has the qualification or not.

Did the MRCGP improve the GP's status, the way their hospital specialist colleagues regarded them? The original debate on the introduction of the MRCGP had alluded to the exam as a means of achieving parity in status for the RCGP and the historically august colleges of physicians and surgeons. Whilst that mutual respect may have been achieved for the college, it has not for its members. Any request for admission of a patient was still likely to be greeted with contempt by a junior hospital doctor. The discharge letter on that same patient was still likely to contain a throwaway line deriding the GP's performance.

Training in hospital-based disciplines has traditionally been based on the triple pillars of 'see one, do one, teach one.' These luxuries were not afforded to a doctor in the community. GPs work in isolation with little opportunity or inclination to learn from their colleagues. The intensity of the working week simply does not allow for one doctor to sit in on another's surgery. GPs have to be self-motivated to learn on the job. The fact that they manage to do so in a challenging environment, with generally beneficial outcomes for their patients, is to be commended. Nevertheless, the structure of the vocational training scheme and MRCGP, with its continuous assessment of recorded evidence, have prepared a later generation of GPs for a lifetime of learning and, inadvertently, annual appraisal.

Is there still a need for the trained GP in primary care? The patients presenting at healthcare centres are increasingly managed by ancillary healthcare professionals who have not undergone the years of rigorous education and training required to become a GP. Again, there is no evidence that the morbidity or mortality of the British population has been detrimentally impacted by this move away from the traditional, doctor-centric model. Thus, provocatively, one could argue that GPs are grossly overeducated for their role in primary care, in which case all that has been written in this chapter will become of historic interest only!

---

[66] www.gmc-uk.org/ethical-guidance/ethical-guidance-for-doctors/good-medical-practice

9

Scrutiny and Regulation

There is no witness so terrible and no accuser so powerful as conscience which dwells within us.

(Sophocles)

9.1 INTRODUCTION

All medical practitioners in the UK are registered with and regulated by the General Medical Council. For most of those doctors, the only contact with their regulating body would be the invoice for the annual registration fee. For a tiny minority, the envelope on the doormat might be of more concern than the size of that fee. The only time that the GMC takes on a face is when doubts arise regarding a doctor's suitability to practice medicine. Such cases are relatively few. In 2018, the GMC felt the need to investigate 1,544[1] out of a total of over 200,000 licenced practitioners.

The GMC attempts to minimise complaints by producing a guide to good practice, pithily titled *Good Medical Practice*, which comprehensively details the parameters for a doctor's behaviour and duties. Details of the history and function of the GMC have been set out in other chapters, and reference to its role in this chapter is limited to that of medical regulator.

Scrutiny of a doctor's performance in primary care is a relatively recent phenomenon. For the first half-century of the NHS, GPs operated with minimal accountability. The administration in place during those decades dealt primarily with overseeing payments for services rendered under the GMS/PMS contracts. GPs had almost total autonomy on how they delivered those services. Had that situation remained unchanged, this would have been a very short chapter indeed! However, and many doctors bemoan the fact, this elysian period of primary care eventually did change. Present-day GPs perceive that every action they take, from entering the surgery in the morning to locking up at night, and for many even outside those hours, is forensically monitored, to a level where they fear the

---

[1] GMC annual report 2018. https://investor.gm.com/static-files/9a63b43f-17c3-47a0-8148-9527a2da1cb3?msclkid=bdf1d38baabc11ec88ef4e335a543b13

DOI: 10.1201/9781003256465-9

dreaded midnight knock on the door becoming a reality. Arguably, scrutiny in all its myriad forms has led to the biggest fall in morale amongst doctors since the inception of the NHS as a public service.

In retrospect, the origins of this intrusive examination of GP performance began with a benign and laudable suggestion, GP appraisal.

Embryonic notions that doctors should have some kind of appraisal process were first mooted in the 1980s, during a time when the thrust of government thinking was towards promoting greater efficiency in the public arena, through the adoption of more accountable working practices from the private sector. Efficiency came about through improved productivity that could only be gauged through regular reviews. With the introduction of other elements of commercial working practice at that time, such as the purchaser/provider split, a system of annual review or appraisal seemed logical.

However, certain fundamental aspects of the employee appraisal process in the business sector had been misunderstood. Not the least of these was that such appraisals encompassed a performance review and setting of targets for the following year, which could be both robustly assessed and rewarded. It was especially the 'reward' element that doctor appraisal would be missing, leaving the participants with a sense of disenfranchisement that took many years to overcome. However, the implementation of any form of appraisal remained in a nascent stage until the turn of the century.

No one, especially patients, ever agonised over a GP's overall knowledge or performance for the first 50 years of the NHS's existence. No one. And that situation may well have lasted to the present day, had it not been for one GP, Harold Shipman.

9.2 SHIPMAN

Harold Shipman (1946–2004) began practice as a jobbing GP in the suburbs of Manchester in 1977. He initially joined a group practice but left in 1993, to set up as a single-handed practitioner. It will never be known for certain, since he never revealed the motives for what subsequently took place, but one theory was that he became psychotically delusional regarding a doctors' duty to relieve suffering. Palliative care segued into murder. Assisted dying, a subject barely raised before, became conflated with murder. Before Shipman, doctors felt duty-bound to help their patients by every means possible, including the liberal use of diamorphine in painful, terminal conditions such as cancer. After Shipman, no doctor dared to act in such a way. The review of the medical records after Shipman's arrest in 1998 revealed that he may have committed over 250 murders, most in patients without life-limiting conditions, who had placed their total trust in him as their 'caring' GP. He was arrested in 1998, tried and found guilty in 2000, and hanged himself in prison in 2004. The case highlighted an extraordinary criminal and moral dereliction of duty by a doctor, both shocking the nation and resulting in much soul-searching in the medical community and government. Answers as to how such a horror could occur in a civilised society were sought through a governmental inquiry in 2000, chaired by Dame Janet Smith.[2] Her inquiry produced its sixth and final report five years later. Within it were several recommendations covering the medical profession. These included:

1. Better training for coroners
2. Revision of the documentation needed for cremation
3. More robust controls on the use of controlled drugs by doctors and pharmacists
4. Closer scrutiny of prescribing data from individual doctors
5. Routine practice mortality monitoring
6. Simplification of complaints procedure
7. A lambasting for the GMC and recommendation that it reform its surveillance of doctors
8. Introduction of checks on qualifications, professional history, and police record of candidates applying for a position in general practice
9. Introduction of GP appraisal, revalidation, and relicensing
10. New powers to enable PCTs (at that time) to suspend or remove a GP from a local performer's list

The narrative report confirmed that Shipman was a devious and unscrupulous character who used his professional standing and plausible caring manner to conceal the traces of his criminal actions. Nevertheless, the inquiry found that he did let his guard slip on several occasions, leaving clues that could and should have been picked up at an earlier stage; two of Shipman's professional colleagues had noticed his inappropriate use of diamorphine but failed to report their concerns. Other people, including a colleague in a neighbouring general practice who countersigned his cremation certificates, eventually noticed the unusually high number of deaths among his patients but the police disregarded their concerns. Only when Shipman forged the will of one of his victims was serious action taken to unmask his activities.

In summary, Shipman was the tragic product of the prevailing mores regarding the medical profession; hubris and absolute autonomy in the doctor, unquestioned respect and trust from the public.

The Smith inquiry concluded that had stronger safeguards had been in place, Shipman might have been deterred from his criminal career or, at the very least, his crimes would have been detected earlier.

During the running of the inquiry and pre-empting its findings, the GMC had independently produced a proposal for the annual appraisal and revalidation of all doctors. Sadly, despite its attempt at appearing proactive, it was excoriated for its efforts, told to beef up its tepid suggestions for appraisal, and introduce mandatory periodic relicensing to practice as the endpoint of a robust revalidation process. These admonitions were made despite the sentiment within the profession that they were unlikely to prevent a repeat of a Harold Shipman in the future.

---

[2] Dame Janet later went on to chair the BBC investigation on the sexual abuse of children. The Shipman Inquiry Report(s) 2002–2005. https://webarchive.nationalarchives.gov.uk/20090808155114/www.the-shipman-inquiry.org.uk/backgroundinfo.asp

Whether the Smith enquiry was the catalyst for tighter GP scrutiny, or the profession was already evolving in that direction was debatable. Either way, the new millennium heralded the end of the cosy bubble of immunity in which GPs had become so used to working.

Prior to the introduction of mandatory GP appraisal and revalidation, the only scrutiny general practitioners faced was financial. The structure of GP payments was based on the submission of an annual report of work done, in effect an invoice, to a primary care organisation. In theory, evidence of that work, especially covering items of service fees, was required to justify claims. In practice, the details were flimsy. Both parties to the contract trusted each other. That cosy relationship changed after the Shipman enquiry.

The DH and the medical profession proceeded to publish a torrent of policy documents to demonstrate how the profession could raise standards and, more importantly, police itself. The first to see the light of day (1998) was the garrulously titled, 'A First-Class Service. Quality in The New NHS, clinical governance set up and promotion of lifelong learning and CPD,' followed quickly by the more modest, 'Supporting Doctors, Protecting Patients.' Both documents concluded that appraisal and revalidation should be compulsory for any doctor wishing to practice medicine in the UK. The following decade saw further publications from various stakeholders:

'Assuring the Quality of Medical Appraisal,'[3] 2005. Produced descriptors of Good Medical Practice.
'Good Doctors—Safer Patients,'[4] 2006. Contained proposals to strengthen the regulatory system, to assure and improve the performance of doctors and protect the safety of patients.
'Good Medical Practice,'[5] 2006. GMC updated contents to include appraisal and revalidation.
'Good Medical Practice for GPs,'[6] 2008, RCGP document updated to reflect revalidation needs of GPs.
'Principles of Appraisal,'[7] 2008. RCGP document set out policy and principles of appraisal.
'Assuring the Quality of Medical Appraisal for Revalidation,'[8] 2009. NHS Revalidation Support Team document set out a quality framework for organisations providing appraisals.

In 2002, annual appraisal became a contractual obligation for any registered GP.

---

[3] www.kingsfund.org.uk/sites/default/files/field/field_publication_file/medical-validation-vijaya-nath-mar14.pdf
[4] Chief Medical Officer. *Good Doctors, Safer Patients.* London: Department of Health, 2006.
[5] www.ub.edu/medicina_unitateducaciomedica/documentos/Good_Medical_Practice.pdf
[6] RCGP. *Good Medical Practice for General Practitioners.* London: GCP, 2008.
[7] RCGP. *Principles of GP Appraisal.* London: GCP, 2008.
[8] NHS Revalidation Support Team. *Assuring the Quality of Appraisal for Revalidation.* London: NHS, 2009.

9.3 GP APPRAISAL AND REVALIDATION

At first, GP appraisal was largely left to its own devices. Unusually, PCTs left the running of the process to their constituent doctors. Appraisers were recruited and trained locally and paid differing rates across the UK. This eclectic system remained in place until 2014 when the administrative structure was unified following a further publication, 'Medical Appraisal Guide,'[9] produced by the NHS Revalidation Team. NHS England and NHS Improvement took overall control of the administration of the process, and a national rate of £500 was set for each appraisal a GP appraiser undertook.

Despite the numerous sources on the subject, the purpose of medical appraisal and process remained somewhat imprecise. The choices included:

- Appraisal is a process of facilitated self-review supported by information gathered from the full scope of the doctor's work.[10]
- 'Appraisal for GPs is a professional process of constructive dialogue, in which the doctor being appraised has a formal structured opportunity to reflect on his or her work and to consider how his or her effectiveness might be improved.'[11]
- A medical appraisal is a process of facilitated self-review supported by information gathered from the full scope of your work. The annual appraisal and supporting evidence are key to demonstrating your GMC fitness to practise whatever your branch of practice.[12]

What appraisal was not supposed to be was:

- *'Just a paper exercise with forms to fill in.'* Appraisal requires appropriate time, resources and support. If these are not available, then it is likely to be ineffective.
- *Synonymous with assessment.* The latter can be defined as 'measurement of an individual's performance at a particular point in time, usually against predetermined standards.'[13]

Regrettably, despite these avowed aims, many front-line doctors viewed appraisals as a time-consuming, box-ticking, mildly threatening exercise.

The content of a GP appraisal covered six domains, defined by the GMC booklet *Good Medical Practice and the Practice Framework for Appraisal and Revalidation.* These included:

---

9 www.england.nhs.uk/revalidation/wp-content/uploads/sites/10/2014/02/rst-medical-app-guide-2013.pdf

10 NHS England. www.england.nhs.uk/medical-revalidation/appraisers/med-app/

11 Department of Health. www.mysurgerywebsite.co.uk/website/IGP367/files/GP%20Appraisal%20Guidance.pdf

12 BMA.

13 Revalidation: prepare now and get it right ruth chambers, Gill Wakley, Alison Magnall. ASIN: B01I155D7A

- *Continuing Professional Development* (CPD). A minimum 50 hours per annum, 250 over five years of education learning using a variety of learning methods: reading, seminars and meetings, online teaching modules and PUNs/DENs (Patient Unmet Needs/Doctor Educational Needs).
- *Quality Improvement Activity* (QIA). Originally specified as a formal clinical audit to be undertaken once during the five-year revalidation cycle, it has since been expanded to include reflective case reviews, review of personal outcome data, small-scale data searches, feedback from any source, learning from continuing professional development, writing or revising practice policy, and monitoring and evaluation of patients on long-term therapies.
- *Significant Events* (SE). Defined as an unintended, unexpected event that may have led or did lead to harm in a patient. The intent was that the doctor should learn from such events, ensuring that they did not recur. Two SEs had to be submitted each year unless none had occurred. It was hard to imagine that any active medical practitioner would pass through a whole year without committing any errors; nevertheless, annual appraisals rarely seemed to include any! Learning events, similar in origin but not harmful in outcome, were added in later years.
- *Feedback from colleagues.* A multi-source questionnaire, completed by colleagues and any member of staff, once in every five-year revalidation cycle. The criteria required a minimum of 15 respondents. Feedback toolkits included benchmarking individual areas of feedback against the local and national norms.
- *Feedback from patients.* A questionnaire, undertaken once in every five-year revalidation cycle from, ideally, 30 consecutive patients seen in clinic. Feedback toolkits include benchmarking individual areas of feedback against the local and national norms.
- *Review of complaints and compliments.* Discussion regarding the former was often welcome by an appraisee. The latter was often ignored.

Evidence, including notes on reflection, had to be submitted for all of the above domains.

The various bodies (NHS England, GMC, RCGP) also advised that the appraisee should:

- Be fully engaged with the process
- Prepare his or her supporting evidence throughout each year
- Book a date for the appraisal with the Local Area Team; some areas allowed choice of appraiser
- Complete the pre-appraisal documents, generally an online toolkit, for presentation to the appraiser at least two weeks prior to the date of appraisal
- Allocate some dedicated time in a 'safe' environment with access to computer, practice, and patient records
- Formulate a personal development plan for the coming year according to SMART principles, i.e. short, punchy, and relevant
- Agree with and sign off on final outcomes report from the appraisal

The acronym 'SMART' became a part of the vernacular, along with 'revalidation' ('what exactly is the difference between revalidation and relicensing?') and 'reflection' (was this not synonymous with everyday 'thinking and worrying'?) of elitist educators driving appraisal to intellectually intimidate the jobbing majority. The concept of SMART had originated in an article in a rather obscure publication, *Management Review*,[14] in 1981, as a means by which management could set out goals and objectives for an employee. It was popularised by Peter Drucker (1909–2005), an Austrian-American business guru considered by many as the godfather of modern management theory.

The acronym stood for the following:

S – specific   Specific tasks and activities; not general statements
M – measurable Can be easily assessed
A – attainable   Should be possible for that individual to achieve
R – realistic   Within the individual's capabilities
T – timed   Within a realistic timeframe of achievement or re-assessment

Later it was joined by E, evaluate and R, revise to become SMARTER.

Front-line GPs were confused by these terms and the need to apply them to their personal development plans (PDPs). Indeed, most could not differentiate between a PDP and a CPD; the work for both overlapped. They also baulked at the need to provide evidence of reflection on every item included in their appraisal submission. Doctors felt that reflection was synonymous with the innate cognitive process that followed every action undertaken during a working day. They had no issues with the need to reflect, only the structuring and documentation of that reflection. To assist them with the latter concern, NHS England recommended a structured reflective template,[15] based on a conference of the National Association of Primary Care, NAPC, held in Leicester in 2007.[16] The same meeting included some helpful advice regarding the standard reflective template (SRTs);[17] use it contemporaneously, be true to yourself and be honest in your comments. After all, the SRT was purely an aid to learning!

However, their advice did not address the main concern of doctors undergoing appraisal; they simply did not see the point. That sentiment was particularly true for long-established GPs who viewed the whole exercise as demeaning and a waste of time that should be spent treating patients.

Despite antipathy to the process, all licenced GPs had to engage in the process of annual appraisal. Recorded evidence initially used a paper-based format, the

---

[14] Drucker P. *The Practice of Management*. New York: Harper, 1954; Heinemann, London, 1955; revised edn, Butterworth-Heinemann, 2007.

[15] www.england.nhs.uk/south/wp-content/uploads/sites/6/2017/07/cpd-structured-reflective-template.pdf

[16] www.nesg.org.uk/nesg-web/docs/filef5ed5cec59b5f498c2d71e2f41263a9b.pdf

[17] www.nesg.org.uk/nesg-web/docs/filef5ed5cec59b5f498c2d71e2f41263a9b.pdf

Medical Appraisal Guide Model Appraisal Form (MAG form),[18] that had been developed the NHS Revalidation Support Team, but this was rapidly replaced by online applications, Clarity,[19] FourteenFish,[20] GPTools.[21] The RCGP developed its own cumbersome form that proved wildly unpopular and was quickly 'merged' with Clarity.[22] MAG was free; fees for the commercial providers reasonable. Overall, the electronic formats provided a more structured offering with all the data and evidence stored on one site, allowing easy access by both appraisee and appraiser.

Regardless of format, each appraisal had to conclude with a statement that:

- An appraisal had taken place that reflected the whole of a doctor's scope of work and addressed the principles and values set out in Good Medical Practice.
- Appropriate supporting information had been presented in accordance with the Good Medical Practice Framework for Appraisal and Revalidation, and this reflected the nature and scope of the doctor's work.
- A review that demonstrates appropriate progress against last year's PDP had occurred.
- An agreement had been reached with the doctor about a new PDP and any associated actions for the coming year.
- No information had been presented or discussed in the appraisal that raised a concern about the doctor's fitness to practise.

Whether the above statements could be made with a clear conscience depended not only on the appraisee's honesty in engaging in the process but also on the appraiser's interpretation of the appraisal discussion. There was a significant subjective element in what should have been an entirely objective exercise. Some appraisers applied the rules less zealously than others!

The appraisee had the right to withdraw consent for including any specific items within the report in the final draft for submission, although the appraiser's report had to note their doing so.

Both appraisee and appraiser had to sign off on the final document before its submission to the local PCT appraisal team or, after 2012, to the regional Responsible Officer (RO) based in the Local Area Team (LAT) of NHS England. The document was confidential, available only to the appraisee and RO. Specifically, it was not accessible to the DH or GMC. The RO was responsible for reviewing the five years of appraisals before submitting their recommendation to the GMC as to whether the doctor was eligible for revalidation. The GMC invariably accepted the recommendation of the RO, thereafter confirming revalidation and relicensing to continue practising as a GP.

---

[18] www.england.nhs.uk/medical-revalidation/appraisers/mag-mod/

[19] https://clarity.co.uk/products/clarity-appraisals/appraisals-for-doctors/

[20] https: //www.fourteenfish.com/

[21] www.gptools.org/

[22] https://clarity.co.uk/products/clarity-appraisals/appraisals-for-doctors/

From the beginning, the DH recognised that GPs would more likely engage in the process of appraisal if they were financially compensated to do so. The appraisee GP principal was subsidised for the time taken at a rate equivalent to three clinical sessions. A rate of £500 applied to GP principals, £300 to GP locum and sessional doctors. Scotland did not reimburse non-principals.

Salaried GPs were not required to financially contribute to be appraised. Funding for appraisal for salaried GPs employed by a GMS practice was via an appraisal premium, included in the practice's global sum. Comparable arrangements were also instituted for PMS practices. Funding for appraising PCO-employed GPs and freelance GPs was via the employer.

Additional criteria introduced as of 2015 required that the ratio of appraisers to doctors in any region should be no less than 1:20 or more than 1:5, with each appraiser undertaking between 5 and 20 appraisals a year, to maintain an appropriate level of quality and consistency. These characteristics, quality and consistency, were benchmarked on guidance provided by the NHS Revalidation Support Team (RST) document 'Quality Assurance of Medical Appraisers.'[23] In practice, they were applied by an appraisal lead, elected from their own, through three-yearly appraisals of appraisers, during which a sample of appraisal reports would be reviewed. The whole exercise, as with GP appraisals, was non-threatening and lacking in censure.

Initially, GPs had the freedom to choose their appraiser, allowing the selection of a colleague whose views on general practice were most attuned to their own. Acknowledging the issues arising from fraternisation, the freedom of choice was removed in 2015, and the appraiser was allocated from a centralised Revalidation Management System.[24] In addition, individual appraisals with the same appraiser could not take place for more than three consecutive years.

How do GPs honestly view appraisal and revalidation? Remarkably little research exists on the subject. A paper published in the journal *Medical Education* in 2003,[25] the first year of mandatory GP appraisal, pointed towards an overall positive view.

Of the 343 GPs sent questionnaires, 272 (79%) replied. Lincolnshire GPs had more positive attitudes towards appraisal than towards revalidation. They welcomed appraisal provided that it had local ownership and took into account their views and concerns on the process. Other factors that correlated with a positive attitude towards appraisal included agreement that the purpose of appraisal is educational and that it should result in an agreed development plan.

[23] www.england.nhs.uk/medical-revalidation/appraisers/qa-guidance-notes/

[24] www.england.nhs.uk/contact-us/privacy-notice/how-we-use-your-information/health-care-professionals/medical-revalidation/

[25] Middlemass J, Siriwardena AN. General practitioners, revalidation and appraisal: a cross sectional survey of attitudes, beliefs and concerns in Lincolnshire. Med Educ. 2003 Sep;37(9):778–85. doi: 10.1046/j.1365-2923.2003.01469.x. PMID: 12950940.

The paper highlighted time involved and lack of resources as the two main concerns of appraisees.[26] Further surveys over the years broadly concurred with these early findings.[27-29]

In 2018/2019, the NHSE/NHS Improvement Survey on medical appraisal,[30] with 13,440 respondents, noted that the majority perceived appraisal as beneficial in improving patient care (88%), promoting quality improvement (91%), promoting personal development (92%), and promoting professional development (92%). The survey, a snapshot of an individual appraisal rather than the process, also reported that 97% of appraisees were happy with the skills of their appraiser. Appraisees welcomed the opportunity to discuss their work and particularly their concerns in a convivial atmosphere with a sympathetic colleague, an opportunity absent during their normal working week. Appraisals gave them the chance to blow off some steam.

The RCGP, ever mindful of any negative comments, set out in 2017 to address concerns regarding appraisal and revalidation in a document, 'RCGP MythBusters,' which addressed any misunderstandings over the evidence required from the appraisee.[31] The text applied a timely brake to the activities of the more fanatical appraisers!

However, appraisals were only a link in the chain towards revalidation and relicensing. Revalidation could not take place without annual appraisal. Relicensing could not take place without revalidation.

9.4 REVALIDATION AND RELICENSING

As of December 2012, every medical practitioner in the UK had to obtain a licence to practice as a clinician. The GMC definition of a licence to practice covered the doctor/patient interaction and, specifically, the authorisation of a prescription and death certificate. Confusion reigned regarding the considerable overlap between the term's 'revalidation' and 'relicensing.' Indeed, despite clarification by the appropriate regulatory bodies, there was no difference. Essentially, one automatically arose from the other.

26 www.ncbi.nlm.nih.gov/pubmed/12950940
27 Colthart I, Cameron N, McKinstry B, Blaney D. What do doctors really think about the relevance and impact of GP appraisal 3 years on? A survey of Scottish GPs. Br J Gen Pract. 2008 Feb;58(547):82–7. doi: 10.3399/bjgp08X264036. PMID: 18307850; PMCID: PMC2233956.
28 Finlay K, McLaren S. Does appraisal enhance learning, improve practice and encourage continuing professional development? A survey of general practitioners' experiences of appraisal. Qual Prim Care. 2009;17(6):387–95. PMID: 20051189.
29 Scallan S, Locke R, Eksteen D, Caesar S. The benefits of appraisal: a critical (re)view of the literature. Educ Prim Care. 2016 Mar;27(2):94–7. doi: 10.1080/14739879.2016.1142772. Epub 2016 Feb 25. PMID: 26915657.
30 www.england.nhs.uk/wp-content/uploads/2019/07/medical-appraisal-feedback-from-gps-18-19-v1.1.pdf
31 https://elearning.rcgp.org.uk/file.php/1/RCGP-mythbusters-dec-2017.pdf

Doctors working in diverse, non-clinical settings, such as pharmaceuticals research, occupational health,[32] general management, and finance, were initially instructed that they also required annual appraisals, to comply with revalidation despite not needing a licence to practice. After an initial panic, each sector developed a process aligned to that in primary care, with their own designated body and Responsible Officer.

Fears regarding revalidation were quickly allayed, once the first cohort of appraisees had passed through the process. The pivotal role of the Responsible Officer remained a somewhat nebulous one to most practising doctors, who were seamlessly relicensed with minimal disruption to their daily lives. Should the RO reserve judgement on revalidation, the doctor was informed of the grounds for the decision and allowed a period of grace, a deferral, to address any shortcomings. On occasion, the RO had no option but to inform the GMC that the doctor had not engaged in the appraisal process, in which case, by definition, the doctor could not be revalidated.

The GMC rarely rejected the RO's recommendation. Rejection occurred where the GMC was confidentially privy to third party information, highlighting concerns regarding that doctor's performance. In such cases, the GMC would defer revalidation and the issuing of a licence until the issues had been satisfactorily resolved. In the year 2018, the GMC revalidated 40,808 doctors, from both primary and secondary care; an additional 7,169 doctors had their revalidation temporarily deferred and 103 were suspended for non-engagement with the process.[33]

There are no definitive figures for the financial cost to the NHS of annual appraisal. A back of the envelope calculation based on the fee of £500 paid to the GP appraiser and around 50,000 licenced GPs would add up to a minimum of £50 million per annum; a not inconsiderable sum for reassuring the public that their doctor was both competent and in good standing with the regulatory body. Its success in this aim has never been tested.

9.5 QUALITY OUTCOMES FRAMEWORK (QOF)

Clinical scrutiny merged with financial, following the introduction of performance-based targets, such as those for chronic disease management and minor operations in the 1980s. Payments for these initiatives were subject to the provision of detailed reports on each clinic.

This situation remained in place until the GMS GP contract of 2004, following which several regulatory bodies introduced means, and metrics to raise standards, improve the patient experience, and disseminate best practice. An early entrant was the Trojan horse of Quality Outcomes Framework (QOF) innocently welcomed by a profession unaware that behind the gift lay the might of Agamemnon's army, a revitalised PCT.

QOF, an innovative element of the GMS contract of 2004, heralded a step change in performance review, one that also carried a significant financial

---

[32] www.som.org.uk/qaas-appraisal-scheme#

[33] www.gmc-uk.org/-/media/documents/annual-report-2018-english_pdf-80413921.pdf

incentive. However, it could never have been implemented without the rapid development and uptake of robust GP IT systems that had occurred in the previous decade. The software allowed easier data input with cross-referencing and remote data capture. The data provided regulators and PCTs with the means to calculate progress against targets and ensuing payments. Since QOF contributed significantly to practice income, ensuring that targets were met became an imperative rather than a luxury. Practices set to with gusto, with the vast majority of UK practices achieving 950 of the available 1,050 points in the first year of QOF implementation.

QOF points generated a payment of around £77.50 per point per annum and, as such, contributed a not-insignificant amount to the practice income. Rapid data acquisition and analysis also had unanticipated consequence, allowing targets to toughened up. Nevertheless, over the following years, the number of points were rationalised and reduced, compensated by the increase in payment per point to £124.60. Chapter 12, 'Finance,' covers further details regarding QOF payments.

Although largely automated, gathering data for QOF required an obsessive, compulsive mindset, frequent internal reviews, and extra staff. It was also a distraction during the average consultation. Most practices designated a partner as QOF lead, to coordinate all these activities. After the initial golden years when GP remuneration increased dramatically through the fulfilment of QOF targets, a universal irritation with the whole process began to set in. Subjects and sections seemed to be arbitrarily added or removed on an annual basis, with minimal, if any consultation with those trying to meet them. All the extra activity appeared to have minimal impact on improving the health of the nation.

A study published in the *Lancet* in 2016, looking into mortality levels between 1994 and 2010, for cancer, ischaemic heart disease, and non-targeted conditions, compared to other similar countries without payment by performance schemes, showed no significant benefits.[34] A systematic review of the literature, published in the *BJGP* in 2017,[35] came to the same conclusion:

> This systematic review found no convincing evidence that the QOF can promote better integrated care, personalised, holistic care, or self-care, or, indeed, improve any other outcomes in people with long-term conditions.

Faceless bureaucrats seemed to dictate to clinicians where they should focus their limited resources. The freeze on GP income had long since absorbed the extra

[34] Ryan AM, Krinsky S, Kontopantelis E, Doran T. Long-term evidence for the effect of pay-for-performance in primary care on mortality in the UK: a population study. Lancet. 2016 Jul 16;388(10041):268–74. doi: 10.1016/S0140-6736(16)00276-2. Epub 2016 May 17. PMID: 27207746.

[35] Forbes LJ, Marchand C, Doran T, Peckham S. The role of the quality and outcomes framework in the care of long-term conditions: a systematic review. Br J Gen Pract. 2017 Nov;67(664):e775–e784. doi: 10.3399/bjgp17X693077. Epub 2017 Sep 25. PMID: 28947621; PMCID: PMC5647921.

income QOF generated in the years following its introduction. GPs became disillusioned with the whole process. To its credit, the DH eventually responded to these concerns. Consultation with front-line stakeholders led to a reduction in the number of domains within QOF to reflect more rational clinical care. In the guidance 'General Medical Services (GMS) Contract QOF' (April 2019),[36] 175 points (31%) of the 559 points in operation at that time were 'retired' and recycled into 101 points of clinically appropriate indicators[37] and 74 points of newly created Quality Improvement Modules, covering prescribing safety and end-of-life care. Whether the changes addressed the failings raised in the *BJGP* article two years previously remained to be seen.

9.6 CARE QUALITY COMMISSION CQC

The CQC was set up in 2009 as a Quango,[38] an executive, non-departmental part of the DH, to monitor standards across the health and social care sectors. It replaced and absorbed the three bodies that had preceded it in this function: the Healthcare Commission, the Commission for Social Care Inspection, and the Mental Health Act Commission.

The CQC's remit was to ensure that hospitals, care homes, dental and GP surgeries, and all health and social care providers in England and Wales provided safe, effective, compassionate, and high-quality care.

The CQC initially received the usual cynical suspicion with which the profession greeted every government initiative. The sentiment was not improved when the body began carrying out its inspections It rapidly became apparent that the CQC inspectors were not only interested in the practice premises and processes but also sought to intrude on clinical practice covering safety, significant events, care of vulnerable groups, and prescribing. The garrulous wording of its mission statement,[39] 'the encouragement of improvement, innovation and sustainability in care, the delivery of an intelligence-driven approach to regulation, the promotion of a single shared view on quality and the improvement of their own efficiency and effectiveness,' only succeeded in furthering the profession's jaundiced view that this was yet another bureaucratic body created to obstruct rather than enhance patient care. However, those practices inclined towards ignoring the body as an irrelevance, found themselves quickly disabused. The CQC had teeth.

---

[36] 2019/20 General Medical Services (GMS) contract Quality and Outcomes Framework (QOF); NHSE, BMA. www.england.nhs.uk/wp-content/uploads/2019/05/gms-contract-QoF-guidance-april-2019.pdf

[37] KISS; QoF indicator changes for 2019/20-overview NB medical. https://nbmedical.secure.force.com/servlet/servlet.FileDownload?file=0151p0000006OVJbAAO

[38] Quasi-autonomous non-governmental organisation. https://www.oxfordreference.com/view/10.1093/oi/authority.20110803100358945?msclkid=67a429f1ab2311ec87f28393941c29b3

[39] Care quality commission annual report and accounts 2018/19. www.cqc.org.uk/sites/default/files/20190812_annualreport201819.pdf

Apart from primary care, the CQC was also responsible for registering and inspecting other health and adult social care providers in the UK. These ranged from individuals caring for a relative in their own home to hospitals with over 1,000 beds. In all, there were 15 regulated activities:

- Personal care
- Accommodation for people who require nursing or personal care
- Accommodation for people who require treatment for substance misuse
- Accommodation and nursing or personal care in the further education sector
- Treatment of disease, disorder or injury, i.e. licensed clinicians
- Assessment or medical treatment for people detained under the Mental Health Act 1983
- Surgical procedures
- Diagnostic and screening procedures
- Management of supply of blood and blood-derived products
- Transport services, triage, and medical advice provided remotely
- Maternity and midwifery services
- Termination of pregnancies
- Services in slimming clinics
- Nursing care
- Family planning services

GP practices were inspected and graded on whether they were safe, effective, responsive, caring, and well-led with each rated as 'outstanding,' 'good,' 'needs improvement,' and 'failing.' The interpretation of these broad terms and domains was alien to most GPs. The publication of quality ratings, online[40] and in poster form, underlined by a traffic-light grading system, created unease in practices where the colour red predominated.

The CQC had the legal power to act where poor care was identified, including the closure of services if necessary. A GP practice could be closed with immediate effect if considered unsafe, a power rarely exercised and only after all other measures at improvement had failed. Such closures created mayhem in the local community, especially in adjacent practices suddenly faced with taking on thousands of disenfranchised patients.

All GP practices had to be registered with the CQC as of April 2013. By 2018/2019, all 6,873 practices in England had been inspected, 5% of which were rated 'outstanding,' 90% 'good,' 4% 'requires improvement,' and 1% 'inadequate.'[41]

Surprisingly, despite the CQC's draconian powers, feedback from inspected practices was mostly positive, with over two-thirds reporting that the visit and inspectors' report had helped them improve the running of their practice and service delivery.

The funding for the activities of the CQC was through fees levied on individual practices. For 2018/2019, the total sum across all sectors of health and social

[40] www.cqc.org.uk/what-we-do/services-we-regulate/find-family-doctor-gp
[41] State of care CQC. www.cqc.org.uk/publications/major-report/state-care

care was £204.3 million, of which £56 million came from primary care. Fees for an inspection, calculated on patient list numbers, ranged from £500 for list size less than 2,000, to £57,000 for lists of 100,000 or more.[42]

Professor Steve Field, previously Chair of the RCGP and Deputy Medical Director at NHS England, was appointed as the CQC's first Chief Inspector of General Practice. The format for inspections was based on a team of three or four inspectors, one of whom was medically qualified, a GP or a nurse, with the other members drawn from practice administration and allied healthcare professions. The inspection team spent up to three days on-site, observing and talking to staff drawn from all areas of practice, including doctors and, crucially, patients. The inspection focussed on five key domains or Key Lines of Enquiry (KLOE), Safe, Effective, Caring, Responsive, and Well-led. Further details can be found on the CQC website.[43]

The inspections were lengthy, rigorous, and forensic in detail, but the final report was formulaic, with much detail cut and pasted, in stilted language.

Common examples of the requirements for individual areas of inspection included:

Care and welfare of people who use services

- A written practice protocol covering consent, which had to be published and displayed for patients to see.
- An understanding of which patients lack the capacity to give consent, such as those patients covered by the Mental Capacity Act or Children's Act.
- A statement that staff had been trained to act as chaperones, causing some bemusement among doctors. What training did they need? The offer of a chaperone and the outcome of that offer had to be recorded in the patient's notes prior to all intimate examinations.

Cooperation with other providers

- A competent referral letter to ensure that the patient or their carer/representative were informed and involved in the decision for referral.
- Training in Caldicott principles on information governance before the sharing of personal data.

Safeguarding patients, children, and adults from abuse

- Ensuring all staff were trained and knew the processes involved in safeguarding children and vulnerable adults. This was duplicated for doctors as a mandatory requirement for inclusion on the performers list and insinuated itself into the annual GP appraisal.
- All staff checked under the Disclosure and Barring Service (DBS).

---

[42] www.cqc.org.uk/guidance-providers/fees/fees-calculator

[43] www.cqc.org.uk/what-we-do/how-we-do-our-job/what-we-do-inspection

Cleanliness and infection control

- A written protocol ensuring that the premises were kept scrupulously clean.
- A risk assessment for infection. This included several dubious unproven requirements, such as the placement of disposable synthetic material curtains around examination couches, despite no research having shown that curtains harboured harmful bacteria in general practice premises; disposable hand towels or air dryers by sinks; and liquid soap dispensers. An empty dispenser was an immediate black mark on inspection. Sinks had to have a graphic poster instructing the user on how to wash their hands, a rather condescending instruction to a professional who had had at least ten years' medical training to stand by that sink!
- Patients with transmissible infections had to be seen in an isolated area. This instruction came to the fore during the COVID pandemic, where patients suspected of a coronavirus infection were seen in a separate room that was regularly disinfected.

Management of medicines

- Medicines on-site had to be in date. A practice was often caught out on this item during a CQC inspection. For many years, doctors had been in the habit of keeping returned unused packets of pills in a desk drawer. These were sometimes dispensed to patients on a trial basis. Such actions, rightly, were considered a major misdemeanour.
- The fridge where medicines and vaccines were stored had to be working properly, with a lock and a visible temperature gauge. Thrice daily, temperatures had to be logged and the temperature range kept within two to eight degrees centigrade. Whole stocks of vaccines had to be discarded following a CQC inspection if the logbook showed temperatures outside this range.

Safety and suitability of premises

- Waste was stored and disposed of appropriately, clinical waste in yellow bags.
- Fire safety was vital. Regular inspections, fire extinguishers in date, fire evacuation notices in place, fire drills, fire doors. Fire safety became mandatory training for inclusion on the performers list.
- Access for the disabled, including ramps, wide doors, lifts, toilets, including provision for breastfeeding and nappy-changing.

Requirements relating to workers

- The right staff were recruited for the right job and that their details and references were checked. Staff had to have a current DBS certificate (as mentioned).
- Every employee had to have a written employment contract, job description, and training. Early CQC inspections found such requirements lacking, not the least for doctors employed on a locum or sessional basis.

Service users

- The CQC was more enthusiastic about patient feedback and patient participation groups than the public. However, the latter were quite keen on using the complaints procedure.

Complaints

- As alluded to above, complaints were important and, therefore, had a whole section to themselves. Perhaps as a throw off from the retail sector, the plaintiff was always considered to be in the right, and thus, all complaints, major and minor, had to be escalated through a rigorous complaints pathway until a resolution was reached. Thereafter, the practice was encouraged to reflect on the process and outcome and ensure that a similar situation never recurred.

Medical records

- The Data Protection Act 1998 and the Freedom of Information Act 2000, and woe betide anyone who forgot them. The only way to avoid future litigation was to ensure that everything was recorded.

Many of the details highlighted above could catch out the unwary or unprepared doctor or practice manager. The fallout could be emotionally devastating when that happened. Doctors are intrinsically perfectionists. They are their own worst critic. They do not cope well with perceived failure.

Anxiety levels were raised before, during, and after a CQC inspection. For the 5% of practices rated as inadequate or requiring improvement, a retrieval exercise followed to reassure patients that such labels did not mean that their doctor was incompetent or dangerous. The subtlety of the message that the CQC rating related to practice administration and function was difficult to communicate to patients. I have personally witnessed senior doctors devastated by a 'bad' CQC report and, whether through frustration or a sense of professional failure, reduced to tears when confronted with even the innocuous label of 'needs improvement.' It is a chastening sight.

As with all regulatory roles, the atmosphere surrounding the inspection of any practice depended on the character of the inspectors. Most were supportive and non-threatening. The role of a CQC inspector had many attractions but little appeal to most practising GPs, who viewed it as akin to that of poacher turned gamekeeper. Open to any registered clinician, the position provided an invitation to gain an in-depth insight into the workings of a variety of GP practices, an opportunity unavailable in any other role. The findings could be fascinating, instructive, perturbing, and humbling. There were many excellent practices, from which a GP inspector could learn and improve their own. Appointments were generally on an ad hoc consultancy basis.

Many of the requirements of the CQC inspection pre-existed in daily practice prior to 2004. The novelty for many practices lay in the provision of written evidence, standard operating procedures. The preparation for the first inspection was time-consuming, distracting, and frustrating but, once completed, little extra effort was required for subsequent CQC visits.

Although the CQC could be the most daunting of regulators, there were other participants in overseeing GP performance and practice; PCT, now CCG and, of course, patients.

9.7 CCG

Since CCGs had been given the budget to run an efficient primary care service, it was no surprise that, thereafter, they sought to understand how and where that money was being spent. Pair that with the increasing pressure on resources, and the result became another layer of practice scrutiny. To date, this has tended to focus on drug spending/budgets, a perennial concern of all PCOs, hospital referral rates, investigations, and non-scheduled hospital attendance, that is, patients self-referring to A&E.

CCGs tended to apply a soft-touch approach to scrutiny, identifying failures in meeting local benchmarks and sending specialists into practices to identify where specific service improvements could be made. As a common example of such provision, a CCG appointed pharmacy advisor might assist in switching a population from an expensive drug to a cheaper but equally effective alternative. Although the logic in doing so might have seemed irrefutable, such actions did lead to patient confusion and irritation, especially if they were switched back to their original brand some months later following a change in a drug company's pricing policy!

9.8 PATIENTS

GPs might have been self-employed, but they were always answerable to their patients. Doctors have always taken their responsibility to their patients very seriously; they have a finely tuned sense of duty. Doctors were and remain 'public servants.'

Patients have always commented on the service they received from their family practice. Mostly, these conversations took place in a chip-shop queue, over coffee, or in the pub. Verbal expressions of gratitude and sometimes a short note or card might be directed to a doctor, nurse, or staff member after a particularly helpful interaction. Conversely, a verbal or written expression of dissatisfaction or a complaint might arise. The last invariably created a profound sense of failure and distress in the recipient. Doctors tend to ignore plaudits but ruminate on criticism. They can be emotionally childlike, welcoming a pat on the head but dreading a scolding.

Prior to 2004, patients had no opportunities for giving any formal feedback, unless a complaint, on the service received. Thereafter, they were given a plethora of opportunities ranging from the immediate, the Friends and Family Test, the local, the Patient Participation Group, and national, NHS Choices and the National GP Patient Survey. And of course, there was always social media!

9.8.1 NHS Friends and Family Test (FFT)[44]

The FFT was a simple, single-question postcard that has sat forlornly on the receptionist counter in every surgery since 2013. Since then, 75 million have been completed, not all in primary care since the cards were also distributed to hospitals and providers in mental health, maternity, community care, emergency care, dental practices, and patient transport. The cards were largely ignored by patients in GP surgeries and only actively promoted by the practice when a CQC visit was imminent.

The tortuous question asks, 'From your own experiences with this service, how likely would you be recommending it to a family member or friend as somewhere where they should come with their health-related problems?' with the Likert scale format for answers ranging from Extremely Likely to Extremely Unlikely and Don't Know.

The results were published monthly and have consistently shown 90% of responses as positive. Whether that has informed the provision of GP services in any way is doubtful.

9.8.2 GP Patient Questionnaire

The GMC patient questionnaire template,[45] recommended for GP revalidation, has a concise 12 questions, the majority dealing with doctor/patient communication.

A patient survey for each doctor became obligatory after the implementation of doctor revalidation requiring one to be completed within every five-year cycle. The comments made on the survey, good and bad, needed to be reflected on by the doctor, often in conjunction with their appraiser and conclusions, if any, drawn and acted on. Most answers were positive and flattering. Despite the numerous opportunities for patients to comment negatively on the service, few chose to do so. None of the anonymised comments had the same, potentially devastating impact on a doctor as that of a direct, personal complaint.

9.8.3 Patient Participation Group (PPG)

PPGs were set up to provide a conduit between service providers and users, allowing the latter to input their views on their local medical services. They were useful in transmitting the views of the community of patients in a non-threatening manner and allowing the practice to be more responsive to those views. They were also helpful in raising funds for the purchase of medical equipment.

PPGs proved an invaluable resource for communication and personnel during the COVID pandemic, helping to disseminate information on vaccination

[44] www.england.nhs.uk/fft/
[45] www.gmc-uk.org/-/media/documents/patient-questionnaire—dc7354_pdf-60283 934.pdf

clinics and providing volunteers, marshals, for managing the clinics' throughput of patients.

9.8.4 NHS Choices

NHS Choices,[46] an online star-based rating system, solicited patients' views on telephone access, appointments, being treated with dignity and respect, involvement in decisions regarding their health, and receiving accurate information.

The facility was poorly advertised, little used by patients and replaced by a convoluted process attached to the GP surgery's NHS website. Unsurprisingly it is even less used now than before. Those that did choose to post a moderated review were expected to receive a response within 48 hours.

9.8.5 NHS GP Patient Survey

The NHS GP Patient Survey,[47] managed by Ipsos MORI, was available in paper format or online. Its 63 questions[48] covered access, appointments, consultation, health, out-of-hours, and overall experience. The website also had a useful tool for GP practices to benchmark their results against their peers.

The survey summary for 2021,[49] published by NHS England, contained reassuring data that tended to support overall satisfaction with the service.

Of the 850,000 responses received, 83% reported having a good overall experience of their GP practice, with 96% saying that they had confidence and trust in the healthcare professional they saw. The metrics were equally good for the consultation but significantly less so for access; 40% of respondents could not get an appointment with the person they wanted or at a time of their choosing. The journey may have been demanding but the final destination was worth the effort.

It is difficult for the profession to evaluate the true worth of patient feedback on the service provided in primary care. The overwhelming positivity of the data could be interpreted as a service with little need for improvement. However, that interpretation does not tally with anecdotal sentiment that patients expressed off the record. The waiting room on a Monday morning often looks like a newsreel of a food lorry in a famine, as frustrated patients jostle to complain about the phone, the paucity of appointments, and the absence of their doctor of choice. The data from patient surveys only succeed in reassuring the paymasters at the Department of Health that their money is well spent, with little need for further funding for primary care. The mandarins at Whitehall are far enough removed from reality to be seduced by such notions. Those on the front line are not.

---

[46] www.nhs.uk/about-us/managing-patient-feedback/

[47] www.england.nhs.uk/statistics/2019/07/11/gp-patient-survey-2019/

[48] www.gp-patient.co.uk/downloads/2019/qandletter/GPPS_2019_Questionnaire_PUBLIC.pdf

[49] www.gp-patient.co.uk/downloads/2021/GPPS_2021_National_infographic_PUBLIC.pdf

9.9 SUMMARY

Doctors who had enrolled as independent contractors to the NHS in 1948 were fortunate to remain 'independent' for much of their working lives. Blissfully closeted in their consulting rooms; they were free to treat their patients as they saw fit, within the bounds of medical ethics. Provided they kept a low profile and did not fall foul of the GMC's code of conduct, they were likely to have spent an entire career free of regulatory worries. However, since the turn of the millennium, and through varied, often subtle means, they and their work have come under increasing scrutiny.

Opinion within the profession over inspection and regulation are mixed. CCG input could well be driving down the drug budget and, in due course, may do the same for unplanned hospital admissions and A&E attendance. QOF has raised standards in patient care, and the CQC has done the same for the state of surgery premises and administration. All this has been achieved at the cost of GP autonomy, loss of self-esteem, lowered morale, and early retirement.

A published study in 2016,[50] albeit one showing the statistical failings of online questionnaires, identified that 82.0% of respondent GPs intended leaving, taking a career break, and/or reducing clinical hours within the next five years. Their reasons included volume of work, intensity of workload, time spent on 'unimportant tasks,' and declining job satisfaction. Further, 28% said that appraisal and revalidation were significant factors in their decision. Supporting these findings are anecdotal reports from appraisals where doctors cite CQC inspections, annual appraisal, and recurrent mandatory training in non-core subjects, such as diversity, manual handling and data security, and even fire safety, as contributors to a sense of worthlessness. Patient expectations and demand are hardly ever mentioned.

To their credit, the various regulatory bodies are mindful of the dissatisfaction within the profession and have sought to address many of the issues raised. Elements of inspection are being watered down. Regular review of QOF data has led to a reduction in the number of descriptors and a focus on those with clearer clinical relevance. Some of the more dogmatic requirements of annual appraisal have been diluted. The CQC has reduced the frequency of inspections for 'good' and 'outstanding' practices to focus, rightly, on those that need improvement. The CQC suspended all inspections during the first year of the COVID pandemic. Likewise, appraisals were temporarily suspended but reintroduced in a modified, light-touch version, the main features of which were the removal of the provision of evidence of learning. Doctors welcomed both moves, in the hope that for appraisals at least, the changes would become permanent.

Medicine is an evidence-based discipline, yet it is difficult to find any consistent evidence of the benefits of regulation and inspection. QOF, designed to lift

---

50 Dale J, Potter R, Owen K, Leach J. The general practitioner workforce crisis in England: a qualitative study of how appraisal and revalidation are contributing to intentions to leave practice. BMC Fam Pract. 2016 Jul 20;17:84. doi: 10.1186/s12875-016-0489-9. PMID: 27439982; PMCID: PMC4955125.

the quality of healthcare provision across the country, has had conflicting data to support it. As an example, rates of unplanned admission to hospital have risen since 2004,[51] with those for COPD emergency hospital admissions increasing by 13% between 2008 and 2014,[52] a disheartening reward for the efforts undertaken by GP practices over that period. The data for CQC inspections is also depressing; 8% of GP practices inspected in 2018/2019 were found to be inadequate.[53]

The only measurable outcomes from GP appraisal and revalidation relate to the data on complaints to the GMC and consequent investigations and sanctions. The former showed an increase for a decade after the introduction of GP appraisal, followed by a levelling off and a slight drop. The number of doctors sanctioned has remained static. Whilst interpretation of such data may be complex, it may show that an annual, intrusive, expensive process has produced little change in public opinion of those providing a public service.

Both national and practice-based patient surveys have poor uptake, are generally flattering regarding care received, provide little in the way of formative advice, and are universally ignored by all but the CQC.

GPs are no longer autonomous, and that loss of independence has led to growing insecurity and a consequent decline in morale. Driven by these factors, GP recruitment and retention is dropping, resulting in increasing, some would say unsustainable, workload pressures on those remaining in post, a situation likely to compromise patient safety. The very regulations put in place to increase patient confidence in doctors have had the opposite effect.

The presence of intrusive scrutiny has become a feature of modern societies. The clock cannot, nor should it be, turned back but, hopefully, what was once a blunt instrument cudgelling many is now in the process of being honed into one identifying and supporting those individuals who are struggling or underperforming. This recognition by regulatory bodies should be encouraged and accelerated before general practice goes into terminal decline.

Ultimately, a doctor will always be answerable equally to their patient and their own conscience.

---

[51] Zhong VW, Juhaeri J, Mayer-Davis EJ. Trends in hospital admission for diabetic ketoacidosis in adults with type 1 and type 2 diabetes in England, 1998–2013: a retrospective cohort study. Diabetes Care. 2018 Sep;41(9):1870–7. doi: 10.2337/dc17-1583. Epub 2018 Jan 31. PMID: 29386248.

[52] www.nice.org.uk/guidance/ng115; www.nice.org.uk/guidance/ng115/resources/resource-impact-report-pdf-6602803741

[53] Secretary of state for health and social care annual report 2018/19. https://assets.publishing.service.gov.uk/government/uploads/system/uploads/attachment_data/file/832765/dhsc-annual-report-and-accounts-2018-to-2019.pdf

10

The BMA and Medical Defence Organisations

Defenders of the Faithful

10.1 INTRODUCTION

The BMA[1] is the registered trade union and professional body representing all doctors in the UK. As it says on its website, 'We look after doctors so that they can look after you.'

The organisation has several disparate divisions covering trade unionism, education, professional standards, and law. It represents the professional, personal, and collective needs of all doctors in the UK, including the third who are not actually fee-paying members. Doctors can opt-in and opt-out of membership at any time as their individual needs change.

The multifaceted nature of the BMA has often led to confusion within the national press and public at large. Is it an altruistic organisation promoting public health or an obstructionist trade union seeking unrealistic living standards for its already wealthy members? The BMA accepts the multiplicity of its brief, stating:

> We promote the medical and allied sciences, seek to maintain the honour and interests of the medical profession and promote the achievement of high-quality healthcare. Our policies cover public health issues, medical ethics, science, the state of the NHS, medical education and doctors' contracts.[2]

10.2 HISTORY

The roots of the BMA lay in the 19th century when, under the energetic stewardship of Sir Charles Hastings (1794–1866), 50 doctors met in the Board Room

---

[1] www.bma.org.uk

[2] https://medical-dictionary.thefreedictionary.com/British+Medical+Association

DOI: 10.1201/9781003256465-10

of Worcester Infirmary on 19 July 1832 to set up the Provincial Medical and Surgical Association (PMSA). The PMSA's stated objectives were to promote the medical and allied sciences and maintain the honour and interests of the medical profession, an aspiration that remains at the heart of the association to this day. The PMSA amalgamated with other like-minded smaller associations to form the British Medical Association in 1856. It subsequently registered as a limited company in 1874 and only became listed as a trade union a century later, following the Trade Union and Labour Relations Act 1974.

The PMSA's and subsequently BMA's initial brief was to identify the profession it was representing. The definition of a doctor at the time was expansive and vague. The task was facilitated following the 1858 Medical Act, which included the creation of a Medical Register, overseen by a General Medical Council, in which only the names of qualified doctors could appear. Prior to 1858, almost anyone could call himself a doctor, and indeed, Charles Hastings himself was operating as a surgeon at his local hospital when still a teenager, with no experience apart from an 18-month apprenticeship as an apothecary.

It was not until the passing of the Medical Act 1886 that all qualified doctors had to be trained in the three disciplines of medicine, surgery, and midwifery, before being allowed to practise on the public at large.

The BMA did not exclusively promote the medical profession. It was also active in initiating and lobbying on many issues that raised the quality of medical care during the late-Victorian period. These included the creation of a register of midwives, the notification of infectious diseases, the exposure of 'quack medicine,' the treatment of alcoholism, legislation on mental health, housing and factory conditions, coroner's law, and death certification.

The first in a long list of political obduracy by the BMA in the 20th century arose in 1911, with the introduction of Lloyd George's National Health Insurance Bill. This set out to provide universal healthcare for every employed person, for the princely sum of 4 pence per week, equivalent to £2.00 in 2019. Thus, even before the NHS, the funding of basic healthcare provision in the UK was already beset by unrealistic fiscal fantasies. The BMA's primary objection (and how often the point has been made) was the lack of consultation between government and profession, prior to the introduction of the bill. Their trepidation was understandable since it would be doctors who would be responsible for the practical delivery of the bill's objectives. Despite the objections and counterproposals of their representative body, doctors, the caring profession, chose to back the scheme and, by 1913, had enrolled in large numbers.

The *Westminster Gazette*, an influential Liberal newspaper of the time, remarked:

> We all admire people who don't know when they are beaten. The trouble with the BMA is that it doesn't know when it has won.

By 1930, BMA membership mainly comprised general practitioners who consequently exerted the most influence on association policy. Working predominantly as single-handed practitioners in their own premises, these doctors greatly valued their independence and used their influence in the BMA to oppose any efforts at diluting it. In particular, they fiercely opposed any kind of salaried service, a suggestion that the Labour-Party-affiliated Socialist Medical Association supported.

In the 1930s, either as a considerably delayed response to the previous bill or a pre-emptive strike against the next, the BMA introduced, with many subsequent revisions, plans for a 'general medical service for the nation,' published just before the Beveridge Report in 1942. The two overlapped in many of their headline aims, most notably in the provision of a universal national health service available to all UK citizens, insurance for the unemployed, and retirement pensions funded by contributions from workers, employers, and the government.

The White Paper 'A National Health Service' was published on 17 February 1944, following which lengthy negotiations ensued with the BMA and other advocates within the healthcare community, including all the royal colleges. The RCGP was absent since it had yet to come into existence.

Whilst agreeing on the broad brushstrokes of the act and lauding its altruistic intentions, the BMA once again objected on the grounds of lack of consultation on matters that were likely to have significant impact on doctors' livelihoods. Not least was the mooted introduction of a salaried service, which a former BMA official described as 'the first step, and a big one, towards National Socialism as practised in Germany . . . under the dictatorship of a "medical Fuhrer",'[3] the latter alluding to Aneurin Bevan, appointed Minister for Health and Housing in the Attlee government of 1945.

The BMA tabled its objections to the Act on 'seven principles':

- No salaried service
- Clinical freedom
- Free choice of doctor for patients
- Free choice for doctors of form and place of work
- Freedom of every registered practitioner to join the public service
- A hospital service centred on universities
- Adequate professional representation on all administrative bodies

Interestingly, the word 'free' appears no less than four times but never in relation to what some would argue is still the fundamental principle of the NHS; free at the point of access.

An editorial in the BMJ from 1946 pulled no punches in describing the dystopian future GPs faced under a socialist healthcare system:

[The GP] will work in a Health Centre owned by the Local Health Authority and be paid, to begin with, partly by salary. He will be unable to start practice or change practice except by permission of a central committee under the direction of the Minister at the Ministry of Health. Owning nothing except the right to work under direction-presumably not even the tools of his craft- and inspired by the prospect of controlled security, what kind of effort will the future general practitioner put forth? Will the kind of regulated service contemplated give the right setting and stimulus to the Jenners, Hunters, Budds, Snows and James Mackenzies of the future?[4]

Stirring words indeed! These concerns were still being heard 70 years later as the edifice of independence was inexorably eroded by newly qualified GPs flocking to salaried positions.

The principles tabled by the BMA were non-negotiable. When put to the vote in February 1948, 9 out of 10 (40,000 out of 45,000) doctors voted against the creation of an NHS, a significant endorsement of the BMA's intransigence on the subject.

The deadlock was eventually broken when the hospital consultants broke rank and accepted the plan with a few changes, such as the inclusion of private hospital beds within nationalised hospitals. Of note, Nye Bevan's infamous quote that he had had to 'stuff their mouths with gold' to gain acceptance, referred to hospital consultants and not doctors in general.

The BMA continued to resist but eventually acceded to the moral case and overwhelming public opinion and, having gained legal assurances that there would be no more talk of a salaried service without a further parliamentary act, put the motion to another vote. This, too, its members rejected, but with a much smaller majority. Bowing to the inevitable, the BMA recommended acceptance of the plan, and by July 1948, 90% of GPs had signed up to join the new NHS. By the end of that year, 97% of the population of the UK had enrolled with a GP. The birth of modern general practice was completed, and the contribution of the BMA to that labour established it as the sole professional negotiating body for ALL doctors.

Although the BMA's stance in the negotiations leading to the formation of the NHS had more than a passing resemblance to the actions of a trade union, the association still eschewed such tawdry company by re-emphasising its lofty roots in improving medical care in general and lobbying government on health issues. Eventually, in 1971, the BMA conceded that it was functioning as a trade union and changed its constitution to comply with the legislation of that time. Within a decade, Barbara Castle, Minister for Social Services, was scolding its negotiators as 'just a middle-class miner' during pay negotiations for junior doctors' pay and conditions. Their recognised dogged and often uncompromising bargaining skills frequently came to the fore in the coming decades, to the particular benefit of the profession in the GP contracts of 2004.

10.3 BMA ACTIVITIES

Beyond politics, the BMA remained active in reporting on an eclectic number of topics of public interest:

---

[4] https://api.parliament.uk/historic-hansard/commons/1946/apr/30/national-health-service-bill

1951   Marriage and divorce
1955   Homosexual offences and prostitution
1959   Marriage (under articles published by *Family Doctor*, a popular health
        magazine published by the BMA, an issue of which was provoca-
        tively titled, 'Is Chastity Outmoded? Outdated? Out?')
1971   Smoking
1980   Global conflict, in particular, nuclear war
1985   AIDS
1992   Genetic engineering

In addition, the BMA lobbied on issues relating to the organisation of health delivery:

1957   The Pilkington Report on Doctors' and Dentists' Remuneration
1962   The Porritt Report for reforming NHS administration, specifically the
        formation of area health boards
1963   The Gillie report on the future of general practice
1965   A Charter for the Family Doctor Service

The British Medical Association and the Royal Pharmaceutical Society also jointly published the *BNF* and the *British National Formulary for Children* (BNFc).

The BMA also provided ancillary services, only available to fee-paying members.

BMA membership increased over the decades, in line with the overall rise in doctor numbers in all specialties. The figure stood at 35,000 in 1932, 110,000 in 1990, and 158,000 in 2020.

BMA standard rate membership subscription for 2019/2020 was £461 for a GP principal. For that sum, members had access not only to the collective representation of the profession in negotiations nationally and locally, but also a wide range of personal services covering:

- Employment
- Appraisals
- Revalidation
- Commissioning
- Contracts
- Ethics
- Fees
- GP practice
- Immigration
- Job planning
- Leave
- Occupational health
- Pay
- Pensions
- Insurance and investments

- Private practice
- Whistleblowing
- Redundancy
- Tax
- Working hours
- The *BMJ* and other in-house publications and learning modules
- Two hotels in central London—rooms available at highly competitive rates!

10.4 BMA ORGANISATION

The BMA has a somewhat complex hierarchical administrative structure, at the top of which sits a board of directors answerable to the BMA Councils representing each of the four home nations of the UK. In turn, they listen and act on the views of the Annual Representative Meeting (ARM) attended by delegates drawn from all divisions and branches of the profession, including consultants, junior doctors, medical students, academia, public health, and general practice, the last represented by the General Practitioners' Committee (GPC).

The upper echelons of the BMA are too remote and of little interest to most GPs. However, that does not apply to the General Practitioners and Local Medical committees, both of which play an important role as the interface between the Department of Health and primary care.

10.4.1 General Practitioners' Committee

The GPC is an executive committee within the BMA, with the authority to deal with all matters affecting NHS general practitioners and prison doctors. It is the only body that represents all GPs in the UK, regardless of whether they are BMA members, on the majority of national bodies concerned with health policy. The Department of Health recognises the GPC as the sole negotiating body for general practice. It is represented in negotiations with ministers and civil servants by a team of eight GPs, elected by the committee and supported by expert advisors in law, finance, and ethics. Committee members are drawn from all branches of general practice in the UK, including GP principals, GP trainees, sessional GPs, the Medical Women's Federation, British International Doctors' Association, prison doctors, and RCGP.

The GPC's extensive portfolio of interests includes:

- Clinical and Prescribing
  - Quality and Outcomes Framework matters relating to drugs, prescribing, vaccinations, and immunisations
- Commissioning and Service Development
  - Commissioning, enhanced services, out-of-hours, new providers, the internal market, the provision by independent GPs of services to community hospitals, and geographically specific services
- Contracts and Regulation

- Regulatory and contractual issues relating to GPs working within the NHS, whether as employees or contractors, to consider matters relating to the interface with private practice, self-regulation, and regulatory and contractual issues relating to prison doctors
- Education, Training, and Workforce
  - Appraisal, continuing professional development, postgraduate training, the role and remuneration of GP educators and trainers, recruitment and retention, and human relations, including practice staff, their recruitment, funding, and development
  - General Practitioners' Defence Fund (GPDF),[5] a public limited company that whose role is to influence, support, and fund LMCs and GPs
- GP Trainees
  - Pay, terms and conditions, and responding to consultations that affect GP trainees and their training
- Joint GPC and RCGP Information Technology
  - GP IM&T
- Joint GPC and RCGP Liaison Group
  - Considers matters of common interest to the BMA and RCGP
- Finance
  - Pensions, tax and accountancy, premises, geography-related costs, dispensing, GPs as sole traders, partnerships, or limited companies
- Representation
  - Monitoring and reviewing the GPC's representative and electoral structures to ensure the adequate representation of all GPs
- Sessional GPs
  - Consider all matters of interest for salaried and locum GPs, collectively known as sessional GPs

GP members, usually with previous LMC experience, are elected to the GPC for three-year terms.

The Welsh and Scottish GPCs are subcommittees of the national GPC but have autonomy on NHS matters exclusive to their countries. The Northern Ireland GPC is independent of the GPC, but with a close working relationship.

10.4.2 Local Medical Committee (LMC)

The GPC is fed by numerous Local Medical Committees, each coterminous with its Primary Care Trust or CCG.

The LMC[6,7] is a statutory body under the NHS made up of practitioners elected to represent all GPs in the locality. GPs need not be subscribed BMA members and, indeed, can be elected officers on the LMC without having any relationship

---

5 www.gpdf.org.uk/

6 file:///C:/Users/Jim/Downloads/Leading%20Medical%20Consensus%20LMCs%20 SCHARR%2020031130.pdf

7 file:///C:/Users/Jim/Downloads/LMC%20-%20statutory.pdf

with the BMA. Thus, the BMA can be seen as representing not only the views of its fee-paying members but also of all other doctors in the profession, and it would not be surprising to find fee-paying members galled by the idea.

LMCs have a venerable history, predating the creation of the NHS by 36 years.

Primary Care Organisations have a statutory responsibility to consult with LMCs on all key issues affecting the latter's stakeholders, primarily contracts.[8]

LMCs are uniquely funded, either by a statutory or voluntary levy, on GP practices rather than individual GPs. The PCO deducts these sums at source from the GMS budget or levied directly from PMS practices. The sum is set at a nominal amount per patient per practice, usually less than £1, and covers administrative expenses, reimbursements for attendance by members at meetings, annual subscriptions to the BMA, and charitable donations to organisations that support GPs and their families.

Elections of LMC members tend to be poorly subscribed. Front-line GPs seem to have little time for the politics relating to their profession, delegating such responsibilities to their practice managers. Their enthusiasm is only piqued when such matters as the 2004 attempt by NHS England to move all PMS practices into GMS contracts and its resulting negative impact on doctors' income. The iniquity of that proposal was softened following the collective front presented by the LMCs and, subsequently, GPC.

10.5 THE *BRITISH MEDICAL JOURNAL* (BMJ)

The intellectual high ground of the BMA is represented by its Science and Ethics arm, at the top of which sits the prestigious publication, the *BMJ*. The *BMJ* evolved from the *Provincial Medical and Surgical Journal*, first published in 1840, which changed its name to the pithier *British Medical Journal* 17 years later.

The *BMJ*, the Koh-i-Noor of the BMA, is the jewel that elevates it from a simple trade union to the heights of academic intellectual respectability. Although not quite as old as its rival, the *Lancet*, both august journals have been at the forefront of medical publishing in the UK and globally, for almost two centuries.

From the beginning, the quality of the submissions to the journal relied on the crusading scholarship of the editor, whose average tenure of 20 years in post provided the academic gravitas for editorials that had a profound influence on the medical profession and society at large. Despite that influence, most GPs looked on the *BMJ* as a journal publishing research of limited value to primary care. Although all BMA members routinely received a copy, the cover was left unturned or, at best, the contents skimmed through much as with a daily newspaper, for topics of interest, mainly job vacancies and obituaries. The *BMJ* editorial committee recognised and responded in 1998 to GP apathy by introducing the suffix 'GP' alongside articles of interest. Nevertheless, anecdotal evidence suggested that the distinctive, duck-egg blue cover that decorated bookshelves in practice common rooms remained as untouched as the outdated *Readers Digest* in the patients' waiting room.

---

[8] www.essexlmc.org.uk/about/

The one copy of the *BMJ* that was likely to be read by all doctors was the unfailingly amusing Christmas edition which tended to include 'papers' on arguably less cerebral topics such as, from the edition of 19 December 2015:[9]

- How to avoid the anger of ghosts
- 'Gunslinger gait'; a new cause of unilaterally reduced arm swing
- Do heads of government age more quickly? Observational study comparing mortality between elected leaders and runners-up in national elections of 17 countries
- Plenty of moustaches but not enough women; cross-sectional study of medical leaders
- Evidence of a Christmas spirit network in the brain; functional MRI study
- Debunking the curse of the rainbow jersey; historical cohort study
- Bloodcurdling movies and measures of coagulation: Fear Factor crossover trial

The *BMJ* was intermeshed within the corporate body of the BMA until 2003 when it was spun off as a standalone, independent subsidiary with its own CEO, board, and administration. The move reinforced the editorial independence of the publication, allowing it to remain one of the world's top four most cited general medical journals.

Having gained its 'independence' in the new millennium, the *BMJ* expanded its offering not only to an online presence but also in such areas as e-learning, where its *BMJ Best Practice, BMJ Learning,* and *BMJ Masterclasses* are widely used and respected as being of genuine educational utility, untainted by commercial bias.

The subscription costs in 2020 for access to all online services and the General Practice print edition was £776 per annum, with a more affordable £138 for the online 'thebmj.com.'

10.6 MEDICAL DEFENCE ORGANISATIONS

Whilst the BMA served the interest of doctors as a whole, other corporations, the medical defence organisations (MDO), protected them at an individual level by providing legal advice, representation, and indemnity for negligence claims made against their members.

As of 2020, five companies were offering this service: Medical Defence Union (MDU), Medical and Dental Defence Union of Scotland (MDDUS), Medical Protection Society (MPS), Premium Medical Protection, and Towergate MIA. The first three are mutual organisations, owned by and serving their members without the need to generate profits. Premium Medical and Towergate MIA are commercial insurance brokers.

Medical personal indemnity insurance was not a legal obligation until the 21st century when it was mandated by the GMC and became a contractual requirement for inclusion on the GP performers list; the GMC's Good Medical Practice stating, in no uncertain terms:

> You must make sure you have adequate insurance or indemnity cover so that your patients will not be disadvantaged if they make a claim about the clinical care you have provided in the UK.[10]

In light of the astronomical costs incurred in defending a complaint, it was fool-hardy for any doctor entering practice to not have indemnity insurance in place. MDOs also provide invaluable assistance in defending their members in other quasi-legal settings, such as GMC fitness to practice hearings.

In summary, the services offered by the mutually owned MDOs are:

- Professional indemnity against claims for clinical negligence
- Support and representation at GMC fitness-to-practise hearings
- Medico-legal advice
- Help at inquests, inquiries, and disciplinary proceedings
- Good Samaritan acts: help in emergencies outside a clinical setting
- Support when faced with media attention
- Risk-management advice and guidance
- CPD-accredited education courses

The MDU, founded in 1885, was the oldest and largest of the MDOs. It had a colourful origin, having been set up following outrage in the medical community over the case of a Dr David Bradley, wrongly convicted of a charge of assaulting a woman in his surgery. Dr Bradley spent eight months in prison before receiving a full pardon.[11] The annual subscription for members was set at 10 shillings (50 pence, equivalent to £65 in 2019). The original fee remained unchanged for 35 years until 1920 when it was raised to the princely sum of £1.

In an increasingly litigious society, the costs of legal proceedings and compensation have skyrocketed. It took 75 years for the MDU to pay out £1 million in compensation to all patients lodging a claim, but by 1988, it had paid out its first claim of over £1million for a single case. Fees had to rise in accordance with outgoings, resulting in an increased and (some doctors felt) unsustainable burden on their income. Concerns regarding GP retention led the government to announce the introduction of legislation enabling the NHS department, NHS Resolution,[12] to cover part of that cost for practising doctors but only for work they undertook in their NHS duties. The NHS Litigation Authority administers the scheme. To cover the fees, a flat rate of 52p per patient per practice was paid to the practice through the global sum. This came into effect in 2019 when all the MDO's substantially reduced their fees by up to half. By 2018, the MDU had over 200,000

---

[10] www.gmc-uk.org/static/documents/content/GMP_2013.pdf_51447599.pdf

[11] www.bmj.com/content/1/1260/403.1

[12] https://resolution.nhs.uk/wp-content/uploads/2019/09/CNSGP-Scheme-scope-table-1.pdf

members, and was opening over 140,000 case files a year, defending and closing over 80% of those without payment of damages.[13]

The MDDUS was founded in 1902, with membership restricted to Scottish doctors and those graduating from Scottish medical schools. These constraints were loosened a century later, to allow membership by any doctor practising in the UK. Subscription fees were lower than those of its rivals, justified by the MDDUS's provocative claim that Scottish born and trained doctors were safer than their English counterparts! By 2018, the MDDUS had over 50,000 active members and was handling 6,000 case files a year.

The MPS was founded in 1892 and has a strong British Commonwealth presence, with a global membership of over 300,000.

Membership fees for all the above providers, including the commercial organisations, are difficult and complex to quantify and depend on the individual working circumstances of the applicant. However, membership fees are income-tax deductible.

Organisations handling medical litigation estimate that, on average, every doctor should expect to defend a case of medical negligence at least twice during a 40-year career. This bland fact can disguise the devastating impact that such cases have on the doctor's emotional, mental, and professional well-being. They are a significant contributor to the high suicide rate in the profession.[14]

Nowadays, all GPs are advised to report any potential complaint to their MDO as soon as it arises from either the public or colleagues. Whether that only succeeds in escalating what is often a misunderstanding to a level where negligence and litigation become inevitable is worthy of debate.

10.7 SUMMARY

The British Medical Association and its publishing arm, the *BMJ*, have been an integral and influential part of general practice in the UK from long before the inception of the NHS in 1948. As its website states, its 'mission' is to 'look after doctors so that they can look after you' (presumably the public), and its 'vision' is to have 'a profession of valued doctors delivering the highest quality health services.'

At times, these laudable aims, partly through their generalisations, have been open to wide interpretation, resulting in waxing and waning opinion amongst rank-and-file general practitioners as to the actual utility of the association. Nevertheless, its history has had undoubted highlights, and few would dispute the influence and dogged hard work that the BMA undertook on work/life-changing issues, such as the 1966 and 2004 GP contracts.

---

[13] www.themdu.com/about-mdu/annual-report-and-accounts

[14] Bourne T, Wynants L, Peters M, Van Audenhove C, Timmerman D, Van Calster B, Jalmbrant M. The impact of complaints procedures on the welfare, health and clinical practise of 7926 doctors in the UK: a cross-sectional survey. BMJ Open. 2015 Jan 15;5(1):e006687. doi: 10.1136/bmjopen-2014-006687. PMID: 25592686; PMCID: PMC4316558.

The association has always been and remains to this day a pick and mix of resources. A profession's department store of products and services that an average GP might not visit for years. Nevertheless, it is reassuring to know that it is there when needed. Overall, the BMA has as much relevance to modern GP practice as it did 150 years ago.

The Medical Defence Organisations, as venerable as the BMA, remain an indispensable part of a GP's freedom to practice without fear of financial ruin. In an increasingly litigious society, that role is as vital as ever. After many years of significant increases in annual membership fees, financial support was provided through NHS Litigation in 2019, ending doctors' concerns that the previously punitive fees were becoming unsustainable.

Overall, both the BMA and MDOs are indispensable in providing support and reassurance to a profession that can at times seem beset by attacks from all sectors of society. They are truly the defenders of the faithful.

11

Administration and Reorganisation

Plus ça change, plus c'est la même chose.

(Jean-Baptiste Alphonse Karr)

11.1 INTRODUCTION

This chapter focusses on the aspects of legislation, management, and administration that have directly impacted the everyday functioning of the average, frontline general practitioner; the précis of innumerable medical and healthcare acts, reports, and regulations, and expanding on the major changes that took place in the GP contracts of 1966, 1990, 1997, and 2004.

The organisation of the NHS has generally retained the tripartite structure it had at its creation when, to achieve the cooperation of the various sceptical professional groups at the time, the Labour administration of Clement Atlee proposed that the management of general practice (primary care), hospitals (secondary and tertiary care), and community care (public health) should be separate, distinct, independent, and individually funded. Despite short-lived attempts to introduce some cross-fertilisation of activities over the decades, these administrative silos were still in place 75 years later.

11.2 PRE-1948

Prior to 1948, no overarching management structure for primary care existed; the overwhelming majority of doctors were essentially autonomous, self-employed small businesses, relying solely on their own commercial endeavours for their income. A.J. Cronin's seminal novel, *The Citadel*, indispensable reading for all doctors, described the life of a newly qualified doctor in the 1920s, and little had changed prior to the creation of a national health service. Cronin told how, depending on personal circumstance and means, doctors could set up their 'plate' and establish a medical practice anywhere they chose and, thereafter, answer to no one but themselves. Despite that apparent individual freedom, primary care as

DOI: 10.1201/9781003256465-11

a business was a closed shop, and most new entrants found themselves becoming indentured 'assistants' to established 'principals,' providing medical services to local communities via Friendly Societies.

Friendly Societies provided an employment-based, contributory, private-health-insurance model of care for company employees. Wives and children were rarely included. Doctors were either employed, as was the case in the big industries, such as mining, or had a formal contract to provide a limited range of healthcare services, for which they were paid a fixed sum per employee. The arrangement was not entirely altruistic. A healthy workforce was a productive workforce. Nevertheless, it was an arrangement from which all parties benefitted.

The populace not covered by such schemes were treated as private patients and charged a fee. Incomes for doctors working under these conditions were unpredictable and low unless they also had a thriving private practice in an affluent area. Levels of outstanding unpaid 'invoices' were high, and doctors baulked, for moral reasons, at the idea of employing debt collectors. GPs enrolled wholeheartedly at the beginning of the NHS primarily for the steady and enhanced income that it offered. However, GPs remained reluctant to give up their independence, resulting in their unique public role as independent contractors providing healthcare services to a single, dominant customer, the NHS.

The organisation of health services prior to the creation of the NHS was fragmented, with public, private, and voluntary sectors involved in delivering a variety of services, often with no communication between providers.

The NHS rationalised the organisation of healthcare in the UK by bringing many of the services previously provided by the various sectors under one umbrella.[1] The civil servants that managed this feat deserved enormous credit for doing so. The administrative structure that they created, from a blank sheet of paper and with uncharacteristic speed, has remained largely unchanged to this day.

11.3 POLITICIANS

There have been 30 Secretaries of State/Ministers of Health since 1948. Some have stood out more than others for the influence they had on primary care. Some have been larger than life characters. Some chose belligerence rather than emollience in their interaction with the profession. Some were energetic in their desire for change; others more conservative. There have been innumerable acts, regulations, green and white papers, and commission reports produced since 1948, many of which have attempted to find the holy grail of fiscal prudence, to expand and improve services whilst simultaneously capping costs. The characters that attempted to square this circle and otherwise remodel and improve the provision of primary care in the UK are listed below, along with further details on some of the more influential publications.

---

[1] www.sochealth.co.uk/national-health-service/the-sma-and-the-foundation-of-the-national-health-service-dr-leslie-hilliard-1980/a-national-health-service/

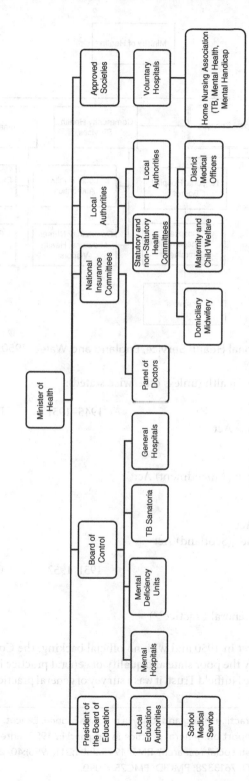

Figure 11.1 The Health Service, England and Wales, 1939.

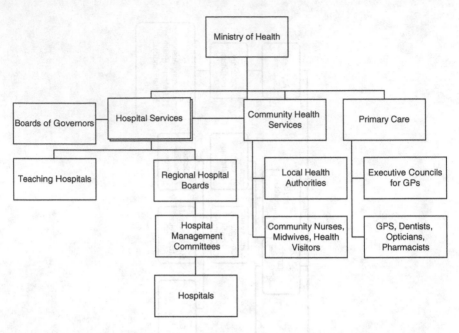

Figure 11.2 The National Health Service, England and Wales, 1950.

Secretaries of State for Health (unless otherwise stated):

Aneurin Bevan	1945–1951	Labour

National Health Service Act
Midwives Act
Medical Act
National Health Service (Amendment) Act
Nurses Act
Children Act
National Assistance Act
National Health Service (Scotland) Act

Harry Crookshank	1951–1952	Conservative

NHS Services Act

(Collings Report on General Practice[2,3])

Published in the *Lancet* in 1950 and with no official backing, the Collings Report was the first to identify the poor state and quality of general practice in the nascent NHS. Sponsored by the Nuffield Trust, it was a survey of general practice in England.

[2] Collings JS. General practice in England today: a reconnaissance. Lancet. 1950;i:555–85.

[3] Petchey R. Collings Report on general practice in England in 1950: unrecognised, pioneering piece of British social research? BMJ. 1995 Jul 1;311(6996):40–2. doi: 10.1136/bmj.311.6996.40. PMID: 7613328; PMCID: PMC2550090.

J. S. Collings, a widely travelled doctor, a GP in Australia before moving to public health in Canada and, thereafter, public health academia in the United States, had never actually set foot in the UK prior to being commissioned to undertake the research.

By today's standards, his survey lacked scientific rigour. It covered 55 general practices where the selection process was unclear. The methodology of data collection eschewed quantitative (since by and large it was non-existent) for qualitative, observational data. Collings visited each practice for between one and five days and sat with doctors during their consultations with patients. It was this invited intimacy that allowed him to make such telling observations:

> I noticed on some occasions that a perfectly serviceable exami-
> nation couch was piled with boxes and bottles; the adherence of
> these articles to the leather cover showed that they had occupied
> this position for some time.

Such couches and scars were still in evidence in some surgeries 50 years later.

The Collings Report arrived at some damning conclusions:

- 'The overall state of general practice is bad and still deteriorating'
- 'The development of other medical services . . . has resulted . . . in wide departure from both the idea and the ideal of family doctoring'
- 'Some (working conditions) are bad enough to require condemnation in the public interest'
- 'Inner city practice is "at best . . . very unsatisfactory and at worst a positive source of public danger"'
- 'Rural practice is "an anachronism" and suburban practice a "casualty-clearing" service'

and recommended that the function of general practice needed defining and that group practice might provide a better service to patients and congenial working conditions for their doctors.

Collings had highlighted the low morale within general practice based on a feeling of marginalisation, low status, denial of access to hospitals, and disappointment with changes brought about by the creation of the NHS. Rather than, being seen by a prickly profession as a criticism of the standard of general practice, Collings was instead lauded for publicising the plight of GPs at that time.

Iain McLeod   1952–1955   Conservative
NHS Act

(Danckwerts[4] 'Report of Working Party on the Distribution of Remuneration among General Practitioners.')

---

[4] Danckwerts Report of Working Party on the Distribution of Remuneration among General Practitioners, https://api.parliament.uk/historic-hansard/commons/1952/oct/30/general-practitioners-danckwerts-award

The Lord Chancellor had appointed Mr Justice Danckwerts to adjudicate the long-running dispute on GPs' income, a small matter that had been glossed over at the launch of the NHS and had festered ever since. Doctors had originally agreed to join the NHS in 1948 only on the arguably naïve understanding that their income would be negotiated once their signatures had dried on the contract. Yet, negotiations had stalled. One outstanding issue remained unresolved, that of the 'betterment' factor: a GP's earnings in real terms, once deductions for practice expenses, estimated at 40%, were accounted for.

Prior to Danckwerts' appointment and binding recommendations, the BMA had been negotiating for four years, during which it was noted that both public and parliamentary opinion had swung solidly to their side. The agreed-upon award would be back-dated and double a doctor's income. In return, it safeguarded the standard of practice by discouraging unduly large patient lists (a maximum of 3,500 patients), improved conditions for practitioners working in disadvantaged areas of the UK, simplified the process for new doctors entering practice, discouraged unethical employment of assistants, and stimulated the formation of group practice. Throughout the report, the principle of independent contractors and payment by capitation remained sacrosanct.

Robin Turton   1955–1957   Conservative
Medical Act

Derek Walker-Smith   1957–1960   Conservative
Mental Health Act

Enoch Powell   1960–1963   Conservative
Mental Health (Scotland) Act
Professions Supplementary to Medicine Act

Royal Commission on Doctors' and Dentists' Remuneration of NHS

The Commission was asked to examine the equivalence of incomes of NHS doctors and dentists with equivalent professions, such as law and accountancy, in the private sector. Amongst its recommendations was the creation of an independent monitoring body to keep remuneration under review. Eventually, in 1971, this body became the Doctors and Dentists Review Board (DDRB).

As an aside, the Commission suggested that a sum of £500,000 per annum be put aside to remunerate 'excellence in general practice.' This would eventually become the seniority award.

Anthony Barber   1963–1964   Conservative
Health and Welfare; The Development of Community Care
Nursing Homes Act

Kenneth Robinson   1964–1968   Labour
NHS (Family Planning) Act
NHS Act; New GP Contract

The GP contract of 1966 cemented the role of the GP as an independent provider of GMS as detailed in the Statement of Fees and Allowances (the Red Book).

Group practice was encouraged through the introduction of the practice allowance which provided funding for improvements in ancillary staffing and premises resulting in a more attractive working environment and enhanced services for patients.

Prior to agreement on a new contract, GPs had threatened industrial action, including mass resignation from the NHS. Their grievances had revisited many of the unresolved issues arising from the Danckwerts Report, including disparity of pay between secondary and primary care doctors and the lack of funding for improvements in primary care.

Richard Crossman   1968–1970   Labour
Chronically Sick & Disabled Persons Act
Secretary of State for Wales took over responsibility for health and welfare in Wales
Ministry of Health and Ministry of Social Security joined to form the
    Department of Health and Social Security (DHSS)
Health Services and Public Health Act

Keith Joseph   1970–1974   Conservative

NHS Reorganisation Act; Democracy in the NHS
National Health Service (Scotland) Act
Chronically Sick and Disabled Persons (Scotland) Act

Barbara Castle   1975–1976   Labour
Health Services Act: 'Priorities for health and personal social services in
    England'
Nursing Homes Act
National Health Service Act: The Way Forward

David Ennals   1978–1979   Labour
'Patients first'
Nurses, Midwives, and Health Visitors Act
Royal Commission on Health Services Act
Medical Act

Patrick Jenkin   1979–1981   Conservative
Health Services Act: Care in the Community

Norman Fowler   1981–1987   Conservative
Promoting Better Health
Access to Medical Reports Act
National Health Service (Amendment) Act: A National Strategic Framework for
    Information Management in Hospital and Community Health Services
Mental Health Act

1987 'Promoting better health': White Paper
A statement of government policy expanding the role of general practice into
   preventive care. The paper provided the foundations for the GP contract of
   1990.

Jon Moore   1987–1988   Conservative
Department of Health and the Department of Social Security split
Community Health Councils (Access to Information) Act
Health and Medicines Act

Kenneth Clarke   1988–1990
National Health Service and Community Care Act
Access to Health Records Act
NHS Management Board reorganised into the NHS Policy Board and the NHS
   Management Executive
Children Act
Working for Patients: The Health Service Caring for the 1990s
Caring for People: Community Care in the Next Decade and Beyond

New GP Contract

The basis for the GP Contract of 1990 was the government's desire to increase
GP involvement in public health and disease prevention. There had been a
growing acknowledgement by health economists that managing ill health at
its presentation was neither clinically effective nor financially sustainable.
A pound spent on preventing disease could save many times that amount for
treating it.

The items of service elements of the Red Book were expanded to include regular health checks, management of chronic disease, such as asthma and diabetes,
and health promotion. Workload increased accordingly as GPs became proactive, rather than reactive, in managing their patients' health. A threat to remove
seniority payments was withdrawn at the last minute.

William Waldegrave   1990–1992   Conservative
Establishment of 57 NHS Trusts, rising to 270 over five years.

Virginia Bottomley   1992–1995   Conservative
Health Authorities Act
A Policy Framework for Commissioning Cancer Services
Developing NHS Purchasing and GP Fundholding: Towards a Primary Care Led NHS

Stephen Dorrell   1995–1997   Conservative
Health Service Commissioners (Amendment) Act
Community Care (Direct Payments) Act
The National Health Service: A Service with Ambitions
Primary Care: Delivering the Future

Frank Dobson   1997–1999   Labour

Abolition of GP Fundholding
Information for Health. An Information Strategy for the Modern NHS.
  1998–2005
A First-Class Service: Quality in the New NHS
Primary Care Groups (481)
Clinical Standards Board for Scotland
National Institute for Clinical Excellence
Commission for Health Improvement
Walk-in NHS Centres
National Framework for Mental Health Services
Devolution of Power to Scotland and Wales
NHS (Primary Care) Act

The NHS (Primary Care) Act of 1997 introduced choice to the way GPs wished to provide medical services. The contents introduced PMS contracts that allocated a lump sum annual budget to GP practices for the provision of all primary care services. PMS practices were ostensibly more independent, allowing for greater flexibility, within limits, in responding to patients' needs. The PMS model differed from that of GMS, which remained funded under the criteria set out in the Red Book. The global sum provided to PMS allowed for the employment of salaried doctors since it did not depend on the basic practice allowance only available to GP principals.

By 2004, nearly half of all GP practices in England and Wales were PMS.

Alan Milburn   1999–2003   Labour
Health Act; Saving Lives; Our Healthier Nation
The NHS Plan
Health and Social Care Act; Shifting the Balance of Power
NHS Reform, and Health Care Act; Delivering the NHS Plan

John Reid   2003–2005   Labour
Health and Social Care (Community Health and Standards) Act; Building the Best Choice, Responsiveness and Equity in the NHS

NHS Improvement Plan
New GP Contract

The GP Contract of 2004 was a significant piece of legislation that has affected the day to day working life of the GP, to the present day. The most significant element of the Act was the removal of the principle of 24 hours a day, 365 days a year doctor's care for patients. Responsibility for out-of-hours care, initially 7.00 p.m. to 7.00 a.m. weekdays and all day Saturday and Sunday, was transferred to the PCT.

The Act retained the founding principle of PMS, payments to practice, not principal, blurring difference between PMS and GMS contracts. PMS practices were encouraged to become GMS.

The 2004 contract accelerated the move to greater accountability and payment by results, through QOF, and cemented the position of health prevention, see 1990, at the core of general practice.

Patricia Hewitt   2005–2007   Labour
Our Health, Our Care, Our Say; Supporting people with long-term conditions
    to self-care
Local Government and Public Involvement in Health Act
Mental Health Act

Alan Johnson   2007–2009   Labour
Our NHS Our Future
NHS Constitution

Andy Burnham   2009–2010   Labour
Equity and Excellence; Liberating the NHS

The Care Quality Commission was created in 2009. Although this had little impact at first, focusing as it did on the inspection of hospitals, social, and secondary care providers, it inevitably extended its remit to primary care. The CQC's influence on raising the quality of primary care provision was to become, arguably, inversely proportional to its reducing morale within the profession.

Andrew Lansley   2010–2012   Conservative
Health and Social Care Act 2012
NHS Mandate

Clinical Commissioning Groups were created in 2012, with the aim of improving locality-based commissioning of healthcare services. The majority of the budget for primary care, 80%, was devolved to the CCGs.

Jeremy Hunt   2012–2019   Conservative
Five-Year Forward View of the NHS in England[5]
Matt Hancock   2019–2021   Conservative
Sajid Javid   2021–   Conservative

Over the lifetime of the NHS, the average tenure of the Secretary of State for Health and Social Care has been two years, with significant legislation affecting some part of the NHS every year. For 20 years (1968–1988), health, the largest employer in the country, was not deemed important enough to warrant its own secretary of state and, instead, had to do with the junior, non-cabinet position of Minister for Health. Not one secretary of state responsible for the overall strategy for health in the UK has ever had any experience of working in the health or social care sector.

---

[5] www.england.nhs.uk/wp-content/uploads/2014/10/5yfv-web.pdf

The outcome of constant change was drily captured in the following quotation attributed to Charlton Ogburn.

We trained hard, but it seemed that every time we were beginning to form up into teams we would be reorganized. Presumably the plans for our employment were being changed. I was to learn later in life that, perhaps because we are so good at organizing, we tend as a nation to meet any new situation by reorganizing; and a wonderful method it can be for creating the illusion of progress while producing confusion, inefficiency and demoralization.[6]

Of the disparate ministers in charge of the NHS, Aneurin 'Nye' Bevan deserves a special mention. No less than the *BMJ* eulogised the man, his attributes, and impact on the nation's health, in its 1960 obituary. As an example of memory mellowed by bereavement, the same journal, in somewhat less generous tones had described Bevan in 1951 as:

vicious in his attacks on the profession, his attempts to sow discord and his rudeness in negotiation would never be forgotten. He never rose above being a clever politician and at critical moments failed to become the statesman. He had done his best to make himself disliked by the medical profession, and by and large, he succeeded.

Much the same epithet could have been applied to every Minister of Health since then, with Kenneth Clarke a particular *bête noire* of the profession. Yet, Bevan, the consummate orator, did distinguish himself as a statesman in his inaugural speech to the medical profession in 1948, in which he said:

My job is to give you all the facilities, resources and help I can and then to leave you alone as professional men and women to use your skill and judgement without hindrance. Let us try to develop that partnership from now on.[7]

The relationship between Secretary of State/Minister for Health, a politician, and the medical profession was always likely to be fraught. The former provided the strategy and framework for the provision of a universal healthcare service within a budget; the latter worked to enact the provisions set out in the NHS Act of 1946, in the best interests of their patients, regardless of cost. The profession carried the plaudits whilst the minister shouldered the blame for the inevitable failings of the service.

---

[6] www.harpers.org/archive/1957/01/0007289

[7] Lancet. 1948;2:24. doi: 10.1016/S0140-6736(48)91807-8

11.4 1948–1973

An extract from the Socialist Health Association 'flyer' of February 1948 gave a taste of the expectations of the new, utopian healthcare service:[8]

> The New National Health Service
> Your new National Health Service begins on 5th July. What is it? How do you get it?
> It will provide you with all medical, dental and nursing care. Everyone—rich or poor, man, woman or child-can use it or any part of it. There are no charges, except for a few special items. There are no insurance qualifications. But it is not a "charity". You are all paying for it, mainly as taxpayers, and it will relieve your money worries in time of illness.
> Choose your Doctor Now
> You and everyone in your family will be entitled to all usual advice and treatment from a family doctor. Everyone aged 16 and over can choose his or her own doctor. A family need not all have the same doctor, but parents or guardians choose for children under 16.
> Your dealings with your doctor will remain as they are now: personal and confidential. You will visit his surgery, or he will call on you, as may be necessary. The difference is that the doctor will be paid by the Government, out of funds provided by everybody.
> Choose a doctor now- ask him to be your doctor under the new arrangements. Many will choose their present doctors. Any doctor can decline to accept a patient. If one doctor cannot accept you, ask another, or ask to be put in touch with one by the new 'Executive Council' which has been set up in your area (you can get its address from the Post Office).
> If you are already on a doctor's list under the old National Health Insurance Scheme, now is the time to decide. Get an application form for each member of the family from the doctor you choose, or from any Post Office, Executive Council Office, or public library. Fill in the forms and give them to the doctor.
> Later, your local Executive Council will send a 'medical card' to everyone who has been accepted by a doctor. If you want to change your doctor, you can do so at any time without difficulty. If you need a doctor when away from your own district, you can go to any doctor who is taking part in the new arrangements. You will not have to pay.

---

[8] www.sochealth.co.uk/national-health-service/the-sma-and-the-foundation-of-the-national-health-service-dr-leslie-hilliard-1980/the-start-of-the-nhs-1948/
https://cdm21047.contentdm.oclc.org/digital/collection/health/id/1400   COPYWRITE STATUS EXPIRED

Help to have the Scheme ready by 5th July by choosing your doctor at once.

For any further information about these arrangements, ask at the offices of the local Executive Council.

The Local Executive Council (LEC) was the administrative layer with prime oversight of primary care at the birth of the NHS. It was a continuation of and conterminous with the National Insurance Committees that had been created following the National Insurance Act of 1911. In addition to medical matters, their responsibilities included oversight of pharmacy, dental and optician services, incorporated into the NHS in 1948.

There were 140 such councils in England and Wales and 25 in Scotland. They were headed by an administrator whose responsibilities included managing the list of registered patients and processing payments to each practice. They had absolutely no influence on the way that a doctor ran his practice. Indeed, since doctors were represented on the committee, the administrator was dismissed as a subordinate whose role was purely to enact their instructions and provide timely payment of invoices. This view was to remain largely unchanged for the following four decades, despite the rare intrusion of management on such matters as the meek suggestion that doctors in practices that persistently outspent their peers on their drug budgets might wish to consider reviewing their prescribing habits!

11.5 1974–1990

That Bevan was a visionary Secretary of State for Health was confirmed in due course by the administrative organisation of the NHS, which remained broadly unchanged until the 1970s. 'The NHS Reorganisation Act, Democracy in the NHS,' introduced in 1973 by Keith Joseph, subsequently knighted, heralded the first of increasingly frequent NHS reorganisations, each with the laudable aspiration of streamlining management, reducing the layers of bureaucracy, and devolving more power to the end-user. Whether they succeeded in doing so is uncertain, but perhaps the fact that they are still trying would suggest that they have not.

The Ministry of Health was subsumed into the Department of Health and Social Security in a first attempt at providing an all-encompassing health and social care service. England was divided into 14 Regional Health Authorities (RHA) with the Secretary of State appointing their members.

Each RHA was responsible for planning regional health and social care provision, with the medical portion delivered through Area Health Authorities (AHAs). There were 90 AHAs throughout England, with a Board whose Chair the Secretary of State appointed and whose non-executive members were appointed jointly by the RHA and local authorities. An executive team consisting of a general administrator, nurse, public health doctor, and finance officer reported to the Board. Note that there were no officers from either primary or secondary care within the team.

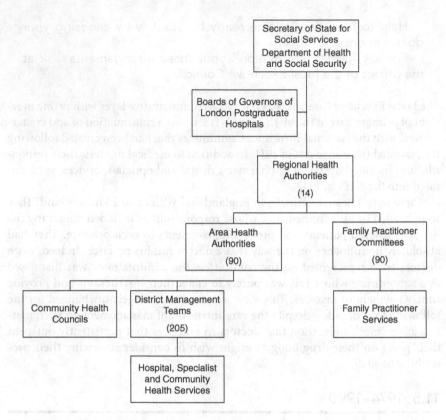

Figure 11.3 The National Health Service, England, 1974.

AHAs were expected to liaise with local civic authorities to provide integrated health and social care for their community. Implementation of policy was through Local Health Authorities (LHAs). Primary care fell under the remit of the Family Practitioner Committee (FPC), which reported directly to the RHA. FPCs managed general practitioners under the provisions of the General Medical Services contract, details of which were set out in the Statement of Fees and Allowances, the 'Red Book.'

The stated aims of the FPC were to ensure that family practitioner services were accessible to all, to improve the quality of service provided, and to be responsive to the needs of the public. However, in practice, they remained the quartermasters of primary care, responsible only for pay and rations.

By the 1980s, central government was increasingly pressuring FPCs to exert greater control over their constituents, a task one administrator likened to herding cats with degrees. The tool for doing so was an increase in the basic practice allowance, from 45% to 60% of overall GP income, allowing less leeway for income from service fee items. The policy had minimal impact on the relationship between GPs and the FPCs since the former retained eight of the 30 positions on the FPC advisory board. Nevertheless, FPCs became increasingly emboldened in setting out local healthcare strategies, moving into clinical and service areas such as:

- Introducing health services to certain vulnerable groups, such as drug addicts, AIDS sufferers, the homeless, and minority ethnic groups. Solution: increased staff training.
- Improving telephone access. Solution: no more than one medical problem could be discussed in each call.
- Improving patient information on services. Solution: practice leaflets.
- Providing additional medical services. Solution: minor surgery with derisory payments.
- Discouraging single-handed practices. Solution: curtail funding for building improvements. Branch surgeries in urban areas were discouraged, but mobile surgeries in rural areas were encouraged!
- Discouraging the use of deputising services. Solution: ignored.
- Training of staff, including doctors, in management skills. Solution: include the subject as one of the three elements of continual professional development attracting payments.
- Reducing prescribing numbers and costs. Solution: public campaign of education on the inappropriate prescribing of medications.
- Raising standards of premises and processes. Solution: none until the advent of the CQC.
- Improving IT adoption and connectivity. Solution: commercial IT providers.
- The submission of an annual report of activities by each practice. Solution: a mandatory requirement if a GP was to be paid.

11.6 1990–2004

In 1990, the FPC morphed into the FHSA, but little changed in either the function or relationship with primary care. The FHSA continued to strive to implement all the aspirations of its predecessor, with barely more success. However, the provisions of the 1990 GP contract gave the FHSA extra control over expenditure, and this was used to drive policies in the following areas:

- Organisation and Administration
  - Practices should be organised to provide safe and effective care. They should have a trained manager and an organogram detailing responsibilities and accountabilities.
  - Medical records should be organised and should include a summary of medical events and a clear record of repeat prescriptions. Access to care should be convenient and mechanisms in place should encourage patient feedback.
  - Urgent cases should be seen on the day of request. Consultation times of at least 7 minutes should be factored into the appointments system.
  - Targets of 80% of the defined population of females between the ages of 25 and 65 years should have a recorded cervical smear test.

- Policies and Procedures
  - Protocols should be formulated and used for chronic disease management of asthma, hypertension, and diabetes.
  - Health promotion and disease prevention in at least three areas, e.g. smoking cessation, obesity.
  - Repeat prescribing, including a practice drug formulary
  - Administration functions, such as making appointments, responding to requests for home visits, coping with emergencies, maintaining confidentiality, and taking messages.
  - Safety, patient and staff safety; spillage of bodily fluids; accident reporting; storing and maintenance of equipment.
- Staffing. Staff Development and Education
  - Every practice should have an adequate complement of staff, with each employee having a clear job description and adequately trained for the duties expected of them.
  - The practice 'core team' should comprise the General Practitioner, Practice Nurse, Practice Manager, reception, clerical, and secretarial staff and dispenser, where appropriate. Each should have the appropriate qualifications for the role.
- Facilities and Equipment
  - These should be of sufficient quality to facilitate efficient and customer-friendly medical care. They should comply with all national (e.g., Health and Safety) legislation, as well as local policies.
  - Emphasis on fewer well-equipped surgeries rather than a large number less well-equipped.
  - Buildings should be sited in a location convenient to their patient population and consider local transport infrastructure. They should be disability-friendly and suitable for prams and pushchairs. People with disabilities should be able to utilise washrooms, with separate washrooms for staff.
  - The waiting room should not be overseen by reception staff.
  - Posters and notice boards should be updated regularly.
  - Telephone calls should be dealt with promptly, and no more than two calls needed to access out-of-hours services.
  - The ambience of the surgery should be welcoming.
  - There should be sound barriers around reception, consulting, and treatment rooms, and screens around examination couches.
  - Heating, lighting, ventilation, fire measures, and dealing with sharps should all comply with the relevant regulations.
  - Drugs should be stored in an appropriate and secure environment.
  - Clinical equipment should include resuscitation equipment, sterilising equipment, peak flow meters, glucometer, sphygmomanometer, scales, a range of vaginal specula and proctoscopes, all of which must be properly maintained and calibrated.

- Self-Evaluation and Research
  - Practices should collect data on service provision, such as consultation rates, referrals, visits, minor surgery, contraceptive care, and compared with FHSA target standards.
  - All clinical members should participate in clinical audit.
  - Regular practice meetings should identify areas of service provision that need improving.

All the above provisions would eventually provide the basis for the Care Quality Commission inspection of GP practices.

The introduction of a more muscular FHSA and the 1990 GP contract signalled a change in the relationship between administrator and doctor. The previous laissez-faire attitude of the former had transmogrified into an Orwellian dystopia for the latter. The FHSA held the purse strings and could easily withhold payments to a practice if it did not comply with what were, after all, reasonable measures put in place to meet consumer demand. The NHS was no longer willing to sign a blank cheque.

Further restructuring of the NHS administration was put in abeyance until the Labour Party landslide victory in the 1997 election, built on the slogan 'things can only get better.'

The incoming young, vibrant Labour administration, frustrated by years in opposition, was only too keen to shine a new light on old practices. The time was ripe for change, and they set about it with gusto. Although their choice for Minister of State for Health, Frank Dobson, a Morris dancer in a suit, was not a figure that inspired innovation, he immediately set about dismantling the existing NHS structure, citing doctrinaire issues over competition and the internal market.

RHAs were reduced in number from 14 to 8 and reported directly to the NHS executive within the Department of Health, reinstated as a separate entity from Social Security in 1988.

The concept of purchaser/provider, introduced by the previous administration, though reviled by Labour in opposition, was nevertheless retained and enhanced by encouraging GPs in geographic areas to group together in Primary Care Groups (PCG), akin to super-fundholding. PCGs reported to fewer Health Authorities (HAs), now responsible for both primary- and secondary care services. Individual fundholding practices were phased out.

A tier of management was removed by the amalgamation of AHAs with DHAs, covering both primary and secondary care and including dental, optician, and pharmacy services.

Another novel introduction that would end up having far-reaching consequences for primary care was the creation of the NICE with the remit of reviewing the evidence base for therapies the NHS used in advising on whether they were clinically and fiscally effective. At that time, GPs paid little heed to it since it was thought that these reviews would focus on new and expensive medicines and clinical procedures used predominantly in hospitals.

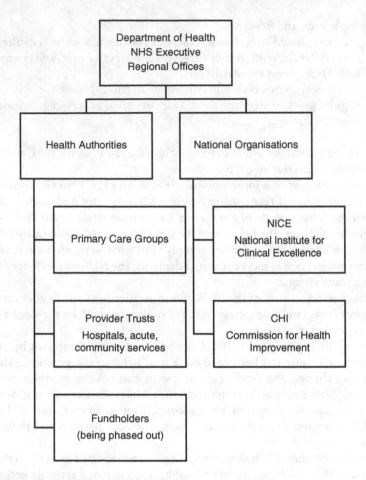

Figure 11.4 The National Health Service, England, 1998.

Fundholding had introduced doctors, the majority of whom had never had more than the most elementary training in bookkeeping, to the concept and practice of managing complex financial matters. However, unlike other commercial ventures, there was a fundamental difference: their income was essentially fixed and came from one 'customer,' the NHS. The only way that they could enhance net income was by reducing expenditure.

PCGs acted as super fundholders and initially were well subsidised. They were expected to operate within an annual budget, managing any overspend without undermining the quality of healthcare provision. The intention was to instil a degree of fiscal responsibility amongst doctors who had now become intimately enmeshed in the structure of their own administration. However, doctors generally uneducated in the finer points of business finance, such as contract formulation and tendering, needed help in such matters, and this could only be achieved by bringing in qualified expertise. Such experts were easily found. They were the newly redundant employees of the recently defunct FHSA. The revolving door of managers never stopped rotating.

PCGs may have been answerable to their stakeholders, doctors and patients alike, but they retained a basic weakness present in fundholding. Doctors were fully committed to delivering clinical care and had no desire to be involved in administration and management. Thankfully, some doctors were attracted to the role, and it was to their credit that they did it in a sensitive, collaborative manner. A growing belief began to build within the profession that doctors could always find ways to get things done, despite limitations of knowledge, experience, and time. This view did not extend to their collective opinion on professional managers. Nevertheless, commercial businesses would have been appalled at the amateur way in which these new responsibilities were assumed. The election of a medical member to chair a local PCG was very much run along the lines of whoever wanted the job could have it. That sentiment gradually changed as more open recruitment procedures were introduced, conforming with those in the civil service. Positions were widely advertised, applications sifted through, short-lists drawn, interviews held, and the outcome remained the same. Any doctor who wanted the job got it since few could be bothered to apply.

Although board and executive members of the PCG administration were salaried, many GPs volunteered their input on such matters as contracting secondary care clinical services. Protocols for secondary care referrals, originating in fundholding, were extended, and expanded. GPs were moving away from individual to collegiate practice. Although encouraged to be more involved, most GPs preferred to remain focused on their own clinical practice and were content to let their more energetic colleagues manage administrative affairs on their behalf.

By bringing the decision-making closer to the front line, the 1998 reorganisation was also intended to improve accountability. GPs could no longer blame a faceless bureaucracy for deficiencies in the service. What used to be remote management was now in their hands, closer to the population their decisions impacted. A local GP would now be directly answerable to a centenarian deemed to be medically unfit for a joint replacement. Chickens now knew exactly in which home to roost!

The Labour administration, emboldened by its first reorganisation, decided to have another go barely two years later.

In 2001, the Health Secretary, Alan Milburn, decided that management structures could be further streamlined, particularly PCGs that varied greatly in the population numbers they covered. PCGs were merged, reducing the overall number by nearly 40% and turning them from 'groups' into 'trusts,' specifically Primary Care Trusts (PCT). GPs took to the policy with such enthusiasm that it took another three years for the policy to be fully implemented. The NHS Executive and Regional Offices were abolished and replaced by 28 Strategic Health Authorities (SHA).

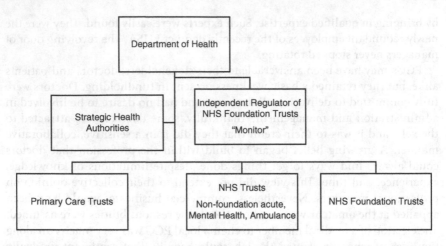

Figure 11.5 The National Health Service, England, 2004.

11.7 2004–2011

PCTs continued to have much the same management structure and, indeed, the same temporarily redundant team as the PCGs and FHSAs that preceded them. However, they were determined to establish their own unique identity to differentiate themselves from their predecessors. They needed a rebrand. The prefix 'NHS' was added to their title. As an example, the West Suffolk Primary Care Group, a mouthful in its own right, became the markedly snappier 'NHS West Suffolk Primary Care Trust.' This latest iteration relied heavily on management consultancies brought in to bring the energy and rigour of the private sector into the bloated, inward-looking public sector.

As implied in the name, the SHAs set the strategy for delivering healthcare in their geographic region and oversaw performance management of local NHS hospital trusts and PCTs.

By 2006, Alan Milburn had long since moved on to sunnier pastures, and Patricia Hewitt, feeling the need to establish her own stamp on the DH, decided that yet another reorganisation would be in order. There were still too many managers, so the number of SHAs and PCTs were further winnowed, the former pared down to ten and the latter to 152. Each PCT now covered a population of around a third of a million, compared to the 100,000 that PCGs covered. In theory, most PCTs (70%) were now coterminous with the local civic authority providing social care, allowing for an organised, efficient, and seamless transition of patients from one to the other. Mergers led to staff redundancies, which led to savings that could be ploughed back into patient services. Yet, the decade in which many of these changes occurred (1999–2009) saw the number of managers increase by 82%, from 23,000 to 42,000![9] And savings were still proving elusive.

---

[9] www.kingsfund.org.uk/projects/general-election-2010/key-election-questions/how-many-managers

PCTs remained extant for a remarkable ten years, during which they were responsible for the management and delivery of the vast majority (over 80%) of the NHS budget. The decade also saw the most significant change in the relationship between general practice and its immediate administrator. The latter moved from an enabling to a directing role. A subtle step change had taken place in general practice, where GPs had become less independent than they realised.

The official responsibilities of the PCT were:

- The implementation and management of the new GP and Dental contracts, including provision for out-of-hours services and practice-based commissioning
- The management of Payment by Results,[10] a system for paying primary- and secondary care providers a standard national tariff for each patient seen or treated
- The purchase of care for local communities from all local providers, essentially secondary care from hospitals
- The provision of community care, district nursing, occupational therapy
- The integration of local health and social care with greater use of private residential and nursing homes
- The improvement in public health, aiming to eliminate inequalities in health and life expectancy across the UK

By 2010, this abridged, and superficially manageable list had been fleshed out and expanded to over 60 statutory duties, nine domains with innumerable subsections within each domain.[11]

The domains covered:

- Overall duties
- Strategic leadership and planning
- Partnership engagement and advocacy
- Providing and securing services
- Monitoring and evaluating
- Accountability and assurance
- Workforce
- Estates and IT
- Service-specific responsibilities

Policy was transmitted from the PCT through meetings of practice managers and, rarely, clinicians. Where the latter were involved, surgery premises would close for a half-day with urgent patient requests handled by locums or out-of-hours services. Despite the novelty of ring-fenced time away from clinical duties, these

[10] https://assets.publishing.service.gov.uk/government/uploads/system/uploads/attachment_data/file/213150/PbR-Simple-Guide-FINAL.pdf

[11] Equity and excellence; Liberating the NHS. 2010. https://assets.publishing.service.gov.uk/government/uploads/system/uploads/attachment_data/file/213823/dh_117794.pdf

meetings were attended with a mood of ennui at best and profound irritation at worst. Underlying this antipathy was a sense that many proposed initiatives for improving the patient experience had been tried before, most with limited success; that the enthusiasm of the PCT officers delivering them was directly proportional to the control that they could exert on front-line staff; that PCT officers had only the most superficial grasp of the policies coming out of Richmond House; and, most importantly to GPs, that their relevance to the real problems in primary care, increasing demand and limited provision, was zero.

So how good were PCTs at making good on their exhaustive list of responsibilities?

A review published in 2018[12] was somewhat damning, citing resistant ingrained cultures, poor management, and poor communication with all stakeholders, public and doctors alike. In short, the principle of devolution of funding and management to meet local needs was found wanting.

External audits of the performance of individual PCTs by national bodies, such as the Commission for Healthcare Improvement (CHI), the Healthcare Commission, the Care Quality Commission, the Audit Commission, and the Department of Health, produced mixed findings.

- With regard to the commissioning of services, a world-class commissioning programme that the DH introduced in 2008 only ran for two years, and although it reported demonstrable improvements (39%) in performance against local priorities, the time was too short to see if this would be sustained.
- Statistics on life expectancy, infant mortality, cancer survival, and hospital-acquired infections showed improvements, but correlation with the work of PCTs was dubious. For example, the use of statins with their known benefits regarding cardiovascular-related morbidity and mortality had increased exponentially following loss of patent and the increased availability of cheaper generics. Annual prescriptions for statins increased from 0.3 million in 1981 to 22 million in 2003 and 52 million in 2008.
- Waiting times for hospital services, including admissions and A&E, had definitely come down, but again, this was likely to have been due to the massive increase in NHS funding under the Labour administration.
- PCTs had managed to balance the books (see the point above) and, indeed, had an overall net surplus, £1.3 billion by 2010.
- PCTs were marginally better at managing community services, such as district nursing, compared to private providers (94% vs 90%) as the CQC reported. In recognition of this finding, the responsibility for providing such services was removed from the PCT in 2013.

PCTs did not enhance their reputation by being seduced by the private sector in employing management consultants to shed new light on old problems. The

---

[12] UK essays. Impact of primary care trusts. Nov 2018. www.ukessays.com/assignments/health-social-primary-care-trusts-impact.php?vref=1

National Audit Office estimated that in 2007, PCTs spent £132.6 million on management consultants. The House of Commons Health Committee report for 2008–2009 was aghast at the unaccountability of these costs and urged the head of the NHS to investigate the figures.[13] The NHS heeded their instruction but with minimal impact on the outlay. By 2014–2015, consultancy costs for NHS Trusts and NHS foundation trusts alone, excluding CCGs, had ballooned to £419 million,[14] equivalent to the cost of employing 10,000 nurses.

An example of whether management consultants gave value for money was provided by Suffolk, where, in 2007, the PCT appointed McKinsey[15] to ascertain the causes impeding patient access to medical services. A team of sharply dressed youths was despatched to various practices throughout the area, where they observed the reception area during a typical working day. Representatives of each practice subsequently attended a half-day workshop involving whiteboards covered with reams of multi-coloured post-it notes. Weeks later, the McKinsey report concluded that the solution lay in increasing the number of phone lines, employing more receptionists, and offering more appointments! The cost of this invaluable advice? Between £350–500,000, the PCT was somewhat reticent about providing an exact figure but professed that it was money well spent. None of the recommendations were implemented, due to lack of funding.

11.8 2012–

The year 2010 brought another election, another government, a Conservative/ Liberal coalition, another reorganisation. Andrew Lansley, who had been waiting in the wings as Shadow Minister for Health for six years, set about dismantling the existing NHS structure, citing doctrinaire issues as reasons for doing so (see Keith Joseph and Frank Dobson above). Lansley's central tenet was to make GPs, those within the NHS most intimately involved in the delivery of healthcare, responsible for administering the majority of the NHS budget. Devolving fiscal responsibility to the coalface would lead to greater efficiencies and improvements in the patient experience. A collateral benefit would be the removal of yet another tier of management, the PCT, which would no longer administer GP budgets. Reducing management levels was politically popular since much of the blame for the previously ailing NHS had been laid at the millipedian feet of the multitude of managers within the organisation.

Lansley's solution was the abolition of all SHAs and PCTs, to be replaced by NHS England Area Teams and CCGs. Local councils reclaimed jurisdiction over public health. A profession that could see no need to dismantle the existing status quo greeted with horror the Health and Social Care Act 2012. Overall,

---

[13] https://publications.parliament.uk/pa/cm200809/cmselect/cmhealth/28/28.pdf

[14] NHS improvement 2017. Freedom of information request. www.england.nhs.uk/wp-content/uploads/2019/10/FOl_NHS_spend_on_external_consultants.pdf

[15] McKinsey & Company, a global management consultancy, founded in 1926, advising on strategic management to corporations, governments, and other organisations.

the current system had become embedded and seemed to be working fairly for doctors and patients alike. Strains that did exist in the relationship between PCT managers and GPs only arose when the former periodically touted 'efficiency' initiatives, a euphemism for cutting costs. Few of these 'innovations in practice' gained traction since most had been tried before and found wanting. Lansley seemed to willfully misinterpret the relationship and functions of manager and the managed, by proposing that the latter could undertake both roles. The profession felt that the proposals in the Act were an unnecessary, destructive, and costly way to address a problem that no longer existed. By and large, PCTs and GPs had learned to coexist in a manner not dissimilar to the Korean armistice, hostile but stable.

Initially, those officers who had volunteered for the new CCG Board shadowed their counterparts in the PCT for a year, in the hope that this would allow for a seamless transition before CCGs took on executive duties in April 2013.

Here is a little historical vignette of how the FPC managed their GPs in the 1980s. There was a falling out amongst the partners in an isolated, rural, three-doctor practice. GP partnerships can be worse than marriages once things start to fall apart. The partners disagreed on several issues, but the main one was ambition. Two of the partners were happy with the existing strategy for the practice, the third was eager to push through a raft of innovations and frustrated by being repeatedly outvoted in practice meetings. Eventually, they decided that the resolution of this situation lay in dissolving the partnership and expelling the dissident doctor. Typical of many practices at that time, there was no practice agreement in place and, thus, no covenants preventing the rebellious doctor from setting up another GP practice in the village. Patients liked and respected him and had no desire to uproot and move away. So, the outcast rented a building 400 yards from his previous practice and stuck his plate on the wall.

The chief executive of the local Family Practitioner Committee had been in post for many years and was contentedly looking forward to a well-earned retirement. He was a highly experienced individual, well respected by the doctors in the district for the sage and calm manner with which he had dealt with their frequent queries and complaints. As the situation in this dysfunctional practice was hurtling towards its denouement, he had to be informed; the prime duty of the FPC was to ensure that there was adequate and safe provision of medical care for the local population. When his attempts at mediation failed, he sanctioned the breakup of the practice. But what to do about the division of patients between the now two distinct practices? His practical solution was to personally go through the filing cabinets of the old surgery, grabbing handfuls of Lloyd George envelopes at random and hurling them into some cardboard boxes. When he thought that he had enough, he carried them around the corner to the new surgery, deposited them on the floor of the waiting room, and with a terse 'that should be enough,' turned around and left. And, thus, the patients were apportioned between the two practices!

Now that was streamlined management!

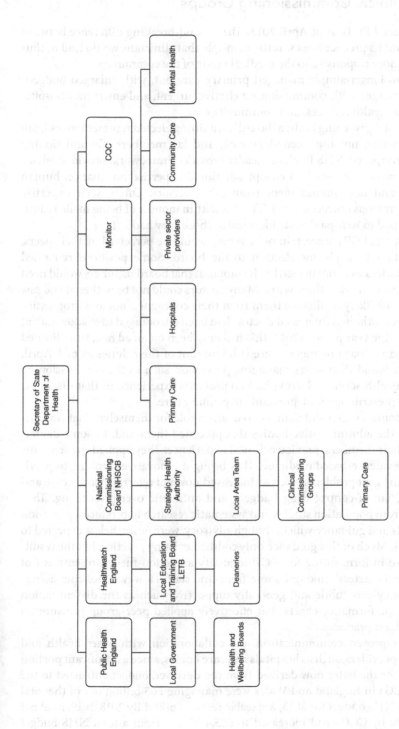

Figure 11.6 The National Health Service, England, 2012.[16]

[16] NHS White paper 2011. https://nhswhitepaper.wordpress.com/2011/08/05/labour-ridicules-david-camerons-nhs-structure/

11.8.1 Clinical Commissioning Groups

CCGs replaced PCTs as of April 2013. The ground-breaking difference between the CCG and its predecessors was the principle that clinicians would lead it, thus making it more responsive to the medical needs of the community.

CCGs no longer simply managed primary care but, with enlarged budgets, were also charged with commissioning elective, urgent, and emergency hospital care, mental health services, and community care.

CCGs had a governing body, a 'board' containing elected representatives from general practice, nursing, secondary care, and lay members. Commissioning Support Groups, via NHS England Leader Provider Framework, provided advice and encouraged the board to co-opt additional expertise on finance, human resources, and data management from other sectors. Often, such expertise resided in previous officers of the PCT who, within months of being made redundant, returned to well-paid posts identical to those they had left.

Initially, local GPs, uncertain of how they would be perceived by their peers, were reluctant to apply for election to the board. Some positions remained unfilled. Matters were not helped by the proposal that board members would need to seek re-election every three years. Many doctors could not be bothered and saw the role as one likely to alienate them from their colleagues, not as a progressive career move. Although interested doctors had been encouraged to shadow staff at the PCT for the year prior to 2013, this had only been on an ad hoc, time-limited basis, so many Board members were still ignorant of their duties as of 1 April. Individuals found themselves managing portfolios, such as the commissioning of mental health services, having had no previous experience in that discipline other than prescribing antidepressants in primary care.

In due course, CCGs did manage to define a role for themselves that was distinct from the administrative bodies that preceded them and, to some degree, based on their members' previous clinical experience. They applied the scientific rigours of evidence-based medicine. They brought innovative thinking to previously intransigent problems, such as increased hospital referrals, both acute and outpatient, out-of-control drug budgets, and antibiotic over-prescribing. They used data from population studies and systematic research to produce a profusion of protocols and guidance which, though advisory, were nevertheless expected to be followed. Much of this guidance only codified existing practice, but the resulting increase in form-filling for a GP to justify an action-fuelled resentment of their 'puppet-masters' amongst some front-line staff. However, policing adherence to policy was subtle and generally supportive, such as the dissemination of practice performance charts that effectively applied peer-group pressure on non-compliant practices.

CCGs improved communication and collaboration with other health and social care providers, such as hospitals and care homes, since a significant portion of income for the latter now derived from the devolved budget entrusted to the former. CCGs in England and Wales were managing £65 billion out of the total £95 billion NHS budget for 2013, a sizeable responsibility! By 2018/2019, total net expenditure by CCGs had increased to £85.4 billion from a total NHS budget of £112.7 billion. Of that total, £7 billion went to primary care, that is, financing the running of GP practices. The net running costs of the CCGs themselves accounted for £1.1 billion.

CCGs were responsible for commissioning health services to meet all the reasonable requirements of patient care, covering:

- Urgent and emergency care, including A&E, ambulance services. and NHS 111
- Out-of-hours primary medical services, except where practices had retained this responsibility
- Elective hospital care
- Community health services, such as rehabilitation services, speech and language therapy, continence services, wheelchair services, and home oxygen services, but not public health services, such as health visiting and district nursing
- Maternity and newborn services, excluding neonatal intensive care
- Children's healthcare services, both mental and physical health
- Services for people with learning disabilities
- Mental health services, including psychological therapies
- Infertility services

All of these were overseen, licensed, and regulated by Monitor,[17] now part of NHS Improvement,[18] which ensured that no actions were taken against patients' interests.

Thereafter, the responsibilities of CCGs and doctors generally covered seven broad headings (my summary comments in italics) including:

- Commissioning
  - *Matching demand with supply*
- Clinical focus and adding value
  - *Prioritising where to match demand with supply*
  - *Engaging with patients and communities; keeping everyone on board when matching demand with supply*
- Delivering quality services and improving productivity
  - *Innovation, quality improvements, and training in matching demand with supply*
- Organisational, governance, and financial responsibilities
  - *Central leadership and control, through protocols and contracts, in matching demand with supply*
- Working and commissioning collaboratively
  - *Ensuring that all stakeholders were committed to matching demand with supply*
- Leading individually and collectively
  - *Good leaders in driving and meeting the above aspirations*

---

[17] www.legislation.gov.uk/ukpga/2012/7/part/3/chapter/1/enacted

[18] www.gov.uk/government/news/monitor-is-now-part-of-nhs-improvement

The following functions remained outside the remit of the CCG:[19]

- Certain services commissioned directly by NHS England
- Health improvement services commissioned by local authorities
- Health protection and promotion services provided by Public Health England

There were 211 CCGs in England in 2013, reduced through mergers to 195 by 2018. Population numbers covered by each CCG varied greatly from 78,000 for Corby to 1.3 million for Birmingham and Solihull.

A representative CCG website, North East Essex Clinical Commissioning Group,[20] with a budget of £437 million for the year 2020/2021, gives a more detailed account of the strategy and activities of an average CCG. The website set out the CCG's vision and values, both peppered with anodyne jargon such as 'service user centred,' 'embedding personalisation of care,' 'inclusiveness,' and 'integrity.' As with much else in NHS management, the text merely laid out in corporate language what had always been an innate activity of the professionals delivering the healthcare of the nation. The commissioning intentions for 2021/2022 were stated in a lengthy, detailed document[21] under the following headings (additional comments the author's) in areas pertinent to GP practices, such as:

- Our integrated healthcare system (ICS)
- Achieving health equality
- Our alliances
- Our localities
- Our CCGs
- Our PCNs
  - Training programmes on clinical leadership
  - Implementation of the NHS Long-Term Plan
  - Integration of mental health services. *In practice, this included funding of many community mental health professionals based in GP practices.*
  - Supporting Social Prescribing Schemes. *An initiative to place an advisor in each practice to perform much the same tasks as the Citizens Advice Bureau[22] did on social benefits and housing.*
- Aligning incentives to deliver change
  - Prioritising and maintaining funding for mental health, *This became an ever-increasing proportion of daily demand for primary care services.*

[19] Clinical Commissioning Groups. Roger Henderson, Cathy Jackson. Nov 2016. https://patient.info/doctor/clinical-commissioning-groups-ccgs#nav-2

[20] www.neessexccg.nhs.uk/

[21] www.neessexccg.nhs.uk/uploads/files/SNEE%20Commissioning%20intentions%20letter%2021-22%20v1.9.pdf

[22] www.citizensadvice.org.uk/

- Quality improvement
  - Focusing on 13 clinical areas, including learning disability and autism, mental health, special educational needs, safeguarding, and dementia
- Strategic Programmes
- Integrated Care (*End of Life, Urgent, and Elective*)
- Mental Health, Learning Disabilities, and Autism
- Primary Care
  - Mainly focusing on integration of GP practices with the primary care network and delivering national service specifications on structured medical review, enhanced health in care homes, anticipatory care, early cancer diagnosis, CVD prevention and diagnosis, and tackling neighbourhood inequalities
- Ambulance 999 Commissioning
- Pathology
- Personal Health Budgets (PHBs)
- Medicines Management and Prescribing. *Ensuring that doctors adhered to guidance and protocols on prescribing*
- Specialised Commissioning
- Enablers (IT, Estates, and Workforce)

The document aimed at keeping all stakeholders, including the public, informed of the activities of the CCG. Whether it succeeded depended on those stakeholders being aware of its existence. Few GPs bothered to read it since, in practice, little of its content directly impacted their day-to-day activities. GPs, apart from those with roles within the CCG, continued to view the activities of their CCG as largely irrelevant to their working lives. An evaluation of GP views of clinically led commissioning in 2017 tended to confirm this view.[23]

NHS England assessed CCG performance annually, grading them under the same categories as those of the Care Quality Commission: Outstanding, Good, Requires Improvement, and Inadequate. Of the 191 CCGs reviewed in 2019/20, 22 were outstanding, 104 good, 56 required improvement, and 9 were inadequate.[24]

Not enough time has passed to judge whether CCGs have been any more effective than their predecessors in delivering 21st-century healthcare at 20th-century prices. Early reports would suggest that they were struggling to do so, with the National Audit Office report for 2018[25] providing some dismal reading.

---

[23] Moran V, Checkland K, Coleman A, Spooner S, Gibson J, Sutton M. General practitioners' views of clinically led commissioning: cross-sectional survey in England. BMJ Open. 2017 Jun 8;7(6):e015464. doi: 10.1136/bmjopen-2016-015464. PMID: 28596217; PMCID: PMC5734491.

[24] www.england.nhs.uk/wp-content/uploads/2020/11/ccg-annual-assessment-report-19-20.pdf

[25] A review of the role and costs of clinical commissioning groups. NHS England National Audit Office, Dec 2018. www.nao.org.uk/wp-content/uploads/2018/12/Review-of-the-role-and-costs-of-clinical-commissioning-groups.pdf

11.8.2 Primary Care Networks

In the meantime, general practice was continuing to adapt and evolve. That old stalking horse of manpower shortages had once again come to the fore. Practices continued to struggle to recruit new doctors. Factors cited included the increasing mobility of newly qualified GPs eschewing partnerships for less constrained and stressful careers as salaried GPs, part-time working, and individuals seeking a portfolio career with more variety in their working week. An improved work-life balance was the mantra of the times. In turn, the drop in GP recruitment placed greater pressure on those still in post, leading to burnout and early retirement.

GP practices sought various means by which they could address workforce deficiencies. Robust neighbours took over some failing practices. Commercial enterprises, such as Virgin and Care UK, took over some practices. Others developed a more collaborative approach in creating 'super-partnerships,' federations, and local primary care networks. All these measures provided no more than a temporary panacea since the underlying problem remained the same, not enough doctors. They also resulted in a dilution of doctor/patient relationships, with the role of the former increasingly replaced by ancillary healthcare professionals, such as nurse practitioners or paramedics.

The division between purchaser and provider became increasingly blurred. Larger practices sought additional income streams by competing with and tendering for services that secondary care had traditionally provided. Umbrella organisations, such as the National Association of Primary Care (NAPC),[26] a division of the NHS Confederation, were created to assist such entrepreneurial practices in achieving these aims.

All of this led to perhaps the most far-reaching changes in general practice that have taken place to date, primary care networks.

The proposal for PCNs first appeared in *NHS Five Year Forward View*,[27] published by NHS England in 2014. The document set out to address the underfunding of the service during the austerity decade, 2010–2020, leading to widespread workforce shortages, budgetary overspends, increased demand on hospital services, and global failures to meet outcome targets, such as hospital waiting times. In return for an extra £20.5 billion five-year funding settlement, NHS England was asked to draw up a long-term plan to improve the service and increase productivity. Primary care was asked to provide 50 million extra appointments a year, and 20,000 extra staff would be recruited to achieve this aim. Funding was provided through a DES, the ring-fenced Additional Role Reimbursement Scheme (ARRS).[28]

---

[26] https://napc.co.uk/

[27] www.england.nhs.uk/publication/nhs-five-year-forward-view/

[28] www.england.nhs.uk/wp-content/uploads/2019/12/network-contract-des-additional-roles-reimbursement-scheme-guidance-december2019.pdf

11.8.3 General Practice Forward View

A strategic plan for primary care, *General Practice Forward View*,[29,30] followed in 2016. The visionary document was well received by the profession since it recognised and sought to address the twin concerns of GPs, burdensome workload and overbearing bureaucracy.

The introduction of GP Forward View by Simon Stevens, CEO NHS, emphasised the vital role of general practice in delivering healthcare to the nation, stating, 'There is arguably no more important job in modern Britain than that of the family doctor,' and went on to include, 'if general practice fails, the whole NHS fails.' Like Cinderella, general practitioners had finally moved from housemaid to princess. Redemption had arrived after decades of underfunding and low morale.

At the heart of the document lay the recognition that GP workload was unsustainable, and that time had to be freed for doctors to undertake their core duty, the holistic care of their patients. Initiatives to achieve this aim included:

Investment

The primary care budget would increase from £9.6 billion in 2015/2016 to over
   £12 billion in 2020/2021, a 14% increase in real terms
£500 million over five years, to help struggling practices
A new funding formula to replace Carr-Hill (see Chapter 12, 'Finance'), to better
   reflect practice workload, including extra for rural practices and those in
   deprived areas of the country
A resolution to the crippling rises in the price of medical indemnity insurance

Workforce

An increase in GP numbers, 5,000 doctors by 2020
35 national ambassadors promoting the role of the general practitioner
A simplification of the routes for retired GPs to return to practice, with the aim
   of attracting at least 500 to return over five years
500 doctors to be recruited from overseas
An increase in numbers of other associate staff: 3,000 mental health therapists,
   1,500 pharmacists, and 1,000 physician associates
Support for existing staff: £16 million for mental health support for GPs.
   Improvement in training for all staff

Workload

An end to hospitals shifting work to general practice
A reduction in the frequency of CQC inspections

---

[29] www.england.nhs.uk/gp/gpfv/about/

[30] Mathers N. General practice forward view: a new charter for general practice? Br J Gen Pract. 2016 Oct;66(651):500–1. doi: 10.3399/bjgp16X687121. PMID: 27688486; PMCID: PMC5033273.

The authors of the report felt that the vessel to deliver these aspirations would be the primary care network, a condensation and collaboration of neighbouring practices embedded within each CCG area. The average PCN would cover 30–50,000 patients. Productivity would improve, driven by economies of scale, adoption of new technologies, and adoption of clinical governance. PCNs would become the sole providers of primary care commissioned by CCGs. The line of reporting would be simplified and shortened. It was a win-win situation for all parties.

In 2018, the RCGP published its assessment on progress.[31] They were not happy. Their survey of GPs revealed that only 17% felt that *GP Forward View* would make a positive difference to general practice in England; a rather depressing 77% expected workload to worsen over the following years.

NHS England was mandated to ensure that all GP practices throughout England became part of a PCN, 1,300 in total, by July 2019. Although this was a voluntary scheme, the financial incentives, as with historical initiatives such as fundholding, were such that few practices chose to opt-out. Over £2.0 billion in extra funding was provided, through directed enhanced payment DES (see Chapter 12, 'Finance') to create and maintain PCN administration and improved patient services.

An update of the GP contract between NHS England and the BMA was negotiated and published in February 2020. This included the delivery of key standards in seven areas (funded by the extra DES), in addition to the previous duties of a GP (my comments in italics). To a great degree, these were a rehash and beefing up of pre-existing QOF indicators.

- Structured medication reviews
  - *Regular revue of polypharmacy in patients with co-morbidities. Rarely leads to a reduction in the medication load. Reviews can be undertaken by pharmacists/clinical pharmacists.*
- Enhanced health in care homes (with community services)
  - *Recognition of the healthcare burden in primary care arising from the increasing numbers of the elderly in care homes. Review and care of these patients had always been patchy and almost an afterthought in many practices. However, by 2018, they constituted over 90% of home visits.*
  - *Inter-disciplinary discussions should be confirmed in a written care plan kept by the surgery.*
- Anticipatory care
  - *Consulting with patients, again mostly the elderly with long-term chronic health conditions, in formulating a healthcare plan for any future deterioration in their condition. In its simplest form, this might be a Do Not Resuscitate directive; on a national level, an Advanced Power of Attorney for health. These discussions should be confirmed in a written care plan kept by the surgery.*

---

[31] GP forward assessment of progress year 2. www.rcgp.org.uk/policy/general-practice-forward-view.aspx

- Personalised care
  - *No change from that already provided.*
- Supporting early cancer diagnosis
  - *Building on the two-week-wait referral system, with the aspiration of expanding primary care access to investigations.*
- Cardiovascular disease case finding
  - *Cardiovascular risk scoring, blood pressure monitoring, pulse taking.*
- Tackling health inequalities
  - *Improving access and help for the homeless, poor, and other deprived groups society neglects. This had already been an element of CQC inspections.*

All of the above had traditionally been an established part of a GP's workload.

As of 2021, GP practices continued to operate independently within their PCN. Anecdotal reports from GPs suggested little observable impact on the functioning of their practice. They welcomed the funding of additional resources in social care, mental health, physiotherapy, and pharmacy but decried the lack of flexibility in allowing for the bespoke, as intended in the NHS plan, needs of their community. The package of help offered was not necessarily the help needed and came with bureaucratic strings attached; additional staff had strictly defined duties, work had to be recorded and justified and they had to be supervised.

PCNs were an example of top-down reorganisation, as opposed to GP federations that had arisen from grassroots. Federations began as a loose liaison between local partnerships, again aiming to develop and share ideas for improved patient services. Over the second decade of the 2000s, they gradually extended their remit to providing services in the community that had previously been undertaken in hospitals, as well as extended, evening and weekend, and out-of-hours services.

GP federations were well regarded by their participants. Their success was based on stakeholder engagement, good communication between practices, excellent IT connectivity, a streamlined management structure, and a not-for-profit business model.

Unlike PCNs, partaking practices funded them, usually through a small annual levy based on the practice list. Additional funding was provided by central innovation funds, such as the Prime Minister's Challenge Fund.[32]

The management structure for a federation was leaner than that for CCGs and PCN, with greater GP participation on the board.[33]

By 2020, the move towards consolidation of GP practices had resulted in CCGs across England overseeing and negotiating with an eclectic mix of primary care providers, including single-handed practices, independent group practices,

---

[32] The Prime Minister's Challenge Fund was established in Oct 2013 with £50 million for NHS England to help improve access to general practice and stimulate innovative ways of providing primary care services.

[33] https://suffolkfed.org.uk/wp-content/uploads/2017/03/Suffolk-GP-Fed-Members-Agreement-2.pdf

commercial practices, primary care networks, and GP federations. The pyramid of NHS administration may have been flattened, but it had also been considerably broadened.

It is difficult to determine whether CCGs have been any more successful than their predecessors in improving the overall well-being of the UK population. No robust quantitative or qualitative evaluations published to date have investigated the effectiveness of CCGs in healthcare delivery. To a degree, they did prove their worth during the COVID pandemic when they quickly responded to a rapidly changing scenario, by organising 'hot' hubs for seeing potentially infected patients and, later, commissioning vaccination hubs.

11.9 SUMMARY

The relationship between GPs and their immediate 'employer' has differed little over the decades, the latter generally having only an intermittent impact on the running of the daily surgery. From the first to the latter half of the NHS's duration, a subtle but significant alteration within that relationship occurred; the administrative arm had reported to the clinical for the first 40 years, the reverse for the past 30. The administrative bodies moved from being an enabler of local medical services to being a director. Doctors working in general practice during that transition found it difficult adapting to that change. Although not necessarily yearning nostalgically for a golden past, many felt that they knew what was best for their patients and resented the PCT and CCG subverting their traditional role of patient advocate.

The first cohort of doctors that joined the NHS did so in a social environment where their vocation, education, and above all, the title 'Doctor' resulted in the general public (including civil servants working in the LEC and FPC) holding them in high esteem and, often, fear. It took a brave clerk to question any financial claim a doctor on the local performers list submitted. Patient list sizes were inaccurate; services performed, unaccountable; duty hours, flexible. The administrators were placed in an invidious role administering a significant number of virtual independent small businesses, run by self-employed contractors who provided services and submitted their annual report on a complex and lengthy template. All saw their job as primarily ensuring payments for those services. As time went by, they became more proficient and, with increasing confidence, slowly introduced the checks and balances essential in any 'purchaser/provider' relationship. Eventually, those administering primary care became as professional as the profession that they were administering.

Inevitably, checks and balances segued into more detailed contracts against which performance was regularly reviewed. The unwelcome intrusion on doctors' working lives by the need for accountability against increasingly defined standards did impact the overall performance of doctors, their staff, and most importantly, their patients. Surgeries operating from domestic kitchens or garden sheds were forced into providing premises suitable for a 20th-century medical service. Provision of primary care was placed on a more professional, albeit increasingly commercial footing.

Successive reorganisations of the lower tiers of the NHS management structure have, over time, led to an increase in micromanagement of GP surgeries and a gradual erosion of the GP's status as an independent contractor. Reasonably in any commercial enterprise, the buyer would require the purchased goods and services to be of a certain acceptable standard. For the first 40 years of the NHS, this principle was not applied, and it took management some time to realise that. When they did, it was with the energy of Communist China embracing capitalism.

Apart from the short-lived experiment of fundholding, most doctors remained committed solely to their clinical duties, devoting little time to administration. A restless, albeit energetic minority did move into management roles, particularly following the creation of PCGs and, latterly, CCGs. They brought with them a practical insight into the role of those whom they were managing. However, few could maintain a dual role for long, and those that chose to move full-time into management soon found themselves immersed in the conundrum of trying to deliver ever-increasing services with ever-diminishing budgets. Nonetheless, some went on to forge highly successful careers in roles such as PCT CEO or CCG Medical Director. Such changes of title tended to rest uneasily on their colleagues at the coalface.

Currently, many GPs are questioning the sustainability of their enshrined role as independent contractors. The profession finds it increasingly difficult to recruit partners, as evinced by the proportion of salaried doctors working in primary care. The next phase of the NHS could well see GPs becoming part of a diverse employed workforce directly managed by a CCG or equivalent, not dissimilar to that currently operating in secondary care. Whether such a move would benefit doctors and patients remains to be seen.

12

Finance

Don't think that money does everything or you are going to do everything for money.

(Voltaire)

12.1 INTRODUCTION

In 1949, the first year of the NHS, UK government healthcare spending amounted to £13.9 billion (adjusted for UK inflation to 2019 levels). This represented around 3.5% of GDP at that time. In 2018, the respective figures were £167 billion and 10%.[1] Spending accelerated between 1997 to 2018 when expenditure, in real terms, nearly doubled. These figures did not include additional expenditure through the private sector via private medical clinics, voluntary health insurance, and charity and employment schemes. When these were factored in, total healthcare expenditure for the UK in 2019 amounted to £214 billion or £3,227 per person.

The majority (98.9%) of the NHS budget is raised through general taxation and National Insurance, with (in England only) about 0.5% arising through prescription charges and 0.6% through an eclectic mix of patient charges, such as on overseas visitors, insurers, car parking, telephone services, dental care, and private treatment on NHS premises.

In 2019, around 80% of the NHS budget for England was allocated to 191 CCGs covering a population of around 56 million. Allocations to the seven local health boards in Wales, 14 Health Boards in Scotland and five Local Commissioning Groups in Northern Ireland occurred separately. Collectively, CCGs in England bore the responsibility (£100 billion) for commissioning local medical services, both primary and secondary care. Each CCG share of the pot was calculated using a 'weighted caption' formula that took into account such factors as general and acute healthcare needs, maternity, mental health, community services, prescribing, geographic isolation, and health inequalities.[2]

---

[1] Office of National Statistics. www.ons.gov.uk/peoplepopulationandcommunity/healthand socialcare/healthcaresystem/bulletins/ukhealthaccounts/2018

[2] Fair Shares. A guide to NHS allocations. www.england.nhs.uk/wp-content/uploads/2020/ 02/nhs-allocations-infographics-feb-2020.pdf

DOI: 10.1201/9781003256465-12

The remaining 20% of the global NHS budget in England covered capital spending and national programmes, such as health screening, education and training for the NHS workforce, and budgets for special health authorities, for example, the NHS Blood and Transplant Authority and the NHS Litigation Authority.

Since 2013, the majority of hospital revenues (80–90%) has come from GP commissioned contracts, with the remainder from NHS England, other NHS Trusts, training levies for medical and non-medical staff, and nurse education services (see Chapter 9, 'Education and Training'), the levy for research and development, and from staff, visitors, or patients for services provided, for example, catering, car parking. or accommodation.

Put simply, through CCGs, GPs in England are responsible for around £80 billion of spending funded through the taxation of their fellow citizens and, of course, themselves. Or, to put it another way, they have around £1,428 to spend each year on the healthcare needs of each and every individual in the country.

12.2 WHAT WAS THE MONEY SPENT ON?

The annual report for 2018/2019 from a representative CCG, North East Essex,[3] detailed a budget of £542 million covering 355,000 people, and 32 GP practices. They spent 46% of the budget on secondary care, 10% on primary care, 10% on mental health and learning disabilities, 12% on drugs and medical devices, with the remainder on community and palliative care, ambulance, and the out-of-hours service.

The distribution of funds by the CCG differed marginally from the PCOs that preceded it. The central tenet of the 2004 GMS contract, the devolution of purchasing power to front-line GPs, was little more than a chimera.

12.3 GP REMUNERATION

Despite being classified as self-employed; the majority of a GP's income comes from a public body, the NHS. Each GP principal has around 2,000 employers, their patients, theoretically contributing individually through National Insurance contributions and general taxation, via one accounts department, the NHS. General practice can be considered as a semi-autonomous department within an organisation, comprising staff, premises, and equipment, responsible for a particular function, the delivery of healthcare to the community.

A GP's income is calculated on the notional sum required for the provision of general medical services and, latterly, personal medical services, based on the number of patients on the doctor's list, the provision of services outside GMS, and the reimbursements for practice premises and administration costs. The proportion that each of these areas contributed to overall income has varied over the years, in particular at times of new GP contracts in 1948, 1966, 1990, and 2004.

---

[3] www.neessexccg.nhs.uk/uploads/files/Annual%20Report%202018.19%20updated%20 28.05.19%20JK%20CREATIVE%20REPRO%20VERSION%282%29.pdf

The headline-grabbing sums of money involved in running primary care hide the immeasurably complex, archaic calculations that eventually lead to an individual GP's take-home pay.

12.3.1 Pre-1948

A limited number of specialised people in possession of certain attributes and skills prized by the general public, doctors, have had their services variously valued throughout history. The contract for payment for services in the UK, up to 1948, generally existed on a personal level, between the individual providing the service and the person receiving it. Payment was in cash or kind. However, prior to the NHS and its founding principle of free at the point of delivery, mechanisms already existed to ameliorate the heavy burden of medical costs, at a time when, almost by definition, those needing the service were least able to afford it.[4]

In the late 19th century, in the spirit of Victorian industrialist philanthropy, 'clubs' were set up for workers to donate a small proportion of their wages to a central pool used to retain a doctor to provide healthcare. Critically, workers, and not their dependents, were covered. Although nearly all women and children were excluded, anecdotal tales abound of conscientious doctors treating individuals and either not charging at all for their services or coming to an agreement on discounts, deferrals, or payment in kind. Doctors were only too aware that when dealing with life and death, one could not have the same hard-nosed commercial attitudes of other professional groups, such as lawyers or bankers.

The Victorian scheme was not entirely altruistic and was more analogous to an occupational health service, fashioned to maintain the workforce in a healthier and, thus, more productive state. The employer and employee both benefitted, as did the doctor who, although underpaid, could at least rely on a regular income paid as a stipend based on the number of employees enrolled in the scheme or, in other words, a capitation fee.

12.3.2 From 1948–1966

It was these locality-based schemes and the principle of everyone contributing regardless of immediate personal need that provided the foundations for the eventual National Health Service and the principle of central funding through a hypothecated tax on employer and employee, National Insurance.

The government had a budget, an annual fixed pool of money or global sum, to pay GPs to look after the population of the UK. Remuneration of individual GPs was based on the simple calculation of global sum divided by the number of patients. Thus, the doctor's income was directly proportional to the number of patients, a situation that encouraged the continuance of the closed shop and resulting large lists.

The system was not ideal and contained inherent inconsistencies, not the least being access to patients. Thus, inner-city doctors in areas of higher population

4 www.bmj.com/content/336/7655/1216

density were likely to have high list numbers and high incomes, albeit with corresponding high workloads, whilst the opposite was true in rural areas. This discrepancy was a source of irritation to both groups of doctors in the early years of the NHS. Other areas of contention included poor infrastructure, no incentives for continuing professional development, and a general feeling of being undervalued especially in comparison to hospital colleagues. This resentment gradually built up a momentum for change in GP remuneration and working conditions, culminating in the 1966 Family Doctor Charter[5] and its intricate offspring, the SFA, the 'Red Book.'

Enacted in 1966, the charter upturned the previous funding formula by introducing a basic practice allowance, a universal fixed sum per GP principal, over and above the capitation fee. Additional funding was added for non-core services, paid by results, under the euphemistic term 'item of service payments,' and the reimbursement at up to 70% of staff costs.

The independent Doctors and Dentists Review Body, set up in 1960 but whose remit was not enshrined in law until 1971, suggested an increase in the global sum of £24 million to cover these added elements, but due to recessionary-driven financial constraints, the sum was reduced to £14 million. Nevertheless, this equated to a not insubstantial 1967 pay raise for the individual GP of around 18%, comparing favourably to the annual 3.5% of previous years. Thereafter, the BMA and the Department of Health negotiated any increase in GP income, under the auspices of the Doctors and Dentists Review Body.

The profession warmly greeted the totality of benefits under the 1966 GP contract, and GPs immediately withdrew their, genuine, threat of mass resignation from the NHS. The imposition of a salaried service, mooted at that time, also receded. GPs fiercely guarded their independence and viewed a salaried role as akin to slavery.

In the year that England won the football World Cup, GPs had an extra reason to celebrate.

Having played such a vital role in brokering the deal between the government and the BMA in 1966, the DDRB continued to operate thereafter as the arbiter of doctors' and dentists' pay. Pay of other staff in primary care was covered by the provisions of the Whitley council[6] for NHS employees, a historic statutory council of employers and trade unions that was a throwback to earlier in the century.

A quasi-independent body, the DDRB was expected to exercise good judgement in determining doctors' pay by comparing it to those in other 'equivalent' professions, such as lawyers, whilst resisting any perverse elements in the general economy. Its deliberations and advice were non-binding, and though it was informally understood that any government would implement its proposals, in several years this was not so, much to the profession's chagrin.

Each year, the DDRB accepted written evidence, presented almost like a sealed bid at an auction, from all parties involved in the negotiations; the Department

[5] Gillam S. The family doctor charter: 50 years on. Br J Gen Pract. 2017 May;67(658):227–8. doi: 10.3399/bjgp17X690809. PMID: 28450339; PMCID: PMC5409444.

[6] www.britannica.com/topic/Whitley-Council

of Health, NHS Confederation, Office of National Statistics, BMA, and British Dental Association. The DDRB subsequently submitted its findings and recommendations to the Prime Minister, who either accepted them or, frequently, diluted or delayed implementation, depending on the prevailing economic climate.

The DDRB looked at the anticipated costs of running a general practice surgery and factored those costs into its annual calculation of what the gross income should be for each GP.

Expenditure was considered under the headings:

- Direct fully reimbursable
- Surgery rent and rates
- Water metering and bills
- Commercial refuse, including hazardous and drug waste
- Employers NI and pension contributions for members of staff
- Employers NI, pension contributions and related costs for GP trainees/registrars
- Dispensed drugs
- Direct partially reimbursable:
  - Staff salaries up to a limit (set by the Whitley scale and, thus, arguably outside the control of the GP employer; see above)
- Indirectly fully reimbursable:
  - Items of service under the Statement of Fees and Allowances

The DDRB calculations also took into account the previous year's reimbursements and GP taxable income, using a sample of GP tax returns provided by the Inland Revenue (now HMRC).

GPs were indifferent to the manner in which the annual uplift was calculated, but they eagerly awaited and were invariably disappointed by the final figure. For much of the 20th century, that figure was synonymous with inflation; for the 21st century, less than 2%.

12.3.3 1966–1990

The 1966 GP contract was a signed compact between GP principal and Health Authority (HA). A full-time GP principal was defined as a doctor available for the provision of healthcare services to the population at hours that were convenient to patients, for 42 weeks a year, a minimum of 26 hours and five days a week. Hours convenient for the patient led to surgeries opening at 8.00 a.m. and closing at 7.00 p.m. Health Authorities could not dictate which days of the week the doctor worked. Nevertheless, most practices voluntarily ran a restricted morning service at weekends. Even without the inclusion of mandatory out-of-hours, the working week amounted to well in excess of 26 hours, a point that paymasters never appreciated. Part-time principals were still entitled to receive the basic practice allowance at a reduced rate of three-quarters if they worked 19–26 hours per week or half for 13–19 hours per week.

Health Authorities accepted that not all GP duties had to be patient-facing, and time was needed for administration, paperwork, and training. A half-day a week was set by for non-clinical activities. Most doctors accepted this, and some partners agreed amongst themselves that this could be increased to one whole day per working week. This was not 'a day off,' although in practice most doctors spent the time away from the surgery, undertaking 'paperwork.'

Annual leave was negotiated between partners and averaged six weeks per annum for holidays and one week for training.

The GMS contract specified which allied health-related activities a GP could be undertaken within the available hours. These included:

- Organisation and training of medical students or prospective GPs
- The provision of other types of medical care e.g. acupuncture
- GMS administration
- Health service appointments, e.g. hospital clinical assistants
- Other medically related appointments with the Crown, government departments, public or local authorities
- GMC issues regarding regulation and performance of doctors
- Medical audits as per the instructions of the Medical Audit Advisory Group (MAAG)

All allowable direct and indirect payments to GPs were laid out in painstaking detail in what became the SFA, a sizeable tome that gained familiarity as the Red Book, due to the colour of its cover. The SFA has endured, almost unchanged, to the present day and is now known as the Statement of Financial Entitlement.

The SFA; 'Red Book' (1966–1990)

The SFA arose following the GP Charter of 1966, which had sought to address four key areas of concern to GPs:

- Improvement in the equipment and staffing of GP premises subsidised by state grants
- A guaranteed minimum income comparable to other unstated professions
- A decent pension on retirement
- Continued GP independence to carry out their duties as they saw fit

In return, GPs were expected to provide a comprehensive medical service to a standard based on what a peer group would find acceptable, a somewhat vague concept best illustrated in minor surgery where the excision of a sebaceous cyst should not result in a disfiguring scar, but neither should it be expected to be invisible.

Prior to 1966, the contract between GP and NHS was comparatively brief and imprecise. After that date, it became a beast of Byzantine detail, covering every activity of a typical GP practice. The Red Book was a weighty tome, 350 pages of tiny script, updated annually with many amendments added during the year. It eventually evolved into a loose-leaf binder format to accommodate the frequent revisions.

Section headings within the Red Book covered:

The Basic Practice Allowances

- Designated area allowance
- Seniority allowance
- Assistant allowance
- Sickness allowance
- Maternity allowance
- Prolonged study leave allowance
- Temporary absence through GMC investigation allowance
- Deprivation
- London initiative zone
- Rural

Item of Service Payments

- Out-of-hours arrangements
- Child health surveillance
- Maternity services
- Contraception services
- Minor surgery
- Chronic disease management
- New patient checks
- Over 75 years old checks
- Provision of medical certificates
- Temporary residents
- Emergency care
- Immediate and necessary treatment
- Arrest dental haemorrhage
- Drugs and appliances

Target Payments

- Cervical cytology
- Childhood immunisation
- Vaccination and immunisation services

Training

- Postgraduate education allowance

Computer

Premises

Rent or mortgage
Rates

Water
Waste

Staff

Salaries
NI
Annual leave
Sick pay

There were innumerable subsections within each of the above sections. Even patients were listed under 12 different categories!

The details of the fees and allowances are covered in greater length by other authors,[7] but an example of the complex calculations contained in the text can be found in that relating to the basic practice allowance.

1.0 The Basic Practice Allowance (BPA)

The BPA could only be paid to a doctor who was a partner (which became synonymous with 'principal') and was intended to compensate the doctor for the provision of General Medical Services but not premises and staff costs.

The BPA for a full-time partner came in at two levels, depending on list size:

- Full   >1200 patients
- Lower >400 but <1199 patients (with incremental increases at 200-patient intervals)

BPA for part-time partners worked on the following equation:

Total practice list size, divided by a number of shares reflecting time commitment of all doctors within the partnership, multiplied by the actual share of each doctor.

Example:

- A practice with a list size of 9,000 patients and 4.5 FTE partners (or 9 × 0.5)
- 9,000 / 9 × 1 = 1,000 (upper stratum of lower-level BPA for the half-time partner)
- 9,000 / 9 × 2 = 1,800 (full BPA for full-time partners)

The BPA calculation encouraged doctors to go into partnership rather than be employees since the former attracted some level of BPA whereas the latter did not. In the example above, the practice would have lost out on three-quarters of the full BPA had it chosen to employ a part-time salaried doctor instead of a part-time partner.

BPA would normally be paid to the practice quarterly, but an interesting anachronism was a provision that up to 20% of BPA could be paid in advance to cover annual leave, with the sum being deducted in instalments from subsequent

[7] Ellis N, Chisholm J. *Making Sense of the Red Book*. Radcliffe. ISBN-10: 1857752910
https://books.google.co.uk/books/about/Making_Sense_of_the_Red_Book.html?id=
ybtLAQAAIAAJ&redir_esc=yls

payments. Accountants frequently advised clients to access this loophole and invest the money or use it to even out cash flow.

The BPA was the key driver of a GP's income and opened the door to other payments in the Red Book, such as:

1.1 Designated Area Allowance
- An area considered to be under-doctored, where list sizes exceeded 3,000 patients per doctor

1.2 Seniority Allowance
For GMC registered GPs, set at three levels.
- Registered 11 years GP 7 years
- Registered 18 years GP 14 years
- Registered 25 years GP 21 years

1.3 Assistant Allowance
An allowance available to full-time single-handed GP's or equivalent partnerships, where the average list size exceeded 3,000 patients, for employing an assistant or salaried doctor. The allowance was relatively small. Recruiting an additional partner made more financial sense.

1.4 Sickness Allowance
The Red Book surprisingly and generously offered to cover some of the costs of the GP, (an independent contractor and not an NHS employee) for locums in case of absence through illness or injury. The allowance was dependent on list size and length of absence and, in practice, was viable only in under-doctored urban areas. The majority of partnerships required a private locum or income-protection insurance to defray the costs of a doctor's ill health. Payments depended on the length of service on a sliding scale and based on the 'normal' remuneration of that GP in the preceding years.

- Length of service 1–2 years = 2 months' full and 2 months' half payment up to 12 months.
- Length of service >5 years = 6 months' full and 6 months' half payment.

1.5 Maternity Allowance
The criteria were much the same as those for the sickness allowance but were not related to list size; a maximum of 14 weeks covered. The doctor had to commit to returning to the practice.

1.6 Education Allowance
Very strict and only available to single-handed GPs working in a designated rural area, to employ a locum to cover the practice whilst they attended an approved educational course. The money covered full locum costs.

1.7 Prolonged Study Leave Allowance
A sabbatical to cover an altruistic aim by the doctor to indulge in a medically related activity to aid their continuing professional development. For example, a GP might wish to study tropical medicine in Barbados.

- Applications had to be submitted to the Regional Postgraduate Dean and approved by the Secretary of State. Few applications were deemed acceptable!
- The fund covered from 10 weeks' to 12 months' absence, for all locum costs for that time. It was unrelated to list size.

The cost of staff accounted for the major outlay in practice accounts. The practice staff reimbursement scheme covered a wide range of roles, including Managers, Administrators, Secretaries, Nurses, Physiotherapists, Chiropodists, Dieticians, Counsellors, Link workers (mental health, social service), and Translators. The Health Authority covered 70% of the salary, superannuation, NI, and other employment benefits.

The partnership had to justify the need for each employee. The Health Authority had the option, widely exercised, to decline to fund a post, an action often taken at the end of any financial year if a budget overspend was looming. Review of staffing levels and costs was undertaken by the Health Authority every three years.

Familiarity with and adherence to the contents of the Red Book became second nature to doctors and their administrative staff. A rolling log of practice activities allowed for a well-organised practice to be suitably rewarded for its services. Recording such activities, onerous in the decades prior to computerisation, was greatly facilitated once computers began to appear in the 1980s.

12.3.4 1991–1997

The GP contract of 1990 included several novel proposals, the most prominent being fundholding. Despite its short existence (it was abolished in 1997), fundholding laid the foundations for PMS, the GMS contract of 2004, and Clinical Commissioning Groups.

The enabling act of parliament, the National Health Service and Community Care Act 1990, was part of Prime Minister Thatcher's philosophy of reducing the role of big government through the stimulation of an internal market as took place in the private sector. It was hoped that by doing so, the service NHS offered would be slicker, cost-effective, and less of a drain on the exchequer. The profession demurred but was ignored. The concept of a commercial market within a state-run healthcare system was anathema to a few, illogical to some, and controversial to all.

In the early waves, fundholding practices were allocated a generous budget solely for the commissioning of services for their patients, both in the community and secondary care. The purchasing fund also included extras to cover administration, accounting, secretarial, management costs, and improved IT, over and above that considered normal in the running of a GMS practice.

Fundholding had a patchy uptake, appealing to the more dynamic, entrepreneurial partnerships. It tended to divide practices within Health Authorities. Those practices that chose to enter the scheme saw benefits in the autonomous budget provision that allowed them to choose how that money was spent on improving patient services. Those with a conservative bent cynically viewed the enterprise as a step towards the privatisation of primary care, providing an incentive to favour PMS practices with cash in hand. Their fears were unfounded; fundholding practices rapidly cleared their waiting lists for elective surgery, such as joint replacement. Where this was so, fundholding practices with a budget surplus altruistically collaborated with neighbouring non-fundholders, temporarily registering their patients in order to quicken their journey to the operating table. Nevertheless, a lingering resentment prevailed for many years between the two arms of primary care.

A review of the outcomes from fundholding, published in the *BJGP* in May 1998, seemed to favour a nuanced conclusion that any benefits of the scheme were, at best, marginal.[8] A later review in 2005, undertaken by the Centre for Health Economics, University of York, was more positive, highlighting benefits including a lowering of elective rates, reduced emergency-related occupied-hospital-bed days, improved coordination of primary, intermediate, and community support services, and better engagement of GPs in the commissioning and developing of care integrated pathways. Despite these abundant benefits, they also noted reduced patient satisfaction![9]

12.3.5 1998–2004

PMS[10] evolved from fundholding, was introduced by a Labour government that had come to power after 18 years of Conservative rule. Frank Dobson, the incoming Secretary of State for Health, set aside his intrinsic socialist inclinations to accept that there was some merit in devolving budgets to those best able to manage them. As such, the philosophy underpinning PMS would endure to the creation of Clinical Commissioning Groups 15 years later. PMS practices never existed in Wales and Northern Ireland and were called Section 17c practices in Scotland.

PMS rather muddied the waters regarding the way GPs were funded. GMS practices, with a central contract, continued to be reimbursed using the Red Book. PMS contracts were negotiated locally between the practice and the local health authority, the PCT, which had replaced the FHSA in 1997.

In essence, PMS fundholding was a contract between a general medical practice, 'the provider,' and PCT, 'the commissioner,' detailing the proposed services, with metrics, that the former was willing to provide in a financial year. A crucial difference between the PMS and GMS contractor was 'the provider' no longer had to be the 'performer,' the individual carrying out those services. Although the

8   Smith RD, Wilton P. General practice fundholding: progress to date. Br J Gen Pract. 1998 May;48(430):1253–7. PMID: 9692288; PMCID: PMC1410181.

9   GP fundholding-the facts Russell Mannion. www.york.ac.uk/news-and-events/news/2005/gp-fundholding/

10 Shapiro J. Personal medical services: a barometer for the NHS? BMJ. 2000 Dec 2; 321(7273):1359–60. doi: 10.1136/bmj.321.7273.1359. PMID: 11099265; PMCID: PMC 1119099.

contract was between a GP principal and PCT, the principal could employ others (salaried doctor, nurse, or any other healthcare professional) to do the work.

The majority of tendered contracts were 'cut and paste' facsimiles and summaries of what had previously been contained in the pre-existing GMS contract and the Red Book. In effect, the Red Book was retired from active service for PMS practices. Remuneration by the Health Authority was based on calculations of historical income for the practice, with a moderate annual uplift. The commencing budget was based on the previous year's GMS claim, allowing for any changes in the practice list size and additions to enhanced services, such as the employment of such clinical staff as a nurse practitioner. The baseline budget covered all previous income and expenses, the basic practice allowance and other elements of the GP Annual Report detailing services that accrued reimbursements from the Health Authority.

Although the financial incentives for PMS practices faded over the years, participating GP principals continued to enjoy a higher 15–20% net income than their GMS counterparts. The difference in income fuelled the PMS practices' reluctance to switch to GMS in the 2004 GP contract and remained in place two decades later.

12.3.6 2004 to Date[11,12]

The new General Medical Services (nGMS) contract of 2004[13,14,15] waved farewell to the Red Book and hello to its replacement, the Statement of Financial Entitlements (SFE). Practice remuneration underwent a paradigm shift, with every GP practice given a personal budget, thus eliminating the many man-hours previously spent on calculating the details required in the annual report. Although the change was dramatic, the process had been evolutionary, arising from the experience gained from PMS (37% of English GP practices) by 2004.

The 2004 contract upended the fiscal arrangement between individual GP principal and Primary Care Trust. Funding became practice, rather than GP principal, based. The allocated resources, the global sum, gave flexibility and autonomy to practices in how they wished to deliver medical services to their patients. They were incentivised to ensure that clinical services were of the highest standard through the Quality and Outcome Framework.

---

[11] https://assets.publishing.service.gov.uk/government/uploads/system/uploads/attachment_data/file/213225/GMS-Statement-of-Financial-Entitlements-2013.pdf

[12] https://digital.nhs.uk/data-and-information/publications/statistical/nhs-payments-to-general-practice/england-2018-19/executive-summary

[13] https://assets.publishing.service.gov.uk/government/uploads/system/uploads/attachment_data/file/213225/GMS-Statement-of-Financial-Entitlements-2013.pdf

[14] https://digital.nhs.uk/data-and-information/publications/statistical/nhs-payments-to-general-practice/england-2018-19/executive-summary

[15] https://app.croneri.co.uk/topics/gp-payments-under-gms-contract/indepth

Although this simplified the way GPs were remunerated, the annually revised SFA[16] still amounted to nearly 100 pages of densely typed script with each paragraph requiring forensic scrutiny for ensuring practice income was maintained.

The directions within the SFE 2004 covered:

1. Global Sum and Minimum Practice Income Guarantee   GS
2. Quality and Outcomes Framework   QOF
3. Enhanced Services   ES
4. PCO-Administered Funds   PCO
5. Premises   Premises
6. IM&T   IM&T
7. Dispensing/Personal Administration of Drugs   Dispensing

To qualify for the global sum, the contractor, the GP practice, had to provide certain services:

Core (Essential) GMS

- Acute illness, health promotion, referrals
- Chronic disease management
- Palliative care

And Additional Services

- Child health surveillance
- Contraception/IUD
- Obstetrics excluding intrapartum
- Childhood vaccinations
- Cervical screening
- Basic minor surgery

All the elements previously present in the Red Book were recategorised for payments under the seven sections of the SFE.

The provision of traditionally accepted General Medical Services was included in the global sum; health promotion and chronic disease management under QOF, the additional services, as above, in enhanced services. PCO-administered funds covered locum, study leave, and seniority payments; rent and waste came under premises, IM&T as before, as was dispensing.

1. Global Sum

The GS for each practice was based on the preceding 12 months' payments to the practice using the Carr-Hill formula,[17] itself based on the number of registered

---

[16] https://assets.publishing.service.gov.uk/government/uploads/system/uploads/attachment_data/file/975395/GMS_SFE_2021.pdf

[17] *New GMS Contract. 2003: Investing in General Practice.* BMA Publications, Supporting Documentation. www.bma.org.uk

patients, the Contractual Registered Population (CRP), but buttressed by the Minimum Practice Income Guarantee (MPIG).[18] It was calculated quarterly and paid monthly.

For those readers who like a little meat in their sandwich, the nGMS[19] contract and its 271 pages were just as finely and prescriptively detailed as the venerable Red Book they had displaced.

The nGMS contract 2004 was underpinned by several DH commitments.

- Investment in primary care over a three-year period, raising total spending by 33% from £6.1 billion to £8.0 billion per annum.
- Application of the Carr-Hill formula to allocate resources. The calculation covered factors that affected GP workload and expenses: patient age and sex, chronic illness, list turnover, population density, and staff costs. The formula was designed to take account of these factors when reviewing resource distribution across the country.
- Temporary MPIG[20] whilst practices transitioned from historic to Carr-Hill remuneration formulae. MPIG was gradually phased out, finally discontinued in 2020.
- Improvements in GP pension arrangements. The successful enhancement of pension provisions allowed GPs to retire at a younger age (late 50s) than previous generations.
- The repeal of the 24-hour duty of care for patients, the element of the contract that most chimed with GPs; 80% subsequently relinquished out-of-hours commitments.

Professor Roy Carr-Hill (1943–) was another of the influential characters who stood out in the NHS's history. Having gained his PhD in Penology,[21] he joined the faculty at the Centre for Health Economics, University of York, in 1983. The institution was a respected think tank on health and social care policies in the UK, whose publications strongly influenced those in the corridors of the Ministry of Health.

Despite welcoming the 2004 contract, GPs were uncertain about its financial implications, partly due to the opacity of the Carr-Hill formula calculation. Loss of income justifiably concerned GPs. Once the formula was applied, 70% of practices found their annual income fell, compared to the previous year's GMS/PMS income. That unhappy situation particularly applied to PMS practices who subsequently threatened to resign en masse from the NHS, supported by the General Practitioners Committee of the BMA. Following further muscle-flexing by the

---

[18] NHS England. 18 Dec 2013. www.england.nhs.uk/wp-content/uploads/2014/02/annex-a-let-at.pdf

[19] Standard medical services contract. https://assets.publishing.service.gov.uk/government/uploads/system/uploads/attachment_data/file/184931/Standard_General_Medical_Services_Model_Contract.pdf

[20] www.england.nhs.uk/wp-content/uploads/2014/02/annex-a-let-at.pdf

[21] The study of the punishment of crime and prison management.

GPC/BMA, the concession of the MPIG under which, as the name suggested, no practice would find itself financially disadvantaged, was added to the contract.

The MPIG ran for as long as the current practice income fell below that of the previous year's GMS (PMS practices rarely required the safety net) income. Initially intended to be a temporary three-year fix, the correction factor of MPIG was eventually discontinued in 2020.

An unwelcome, though initially overlooked feature of the Carr-Hill formula was the demand for data on many aspects of a GP's workload, such as the duration of a surgery consultation or home visit, even splitting the latter into whether those visits took place in the patient's own home or a nursing home. Automated data capture by PCTs was facilitated by developments in practice computer software. To some degree, Carr-Hill resulted in a step change in the scrutiny of those working in primary care.

2. Quality and Outcomes Framework, QOF

Another revolutionary concept pioneered in the 2004 contract was the proportion of practice income that would be made through payment by results, part of which came from the introduction of the Quality and Outcomes Framework.

QOF evolved the performance-based metric of remuneration, piloted in the 1990 contract, which attracted payments for specific activities, such as child health surveillance, minor surgery, and chronic disease management. QOF was aimed at raising the quality of general practice across the UK in line with nationally agreed, evidentially based frameworks in four key domains: clinical, organisational, patient experience, and additional services. QOF allocated points for the achievement of prescribed, aspirational, milestones and, to quote the catchphrase of many a TV game show, points meant prizes. The prizes were funded through the addition of £1 billion of new money to cover the costs if every practice in the UK hit the maximum target. This equated to a tempting and potentially attainable increase of 30%, up to £42,000 per GP principal, over their previous year's gross income. The sum became a reality in the first year following implementation, as GP practices across the UK achieved an average 91% of the available points with minimal effort.[22] These results were interpreted as reflecting either weak performance targets, more diligent recording of performance, or a confirmation of quality improvements that had previously existed in primary care. However, most of the profession felt the likely explanation was government ignorance of how effective NHS primary care had been at delivering healthcare in the UK!

The QOF was and remains a voluntary programme that provides financial incentives for general practices to meet performance criteria in four domains. Initially, in 2004, these were:

- Clinical Standards, covering ten disease areas with 80 indicators
  - Coronary heart disease
  - Stroke and transient ischaemic attacks (TIA)

[22] https://files.digital.nhs.uk/publicationimport/pub01xxx/pub01946/qof-eng-04-05-rep.pdf

- Hypertension
- Hypothyroidism
- Diabetes
- Mental health
- Chronic obstructive pulmonary disease
- Asthma
- Epilepsy
- Cancer
- Organisational Standards (43 indicators)
  - Records and information
  - Communicating with patients
  - Education and training
  - Medicines management
  - Clinical and practice management
- Patient Experience Standards (4 indicators)
  - Patient survey
  - Consultation length
- Additional Services (8 indicators)
  - Cervical screening
  - Child health surveillance
  - Maternity services
  - Contraceptive services

An example of a clinical domain, COPD, for 2004, was as follows.

Clinical Domain—COPD

Indicator Points Payment Stages	Points	Pay stages
	Points	Target
Records		
COPD 1. The practice can produce a register of patients with COPD Initial diagnosis	5	100%
COPD 2. The percentage of patients in whom diagnosis has been confirmed by spirometry including reversibility testing for newly diagnosed patients with effect from 1 April 2003	5	25–90%
COPD 3. The percentage of all patients with COPD in whom diagnosis has been confirmed by spirometry including reversibility testing	5	25–90%
Ongoing management		
COPD 4. The percentage of patients with COPD in whom there is a record of smoking status in the previous 15 months	6	25–90%

COPD 5. The percentage of patients with COPD who smoke, whose notes contain a record that smoking cessation advice or referral to a specialist service, where available, has been offered in the past 15 months   6   25–90%

COPD 6. The percentage of patients with COPD with a record of FEV1 in the previous 27 months   6   25–70%

COPD 7. The percentage of patients with COPD receiving inhaled treatment in whom there is a record that inhaler technique has been checked in the preceding 27 months   6   25–90%

COPD 8. The percentage of patients with COPD who have had influenza immunisation in the preceding 1 September to 31 March   6   25–85%

Points were weighted and allocated to individual subsections within these domains and totalled 1,000 points, with another 50 points for maintaining improved access for patients.

Each point was worth £75 to the average UK general practice, based on each GP having a list size of 1,800 registered patients. Payments were made in two stages; aspirational monthly, based on the points practices believed they would achieve, and annually, based on what was finally achieved as of 31 March each year.

GPs were allowed to exclude patients from eligibility for specific indicators on several grounds, including failure of the patient to respond to repeated invitations to attend for a health review and unsuitability of an indicator due to patient terminal illness, extreme frailty, allergy, adverse reaction, or contraindication.

The IT providers of clinical software updated their offering to track QOF points and automatically feed the figures to the PCT. Included in these updates were 'pop-up' prompts, an irritating distraction during a standard consultation. Staff were reallocated to QOF related tasks, pursuing patients, updating records, and monitoring progress. A lead partner was charged with overseeing the whole process and cajoling colleagues to comply. Efforts were redoubled in the final quarter of the financial year to maximise points in all domains. Overall, these measures proved financially fruitful.

The complexity of the calculations underpinning reimbursement could tax the great mathematicians from Newton to Nash. Thankfully, a summary guidance, from Sheffield LMC, 2013,[23,24] provides a clearer understanding.

Initially, the PCO checked the veracity of QOF performance and claims through the practice submission in its annual report, but this was eventually replaced by computer-generated monthly reports. Major discrepancies in claims

[23] https://sheffield-lmc.org.uk/website/IGP217/files/Primary%20Care%20Networks%20&%20The%20Future%20-%20GPC%20Presentation%20(17Feb20).
[24] www.sheffield-lmc.org.uk/website/IGP217/files/103%20QOF_Payments.pdf

were infrequent and, when present, were followed up by practice visits from teams comprising a PCO management representative, a clinician, usually a GP or other healthcare professional, a patient representative, and an optional member of the Local Medical Committee. The PCO had to give the practice two months' notice of such visits. The discovery of fraud or other illegal activities resulted in referral to the NHS Counter Fraud Agency, CFA. In 2019, the CFA estimated that £88 million had been lost annually in general practice through fraudulent activities, including list inflation, claims for services not provided, quality payments manipulation, conflicts of interest, and self-prescribing.[25]

Over the following years, QOF became a labile entity, as existing domains were retired, added, or renamed. Points changed, as did their monetary value. By 2020/21, the original QOF domains had been streamlined and relabelled as:

- Clinical   20 clinical standards, 401 points
- Public health   5 clinical standards, 160 points
- Quality improvement   2 standards, 74 points

The average practice achieved 534 out of the 559 available in 2019/20, with each point worth £187.[26]

In 2008, Dr Brian Hutchinson, Editor in Chief of *Health Policy Journal*[27] provided an early critique of QOF. The paper identified several benefits from the introduction of a financially incentivised programme for performance but also had some reservations. Concerns covered the protocol-driven management of medical conditions, the move from a patient-centred agenda towards a QOF-orientated agenda, divisions between staff regarding recognition and payment for efforts in achieving maximum points, and 'gaming' the system, leading to unreliable data. A systematic review published in the *BJGP* 2017 suggested that little had changed over the previous decade and suggested that there might be better ways other than financial incentives to motivate primary care teams to deliver high-quality care.[28]

3. Enhanced Services

As with QOF, the provision of Enhanced Services was optional, though most had existed in GMS/PMS contracts prior to 2004 and were, thus, familiar to all practices.

Enhanced services were remunerated in three ways:

[25] www.england.nhs.uk/wp-content/uploads/2013/06/tackling-fraud-bribery-and-corruption-economic-crime-strategy-2018-2021.pdf

[26] https://digital.nhs.uk/data-and-information/publications/statistical/quality-and-outcomes-framework-achievement-prevalence-and-exceptions-data/2019-20

[27] Hutchison B. Pay for performance in primary care: proceed with caution, pitfalls ahead. Healthc Policy. 2008 Aug;4(1):10–22. PMID: 19377337; PMCID: PMC2645205.

[28] Forbes LJ, Marchand C, Doran T, Peckham S. The role of the Quality and Outcomes Framework in the care of long-term conditions: a systematic review. Br J Gen Pract. 2017 Nov;67(664):e775–e784. doi: 10.3399/bjgp17X693077. Epub 2017 Sep 25. PMID: 28947621; PMCID: PMC5647921.

3.1 National (NES)

PCO commissioned services, from any provider covering anticoagulant monitoring, intrapartum care, minor injuries, IUCD fitting, drug and alcohol misuse.

Over the following decades, additional enhanced services beyond those pre-existing were introduced, including:

- *Patient participation.* The creation of and liaison with patient participation groups.
- *Extended hours.* Weekday early morning and evening, and weekend surgeries.
- *Alcohol reduction.* Recording of patient daily alcohol intake and advice.
- *Learning disabilities health check scheme.* Keeping a register of the population with learning difficulties. Liaising with social services as appropriate.
- Annual review of patients with complex medical and social needs, frailty, and frequent attenders.
- *Proactive detection of patients at risk of dementia.* Application of screening tools, such as the Mini Mental State Examination (MMSE). Early referral to specialist services.
- Enhanced IT systems to enable patients to book appointments and request repeat prescriptions.

Both the COVID-19 vaccination programme and follow-up of long COVID cases in 2021 were funded through NES. National pricing, terms and conditions applied. Work undertaken under an NES was funded by NHSE.

3.2 Directed (DES)

Services that the PCO was legally obliged to commission included maternity, influenza, pneumococcal and childhood vaccination programmes, learning disability health checks, and minor surgery. All had previously been a historic staple of general practice. Payment for work completed was based on national pricing, terms and conditions.[29] As expected, the calculations were complex. Primary Care Networks were funded under a special DES, following the publication of the GP, Five Year Forward Plan. Work undertaken under DES was funded by NHSE.

3.3 Local (LES)

Services negotiated and commissioned by the PCO in response to specific local needs. Subjects qualifying for funding had to differ from those under DES and NES and not be included in the Statement of Financial Entitlement. Examples included management of leg ulcers, monitoring of rheumatology drugs, and chlamydia screening. A typical CCG might have more than 50 individual schemes covered by LES. Work undertaken under LES was funded by CCG.

---

[29] Network contract directed enhanced service: guidance for 2019/20 in England. www.england.nhs.uk/wp-content/uploads/2019/12/network-contract-des-guidance-v3-updated.pdf

4. PCO-Administered Funds

PCO-administered funds covered:

- Locum payments for: maternity, paternity, and adoption leave
- Sickness leave and long-term sickness
- Suspended doctors facing tribunal hearings
- Prolonged study leave
- Seniority (for GMS/PMS Principals only)
- Doctors' retainer scheme. This was effectively discontinued for new applicants, but payments did continue for those doctors already on the scheme as of 2004.

Payments were discretionary, individual, and locally negotiated. An example would be locum payments which were set at £950 per week for a full-time locum.

5. Premises

On 1 April 2004, the National Health Service (General Medical Services—Premises Costs) (England) Directions 2004 replaced the sections of the SFAs, covering costs relating to practice premises.

The Directions were substantially the same as those that had preceded them in the Red Book, and PCOs were forbidden to flout them.

A business plan stating the details for new or additional premises, architectural plans, and preliminary costings had to be submitted to the PCO, which had to sign off on the project before it could proceed.

Prior to the GP contract of 1966; the funding of GP premises was essentially the same as that which had preceded the formation of the NHS; the money came from the doctor's wallet. In reality, the surgery was often a residential property where the doctor both lived and worked; financed by a mortgage loan. As the interest on the mortgage was a non-reimbursable expense that ate into a doctor's income, investment in the premises was minimal and buildings were left to languish into genteel decay.

The 1966 Contract was negotiated partly to address the problem of ramshackle facilities. GPs were financially encouraged, through partially reimbursable loans, to update or build new surgeries that reflected a modern healthcare system and provided a professional clinical environment for the patient and clinician. Both loan and repayment were funded through the public purse in the budgetary merry-go-round the NHS still favours to this day. The General Practice Finance Corporation (GPFC),[30] a statutory body set up in 1967 to raise the money from the public purse for investment in primary care infrastructure, provided the loans. Over the following two decades, the GPFC raised and lent £100 million, equivalent to £1billion as of 2019, allowing for inflation, to 8,000 doctors to build, improve, or rent their premises. The GPFC was the lender of choice for such projects. To obtain a loan, a practice had to adhere to strict guidance covering building plans submitted for approval. The GPFC's remit to improve the environment

---

[30] www.bmj.com/content/bmj/1/6173/1294.full.pdf

in which society's patients were seen was transformational in enhancing the patient experience in the late 20th century.

In the 1980s, under a UK government seeking to roll back state activities in public services, the GPFC was allowed to expand its inventory of loans to £250 million by partnering with the commercial financial sector. As expected, the BMA was aghast at what it saw as the encroachment of the private sector on the NHS, a misplaced concern. However, the policy heralded the demise of the GPFC as aggressive lenders from the commercial banking sector, eying an opportunity for a secure investment with guaranteed returns, eagerly moved to finance surgery infrastructure schemes. The policy also allowed GPs to shop around for loans, often succeeding in obtaining favourable interest rates allowing for an excess on the income from cost/notional rent. In short, GPs could improve cash flow and income whilst watching the value of their assets increase. Surgery properties provided the perfect investment, cost-free with a sizeable lump sum on retirement.

By 1990, the dingy, decrepit, decaying structure of the 1950s had become a modern medical centre, a tangible asset. Property prices were booming. Everyone was a winner, provided partnerships remained stable and long-lasting. However, much as with a Ponzi scheme, early entrants were those who were most likely to profit. New partners 'bought in' to a practice and thereafter owned a share of the equity. When property was cheap, that was not a concern, but as prices ballooned, so incoming partners were put off by the high cost of entry. Stories flourished in the medical press over unrealistic valuations and incumbent partners' expectations and, not to put too fine a point on it, greed. Retiring doctors seeking to realise their share of the assets found it increasingly difficult to do so, as replacement partners baulked at the price of acquiring those assets. The means of addressing the problem led to several solutions.

- Maintenance of the status quo but with staged purchase of equity over time as the incoming partner's income increased. Young doctors remained unimpressed. The sums involved were daunting, especially when coupled with purchasing a home. Nevertheless, the economic case for purchasing a stake in the building was compelling for those thinking of a long-term commitment to the partnership.
- Sale of the property and freehold to an investor or property developer, who would thereafter act as landlord, accruing all income arising from notional rent. The partnership became a tenant with this popular option, but it was insecure since a landlord could choose to evict the tenant at any time if they found a more profitable use for the site. In such cases, the developer often sweetened the deal by moving the practice, and their rental income, to new build medical centre on a less valuable, sometimes geographically remote, site.
- Mixed public-private partnerships (PPPs), such as the Local Improvement Finance Trust (LIFT), were introduced with government support in 2000. They were sanctioned and managed through the PCT to improve healthcare facilities in mainly socially deprived areas. In 2013, the portfolio and head

tenancy of the primary care properties under its jurisdiction were transferred to Community Health Partnerships (CHP).[31] The corporate governance of CHP was unusual in that the company was wholly owned by the Secretary of State for Health and Social Care who retained 40% of the equity in each LIFT company with the remaining 60% held by the private sector in return for financing the projects. By 2013, more than 350 facilities had been developed under LIFT and CHP with total a total capital value exceeding £2.5 billion. The benefits and drawbacks to doctors working within the scheme were similar to those of the original health centres of the 1970s.

- Private sector, including public limited companies, as property developers operating on an invest and leaseback principle.

Not all GPs had the option of owning their surgery buildings. Those working in local authority health centres, around 500 in the UK in 1980, continued to be obligated to their landlord. Labour governments of the 1960s felt that the purpose-built and centrally funded facilities were sympathetic to a socialist philosophy. However, budgets were not ring-fenced, and, over time, many fell into disrepair, to the despair of those working in them. The main advantage of the system was the absence of personal investment by the GP.

6. IM&T

PCOs took over the purchase, maintenance, upgrade, running, and training costs of IM&T, replacing the previous system of practice reimbursement for such items. In return, GPs lost any flexibility regarding their choice of provider. They could still choose and personally fund their preferred system but, naturally, few chose to do so. Practices continued to be responsible for consumables, such as inks and toners.

7. Dispensing

In England and Wales, the mechanism for payment to dispensing practices changed in April 2006. The on-cost and container allowances were abolished and replaced by an enhanced professional fee for each dispensed item.

The Prescription Pricing Division in England calculated the sums due to doctors in fees and allowances for dispensing and personal administration, and these were then paid to the practice through the Exeter system.[32] Similar arrangements applied in Scotland and Northern Ireland. It was advisable for dispensing practices to register for VAT purposes with HMRC, to reclaim the VAT, no longer covered by the DH.

Payments under the GMS contract 2004 remained opaque, particularly as certain elements varied each month.

An example of the paper-based monthly statement can be found in a clearly laid out summary, by an LMC, on GP practice funding in 2006.[33]

---

[31] https://communityhealthpartnerships.co.uk/

[32] www.dispensingdoctor.org/wp-content/uploads/2014/10/DDADispensingGuide-WEB.pdf

[33] www.barnsleylmc.co.uk/gpfocuspracticefund.pdf

As of 2020, NHSE could access many (QOF, DES, vaccinations) of the details pertaining to payments remotely by direct data capture using customised finance software (CQRS,[34] Calculating Quality Reporting Services). They were thus able to produce precise quarterly accounts, greatly facilitating practice cash flow whilst simultaneously reducing the burden of invoice submissions by the practice.

12.3.7 GP Earnings

A GP's income depended on many factors, including:

- Age
  - Older doctors accrued a seniority payment. This was taken individually but sometimes included in the overall partnership profits.
  - They were more likely to have an equity stake in the building, accruing reimbursement of rental.
- Gender
  - Gender per se was not an issue, more the fact that female GPs were more attracted to a part-time role than their male counterparts.
- Full or Part Time
  - Self-explanatory
- Principal or Salaried
  - A GP principal shared the partnership profits whereas a salaried doctor was paid a fixed salary. The disparity between the two sources of income was often significant. Full-time salaried GPs in PMS practices earned around 50% of the income of their employing GP principal.
- Locality
  - Doctors practising in socially disadvantaged urban areas often had larger lists than their colleagues in rural practices.
- GMS or PMS
  - As previously mentioned, PMS practices earned more than GMS. For the decade 2002–2012, the net income before tax of the average GP was around £10,000 more per annum in a PMS than GMS practice.
- Dispensing or Non-Dispensing
  - On average, GPs earned £20,000 per annum more in a dispensing than a non-dispensing practice.

Put another way; a doctor driving a Ferrari, was likely to be a male GP principal in a rural PMS dispensing practice.

---

[34] https://digital.nhs.uk/services/calculating-quality-reporting-service

Over the decades, average annual net pre-tax earnings for a full-time GP principal in England, adjusted for UK inflation to 2019 figures, were around:[35]

- 1960   £50,000
- 1970   £70,000
- 1980   £50,000
- 1990   £75,000
- 2000   £90,000
- 2010   £99,000 GMS,   £113,000 PMS[36]
- 2018   £117,300[37]

The average income for a salaried GP in 2018 was £60,600.

The figures for Scotland showed lower earnings per GP principal but higher for salaried than those for England!

As of 2016, the government mandated that GPs should publish, on their website and surgery premises, the average income of the doctors working in the practice. This was driven by populist stories in the national press regarding excessive GP earnings of £200,000. The policy was justified as transparency, allowing the public to see where their taxes were being spent. Doctors reacted in horror to this edict as a typical GP website clearly showed at the times.[38] In practice, the demand turned out to be not as alarming as it first appeared. Factoring in the number of part-time and salaried doctors, the average figure quoted was rarely above £50,000.

In 2017/2018, around 12% of the GP workforce earned more than £100,000 a year, with one individual earning £600,000. The extremely high earners were almost exclusively executive managers of groups of practices staffed almost entirely by salaried doctors and with minimal personal clinical involvement.

Salaried GPs were almost unheard of prior to 1998 and the introduction of PMS contracts, which allowed practices the flexibility of a budget unrelated to the number of GP principals in the practice, the basic practice allowance they brought in, thus freeing them to employ non-partners.

Salaried positions were often preferred by those wishing to work part-time and this was reflected in the significantly reduced income compared to that of GP principals.

Salaried doctors were not solely employed in GP surgeries but also, increasingly, in other primary care providers, NHS Walk-in Clinics, PCO/CCGs, APMS providers, Darzi Clinics (which ran briefly from 2006 to 2010) and OOH services.

Their role and duties within a practice are covered in greater detail in Chapter 2, 'The Practice Team.'

[35] Moberly T. Data chart: how GP pay has risen and fallen over 60 years. BMJ. 2017 Sep 27;358:j4385

[36] https://digital.nhs.uk/data-and-information/publications/statistical/gp-earnings-and-expenses-estimates/gp-earnings-and-expenses-2010-2011

[37] GP earnings and expenses estimates 2018/2019. NHS Digital. https://digital.nhs.uk/data-and-information/publications/statistical/gp-earnings-and-expenses-estimates/2018-2019

[38] www.westendsurgery.co.uk/net-gp-earnings

The enforced deal between the government and the medical profession at the inception of the NHS in 1948, whilst providing an element of job security and steady income, was resented by the profession for the relatively low sum at which that income was set.

Following the 1966 GP Contract, both income and working conditions improved, but GPs continued to feel undervalued vis a vis comparative professions, such as lawyers, accountants, and dentists. This grievance was further exacerbated by the onerous responsibilities and long hours associated with the job. Nevertheless, a newly appointed GP principal in the 1970s was likely to be pleasantly overwhelmed by the huge jump in disposable income compared to his or her last hospital post. Suddenly, they could afford a second car for the family, and an annual holiday abroad. Times were good.

However, income remained static thereafter. Aspirations regarding private education and university fees for any children had to be balanced against savings in other household expenditure. Dissatisfaction built up as social peer groups, hospital consultants, dentists, and pharmacists stampeded into share portfolios, holiday homes, and boutique businesses for their spouses. GP pay was just enough to prevent desertion from general practice but was a poor return on the investment of emotional, mental, and physical capital.

The GP contract of 2004 changed everything. Overnight it seemed that general practice had entered a portal into the Promised Land. The combination of no night and weekend work coupled with a dramatic (30–40% over two years) increase in income at one stroke rectified all the injustices of the preceding quarter-century. Now it was hospital colleagues who were left envious. The contract was a vindication of the career choices made, for whatever reason, decades earlier.

Sadly, the euphoria was fleeting. Gloom once again stalked the land of primary care as the following decade saw incomes retreat, due to a combination of static budgets and increased expenditure. Nevertheless, in 2020, British GPs were amongst the highest paid in Europe, though the work itself was not entirely equivalent.[39] However those earnings were trumped by any savvy GP trainee entering primary care as a locum where earnings were up to £800 per day, equating to £140,800 per annum for a 4-day week, 44 weeks a year, clinical duties only.

12.4 SESSIONAL GPS

Manpower shortages have been a constant throughout the NHS's lifetime. Finding a replacement doctor at short notice for holidays, sickness, or maternity leave had always been problematic. Locum doctors filled the gap, although prior to 2000 few were available since most GPs were established, full-time principals.

Locum (sessional) GPs worked independently or through an agency, latterly 'chambers,' mimicking the legal profession's model. They were paid hourly or per session. Market forces prevailed, with rates varying across the country, driven by supply and demand.

---

[39] www.eafinder.com/updated-salary-structure-of-medical-doctors-in-europe/

It is unclear how many sessional GPs work in the UK, partly due to the peripatetic nature of the work. Figures for 2018 from the National Association of Sessional GPs (NASGP),[40] using surveys by NHS Digital, estimated that there were around 20,000 doctors, out of a total GP workforce of 62,303, working as locums in England and Scotland, 32% of the total workforce. The entirety of the work undertaken by locums was even more difficult to gauge. NASGP figures suggested that the average locum worked five sessions per week whilst NHS Digital estimated that a headcount of 2,630 GP locums equated to 970 FTE GP locums! Locums saw around 20% of the 300 million GP appointments in England for that year.[41]

It should be no surprise that the majority of newly minted GP trainees now choose to be sessional rather than principal GPs, citing work/life balance and pay as being the main factors in their choice.

12.5 PENSIONS

As with other aspects of remuneration, pensions reflected the unusual model under which GPs work; independent contractors, self-employed but with one dominant 'notional' employer, the Department of Health. GPs did not have a private pension plan as one would have expected of the self-employed. Instead, they contributed to a bespoke NHS defined benefit scheme that differed, until 2015, from their hospital colleagues; the former was based on lifetime earnings. To further complicate matters, the GP's lifetime earnings included those earned in hospital training posts prior to entering general practice.

The NHS pension scheme (NHSPS) is unique and has been in place since 1948. It is the only occupational pension scheme in the UK available to the self-employed. The original features have been modified many times in the past 70 years. Not all of the amendments were trouble-free or greeted enthusiastically by doctors, but by and large, the provisions have been generous compared to other public sector workers.

Following one such amendment in 1971, Hansard[42] recorded this rather distressing picture of the average GP of the time:

> There is precious little encouragement to become a doctor or a nurse or a medical auxiliary in Britain today. Most of us have been lobbied by doctors in our constituencies. They are usually pale young gentlemen who come clutching red dyed bank statements, with horrifying stories of medical moonlighting and the ways in

[40] Locum GP workforce numbers out for the count. NASGP. www.nasgp.org.uk/news/locum-gp-workforce-figures-out-for-the-count/

[41] NHS Digital. https://digital.nhs.uk/data-and-information/publications/statistical/appointments-in-general-practice/oct-2018

[42] https://hansard.parliament.uk/Commons/1966-11-22/debates/0d74fe3a-b30b-4ac9-a720-7d391a813159/NationalHealthService(SuperannuationRegu-Lations)?highlight=there%20precious%20little%20encouragement%20become%20doctor%20nurse#contribution-7abf807c-a9b6-4a85-a34b-7e78f8836b9b

which they have to supplement their inadequate incomes . . . There is another point to be made about the older doctor. It is not wise to throw him on the scrap heap promptly when he reaches retiring age. If he is hale and hearty, he still has many contributions to make in a field which is not overstaffed, to put it mildly. Do these Regulations provide sufficient encouragement for the G.P. of pensionable age to go on working? I rather doubt it.

Sadly, elderly GPs, seemed to welcome being thrown on the scrapheap when they finally reached retirement!

Superannuable income was broadly defined as the net profit derived from earnings for NHS activity. A certificate of superannuable NHS earnings had to be submitted annually to the PCO, currently CCG. This was a legal document. Doctors had to ensure that it was completed accurately and that it truly reflected those earnings as they appeared in their annual tax returns.

Under the 1990 GMS Contract, the income deemed to be superannuable was that arising from the individual GP's share of the practice profits where items of service were calculated at 66% superannuable; target and seniority 100%; other reimbursements, such as for staff, drugs, and equipment, 0%. PMS practices differed in that the superannuable payments were based on the year's practice income divided by the number of FTE GP principals.

The 2004 Contract broadly followed the guidance for existing PMS practices which, in summary, were NHS profits minus expenditure.

The salient points of the GP superannuable scheme are summarised below.

- As a defined benefits scheme, the pension was dependent on the money accrued through career average earnings.
- The total in the pension pot should not exceed £1.073 million (2021). Any contributions in excess of that total were taxed at a prohibitive 55%, paid as an unwelcome lump sum.
- The pot to support GP pensions was mutually funded. The contributions supporting the scheme, the 'income,' came from existing working GPs. The arrangement was secured in law and guaranteed by HM Treasury.
- Major revisions to the pension scheme were made in 1971, 1995, 2008 and 2015.[43]
- A GP commencing practice after 2008 contributed 5% of superannuable income below £16,000, rising in tiers to 14.5% on incomes of £111,000 and above.
  - These are tiered, not graduated, increases. A move from one band to another incurred an increase in the total superannuable income, not just the sum in the new band.
  - The employer, currently the CCG, contributed 14%.

---

[43] www.nhsbsa.nhs.uk/sites/default/files/2021-07/NHS%20Pension%20Schemes-an%20overview-20210706-%28V6%29.pdf

- Prior to 2008, 'added' years could be purchased any time before retirement. They were cheaper the younger the applicant. The cost was tax deductible and, thus, they were considered a sound investment for the more foresighted practitioner.
- Those doctors joining the scheme after 2015 had their annual pension calculated at 1/54th of each year's superannuable pay with the annual uplift is in previous schemes.
- To compensate for inflation, each year's contribution was subjected to a 'dynamising factor.' In essence, this was a percentage uplift, primarily based on the average increase, in percentage terms, in net income for all GPs in that year but, on occasion, an arbitrary figure negotiated between the DH and BMA at times of major contract changes.
    - Since the uplift was added consecutively each year, compound interest was applied. As an example, superannuable earnings in 1981 of £13,213 would be dynamised up to £66,582 27 years later.
- The dynamising factor was withdrawn and replaced with the Retail Price Index (RPI) in 2008, and subsequently by Consumer Price Inflation (CPI) in 2010, but otherwise the incremental calculation remained the same as under the dynamising factor.
- Prior to 2008, the minimum age at which a doctor could draw a (reduced) pension was 50. That increased to 55 after 2008. However, the minimum age to draw a full pension fell from 65 to 60.
- Doctors could draw their pension and return to work immediately following retirement, providing that:
    - They ceased all work for 24 hours.
    - They worked no more than 16 hours per week for the calendar month following their retirement date. Thereafter, they could do what they liked.
    - If the doctor continued to work and draw a pension, then incomes from both were aggregated and likely to fall into a higher taxation band.
- On retirement, GPs could draw their pension with or without a tax-free lump sum. The level of the lump sum varied under the different revisions of the scheme. The annual pension thereafter was, as expected, higher if the GP declined the option of taking a lump sum.
- A 60-year-old GP retiring in 2020 after 30 years of service could expect to receive an annual pension of around £50,000. As a historical comparison, a GP retiring in 1966 after 18 years of NHS service could expect to receive a pension of £788 (£14,000) per annum.[44]
- Following death, including death in service, 50% of the annual pension continued to be paid to the spouse or civil partner.

---

[44] Hansard HC Deb. 22 Nov 1966, vol 736, cc1335–56. https://api.parliament.uk/historic-hansard/commons/1966/nov/22/national-health-service-superannuation

- Retirement on ill health grounds could take place prior to age 60. Medical proof of career-ending ill health had to be provided. A 'consideration of entitlement to ill-health retirement claim' form (AW33E) had to be submitted to the PCO.
- NHS Pensions are currently based in Newcastle, England. They provide an excellent service and are helpful in providing both an estimate of prospective pension and a breakdown of the calculation.

This all applied to GP principals, considered Type 1 beneficiaries under the NHS pension scheme. Salaried and locum doctors were termed Type 2 beneficiaries, but the principle of defined contribution still applied. Type 2 beneficiaries had to submit a form for gross annual earnings, but only contributed on 90%; 10% was considered to represent expenses.

Employers contributed 14.38%, topped up to 20.68% by the Treasury following further amendments to the scheme in 2020. The final pension on retirement depended on whether the doctor was a member of the NHS pension scheme in 1995, 2008, or 2015. That was calculated in the same way as for GP principals for 2008 and 2015, with a different method from 2015, where 1/54th of each year's earnings went towards the pension with each year revalued (dynamised) by the consumer prices index plus 1.5%.[45]

The combination of punitive taxes, 55% on pension pots that had exceeded the life-time allowance, £1.07 million in 2021, provided a compelling case for GPs currently in practice to retire at an earlier age than previous generations. It was simply financial suicide to remain in a full-time post. Not all were lost to active practice, many choosing to draw their pension whilst returning to practice as sessional doctors.

The NHS Pensions Agency (England and Wales),[46] now part of the NHS Business Services Authority, as of 2017 had:

- Membership
- 1.5 million actively paying into the scheme
- 900,000 pensioners
- 600,000 deferred members, those who have ceased paying into the scheme but had yet to draw their pension
- £4.2 billion per annum contributions made by members
- £6.2 billion per annum contributions made by employers
- £7.7 billion that year's total payment to retirees
- £2.2 billion that year's sum taken as a one-off tax-free lump sum

The scheme had £0.5 billion excess income over total expenditure, £22 billion over the preceding 15 years. To paraphrase Mr Micawber in Charles Dickens' *David Copperfield*, 'Annual expenditure 9.9 billion pounds, annual income 10.4 billion pounds, result, happiness.'

---

[45] www.bma.org.uk/pay-and-contracts/pensions/being-a-member-of-a-pension-scheme/the-nhs-pension-scheme-as-a-sessional-gp

[46] www.nhsbsa.nhs.uk/nhs-pensions

The sum of all the above figures meant that any GP who had worked under the NHS for 35 years or more could look forward to a very comfortable retirement.

12.6 SUMMARY

It is a truism that whilst GPs do 90% of the work, they receive only 10% of the budget of the NHS, a fact that has perpetually rankled those at the Royal College of General Practitioners, BMA and most GPs. GPs have long known that they are overworked and underpaid. They have no illusions that the situation will change under the aspirations set out in the current GP Five Year Forward plan, but they live in hope.

General practitioners are self-employed independent contractors who provide medical services to the NHS. The operative word here is 'contractor' and the inference of contract. Since the foundation of the NHS, negotiations between the BMA and Department of Health have led to a handful of contracts, 1966, 1990, 1997, 2004, that significantly impacted the lives of their represented GPs.

Each contract was fiercely contested at the time, but each improved the working conditions of doctors delivering primary care and the quality of the environment in which that care was delivered. They have also had the corollary of improving doctors' incomes to varying degrees. In return, each substantive contract has increased government expectations, and those of the population, of the services expected and scrutiny of that provision.

Funding of the NHS, in inflationary terms and as a proportion of GDP, has increased each year, almost without fail over the past 70 years. During that time, there have been peaks, as during the Blair/Brown administrations of 1997–2010, and troughs, as in the following decade. The NHS spent an inflation adjusted £11.4 billion in 1948; £153 billion in 2018,[47] a ten-fold increase in real terms. As a proportion of GDP during that time, the increase has doubled from 3.5% to 7.1%.[48] In terms of total healthcare, including social care UK spending in 2017, at 9.9% of GDP, placed the UK just above the of OECD average.[49]

In 2018, CCGs were allocated £75.6 billion, £11 billion of which went into commissioning medical services from their GP practices.[50] All these sums were not insubstantial, but they have never been enough to meet the healthcare needs of the British population.

Data on the average income of a GP principal was first collected by the DDRB in 1957 when, adjusted for inflation, the sum was around £50,000. Sixty years later, that had risen to around £100,000. As a comparison, a British Member of

---

[47] House of Commons. NHS expenditure, 17 Jan 2020. https://commonslibrary.parliament.uk/research-briefings/sn00724/

[48] Nuffield Trust. 70 years of NHS spending. 21 Mar 2018. www.nuffieldtrust.org.uk/news-item/70-years-of-nhs-spending

[49] www.ons.gov.uk/peoplepopulationandcommunity/healthandsocialcare/healthcaresystem/articles/howdoesukhealthcarespendingcomparewithothercountries/2019-08-29

[50] https://commonslibrary.parliament.uk/research-briefings/sn00724/#:~:text=Expenditure%20on%20the%20NHS%20has,on%20health%20in%20the%20UK

Parliament's basic salary increased from £17,000 in 1946 to £82,000 (plus expenses) in 2020.[51] British GPs are at the upper end of the pay spectrum compared to their European counterparts. General Practice, despite being an extremely demanding role, continues to be relatively financially rewarding.

The means by which GP principals have been paid has changed little over the decades. The substantive changes have been the shift from per capita to a performance-based model and from personal to practice-based budgets. As independent contractors, GPs have submitted invoices to their contractor, the Family Health Service Authority in early years, Clinical Commissioning Groups of late, and been paid accordingly. The process of invoicing payments has been simplified, following the introduction of annual global practice budgets and integrated computerisation.

The infrastructure of primary care has seen an accelerated trend from owner-occupied to lessee. Increasingly, doctors attend a place of work much as any office worker might.

The demographics of the GP workforce have changed with a shift from male, self-employed, full-time to female, salaried, part-time work. The number of GP principals had fallen to less than 50% of the total workforce by 2020. Younger GPs are shying away from the onerous responsibilities of partnerships. The combination of these factors will inevitably lead to a totally salaried service, ironically fulfilling the aspirations of Nye Bevan and the founding fathers of the NHS, albeit three-quarters of a century later.

[51] www.theipsa.org.uk/mps-pay-and-pensions

13

The Future

> Prediction is very difficult, especially if it's about the future.
>
> (Niels Bohr)

13.1 INTRODUCTION

The art of fortune-telling is dependent on the deft acquisition and interpretation of clues from the present and past, to formulate an 'authoritative' prediction of the future. This chapter is no more prescient in arriving at answers than that of a conversation taking place over a couple of rounds of drinks at the pub would be. Thus, I apologise if, at times, the vocabulary seems somewhat definitive. My excuse is merely to define resolutions around which a debate may take place.

General Practice is in crisis. That cry rings throughout the medical press, is echoed in the national press, and reverberates through the corridors of government. Yet, it is a statement not unique to our times; one that has been a recurring theme throughout the lifetime of the NHS. When the cry turns into a roar, the Department of Health and the BMA tend to lock horns and eventually thrash out a compromise, often in the form of a new GP charter or contract, that temporarily allows the service to limp on until the next 'crisis.' This recurring scenario is unlikely to change in the future. Yet, a case can be made that since the beginning of the new millennium, there has been a fundamental and accelerating shift in all aspects of general practice, very different from those previous.

If GPs are asked what they would most like to see change in the future, then the overwhelming reply would be one word: workload. Their response is unsurprising since all healthcare professionals have been complaining of unsustainable workloads since the inception of the NHS 75 years ago.

The citing of workload as the primary factor affecting a doctor's daily life does not imply that they are in some way work-shy or have unrealistic aspirations for an idyllic work-life balance. When doctors ask for a reduced workload, they do so in the vain hope of providing their individual patients with the time needed to fully resolve their presenting problems; the time to fully address the patient's medical, psychological, and social concerns in a truly holistic manner; the time to resolve issues rather than postpone them. In other words, the time to practice the medicine they were taught at medical school.

Is the attainment of this aspiration likely in the future?

13.2 PATIENTS

The composition of people sitting in a GP surgery waiting room varies by location of that surgery and by the usual demographic indices of age, gender, education, and socioeconomic grouping. Southern shire practices in relatively affluent areas tend to see a different case-mix of pathology from those working in northern deprived conurbations. In a utopian world, one would hope that governmental social and economic policy would level this playing field, but to date, such thoughts remain firmly rooted in the minds of idealistic dreamers. Thus, GPs will continue to provide bespoke services that meet the needs of their idiosyncratic populations. However, some aspects of the patient population do traverse geographic boundaries.

The old and the young, who currently make up the bulk of those seen in GP surgeries, will continue to dominate. The explosion in readily available information and a plethora of choices will feed into relatives' natural anxieties, to the point where they can only be assuaged by the emollient words emanating from a professional's mouth. However, especially with children, parents will increasingly question whether that mouth should belong to a generalist doctor or a specialist paediatrician. Many countries around the world, even those with a comprehensive state health system, exclude paediatrics as well as maternity care from the services provided in primary care. This may well apply to future childcare under the NHS. The converse will be true for the increasing percentage of elderly people in this country, allied as it is to complex co-morbidities and polypharmacy. In such situations, the generalist comes to the fore. As the percentage of the elderly in the population increases, so will the numbers attending GP surgeries.

The move to treat people outside of hospitals, either within or close to their homes, is gaining traction, partly driven by the potential for savings within a constrained budget. Clinical pathways to access secondary care will become more rigid and GPs may find that increasing time is spent explaining to a patient why they cannot have the treatment that would benefit them. On the other hand, the avowed absence of age discrimination will lead to a greater number of nonagenarians having cardiac surgery or renal dialysis, and the family doctor will have to deal with the outcomes of these major clinical interventions.

Those of adult working age who have adopted the public health messages on lifestyle will only attend a doctor for acute conditions. Their wish to be seen quickly and at a time and place of their own choosing will drive the fragmentation of primary healthcare delivery, especially in cities, where a mix of NHS and private clinics will be conveniently sited at train stations, supermarkets, and shopping centres. Many will manage their own symptoms with the aid of health apps and online portals.

If prophecies regarding robotics and automation are to be believed, and here, one must remember that similar predictions were made following the industrial revolution of the 19th century and computerisation of the 20th, then much of the populace will be either underemployed or unemployed, with increasing amounts of leisure time. Whether such a situation leads to increasing dissatisfaction with life in general and deteriorating mental health in particular, is open to debate. If proven so, then mental health will become an increasing part of the GP's workload.

The column inches devoted to medical research and healthcare in the national press and online is unlikely to abate, and this will lead to increased levels of anxiety in their readership. Medical stories, both good and especially bad, make good copy. Sadly, they often also include vilification of the profession with resulting fall in morale, early retirement, and poor recruitment and retention. One can only hope that in due course, reporters will see that their articles are socially counterproductive, leading to more balanced reporting and, one hopes, less vexatious complaints.

13.3 THE PRACTICE TEAM

Two factors will drive the mix within the practice team: the need to find cheaper replacements for doctors and the consolidation of practices into ever larger groups. The proportion of non-medically qualified healthcare professions within the groups will increase, leaving a diminishing number of doctors to deal with secondary referrals from colleagues without a formal medical degree. Doctors will be present to oversee and instruct.

The spirit of the practice team will be diluted by the increasing number of employees working on various sites, resulting in the loosening of social bonds.

Medical secretaries will be replaced by dictation and transcription commercial businesses.

The drift towards an entirely salaried profession will accelerate. This will spread from urban conurbations to the countryside as existing GP principals retire and like-for-like replacements fail to appear. There will be a nationwide standard salaried GP contract prescriptively governing the doctor's duties. General practice will become a job rather than a vocation.

13.4 THE WORKING WEEK

Whilst the structure of the working week will remain largely unchanged, remote consulting using mobile phones, video calls, and email communication will form the majority of 'surgery' appointments. The COVID pandemic of 2020 led GPs to move 80% of their consultations online, and the public was, at least initially, accepting of the change, convenience and fear of infection trumping the desire for personal contact. Telemedicine will likely continue to provide a significant proportion of consultations in the future, and in turn, that will allow doctors to practice from their own home which, ironically, would be a reversion to the practice of the NHS's early years. Finding the right balance between remote and face-to-face consulting remains in its infancy but will improve with experience.

The insatiable appetite of bureaucracy for accountability will require more time allocated to administration and paperwork.

In order to reduce the levels of medical litigation, consultations will routinely be audio- or video-recorded.

13.5 OUT-OF-HOURS

Having relinquished the onerous duty of 24-hour care of their patients for nearly two decades, GPs would unlikely return to bearing a mantle that had previously been so suffocating. Since the GP contract of 2004, 'the out-of-hours' service has become an entirely separate entity that is only likely to evolve further.

Logic would dictate a greater integration between OOH care previously thought to be the remit of primary care with that of secondary care. OOH centres will be sited alongside or within hospital A&E units, and those working within them will closely interact with their hospital colleagues. The numbers of patients seen in such units will inevitably increase, due to public health messages encouraging people to seek help immediately for early signs of disease and societal changes seeking instant gratification.

Some GPs will specialise in acute medicine, and either be solely based in acute-care units or rotate through them as part of locality-arranged schemes. General practitioners will develop more flexible working patterns as the bonds of practice-based partnership are loosened.

The number of patients visited within their home will continue to diminish. Hospital transport will include autonomous cars despatched to bring sick patients to a central hub. Self-monitoring equipment will allow patient management at the end of the phone or computer tablet, much as takes place currently with cardiac pacemakers.

13.6 IM&T

Technology, particularly as a tool in the dissemination of information and social networking, will continue to have a dramatic impact on the way the public interacts with healthcare providers. Patients are increasingly accessing websites, albeit some of dubious provenance, in ways that were not available in the 20th century when, apart from the home-help primer, medical information was under the sole and jealously guarded dominion of the medical profession. The image of the middle-class patient attending a GP consultation armed with sheaves of printouts from a Google search has long since ceased to be a cliché. Patients are already doing some of the legwork required in researching their symptoms and are increasingly being encouraged to do so.

Common chronic conditions, such as diabetes, hypertension, hyperlipidaemia, and asthma, will be self-managed, with the help of sophisticated, miniaturised machines, improving symptoms, control, and complications.

The current multitude of sources providing contemporary medical information to GPs; *BMJ*, BJGP, Pulse, NICE, Univadis, will be rationalised to one central resource.

The process of and arrival at a medical diagnosis has a natural affinity with that of a computer algorithm. Watson (IBM) and DeepMind (Google) are already operating at the level of a final year medical student. Neural networks and artificial intelligence will allow machines to perform all the mental processes of a consultation, temporarily lacking only the emotional and intuitive aspects.

The near future will see patients completing online questionnaires regarding their symptoms, an immediate analysis of which will guide their following actions. They currently do so on the NHS 111 website. Computer algorithms will direct patients, where appropriate, to specialist care, saving time, resources, and bypassing GPs altogether. GPs will embrace this process, with its provision of a non-threatening second opinion, as an aid in increasing productivity and reducing medical errors.

The 'art' of medicine, the role of 'intuition' in medical practice, will become an irrelevant part of medical history, viewed in much the same way as bleeding by leeches.

13.7 DISEASES AND AILMENTS

The conditions presenting in primary care will remain unchanged, but their numbers will be influenced by the social and mainstream media. The proportion of mental health, gender dysphoria, medically unexplained physical symptoms, and long COVID is likely to increase in the medium term.

Acute presentations in all age groups will be increasingly seen in A&E departments.

13.8 DRUGS AND THERAPEUTICS

Therapeutics research, whether in pharmaceuticals, devices, or diagnostics, will continue to be concentrated on secondary care, although some novel drugs, antibacterial, anxiolytics, and analgesics, will slowly be introduced into primary care.

Point of care investigations will become more available as technology drives down the cost of machines. The same will apply to patients monitoring their chronic conditions. Patients will be encouraged to undertake genome mapping once the wider ethical issues have been overcome.

13.9 GP EDUCATION AND TRAINING

The undergraduate medical curriculum will consist of a shortened course covering the basic sciences of medicine before splitting into generalist and specialist arms.

Postgraduate GP vocational training will be longer, four years, and include training in topics such as mental health, sexual health, administration, management, and finance. The MRCGP examination will remain the entry point to independent practice.

Established GPs, whether principals or salaried, will be urged to subspecialise, with some seeking to move full time into managerial roles. Those continuing in clinical roles or medical education will be required to undertake more intensive training, some through sabbaticals. Commercial suppliers will provide a proliferation of training courses, endorsed by the RCGP, and the acquisition of diplomas and certificates will become more widespread. GPs will be at the forefront of clinical research, increasingly running Phase-4 studies for pharmaceutical companies as well as driving up standards in primary care, through the sharing of data on clinical interventions and outcomes.

13.10 SCRUTINY AND REGULATION

The licensing, revalidation, and appraisal of doctors will remain unchanged following a relaxation of requirements during the COVID pandemic.

CQC inspections will become less frequent as more practices achieve higher standards.

The number of cases of GP misdemeanours referred to the GMC will increase, due to an unforgiving public frustrated by the barriers to accessing medical care.

The breakdown in understanding and support, previously inherent in any GP partnership, will result in increased whistleblowing referrals, as independently minded practitioners deviate from protocols and guidance.

13.11 BMA

The role of the BMA through the Local Medical Committees and General Practitioners Committee will remain, as they have throughout the lifetime of the NHS, the advocate and protector of the profession.

The medical defence unions will be more proactive in preventing medical litigation through mandatory training courses in conflict resolution and defensive medicine.

13.12 ADMINISTRATION

The Department of Health will continue to search for ways to reduce costs by streamlining the management structure of the NHS. This will lead to further reorganisations, many repeating past mistakes.

Primary care will become fully integrated with secondary and social care, to finally provide a seamless service across all sectors.

The private sector will take up a greater burden of the primary care workload as an increasingly affluent public seeks alternatives for the reduced access and impersonal care offered by the NHS.

13.13 FINANCE

The funding of the NHS will continue to struggle to meet the demands on the service. Patients will only be able to access some medical and surgical care through paying privately. That will include payments to their GP for non-core medical services, such as minor surgery.

Patients will be charged a nominal fee to make a GP appointment. This will not apply to children, the aged, and those receiving social benefits, the majority seen in general practice. The policy will irritate the working population, contribute little to the coffers, and be expensive to administer.

Savings through a reduction in surgery headcount will be encouraged by a reduction in the reimbursement of staff costs partly driven by patients moving to online facilities for registering, booking appointments, and requesting prescriptions.

13.14 SUMMARY

General practitioners love to moan. They moan at home and at work and anywhere out of their patients' earshot. They moan about patients; too many, not attending appointments, arriving with a list of complaints, not complying with instructions, and having to be admitted to hospital. They moan about colleagues; slow, lazy, ignorant, feckless, and irresponsible. They moan about hospitals; obstructive, long waiting times, ridiculous referral protocols, and discharging patients with unresolved problems. They moan about governments: out of touch, underfunding, unrealistic targets, and repeated reorganisations. There is nothing that a GP will not moan about, and yet, there they are, day in, day out, facing patients in the surgery or online, totally focused on why that person has come to seek their advice. They are not hypocrites, they are just carrying out their vocation, solving people's problems. And in those few precious minutes, they are as one with the patient and truly alive. The interaction is the sole purpose of their working existence. It is why they became a general practitioner. All the emotions that take place outside the consulting room are simply ways of letting off steam, compensatory mechanisms for relieving the stress, anxiety, depression, the strain of repeatedly absorbing another person's problems, compassion.

General practice provides a career that is fulfilling and rewarding. There are few other opportunities in life that allow an individual to be a respected and intimate confidante in helping their fellow human beings, at a time when they are at their most vulnerable. That a doctor is left to do so in relative peace, unanswerable to anyone but conscience, is often unrecognised by the profession but is a testimony to the faith invested in them by their patients. Few things in life are as rewarding as helping a seriously ill patient get better. Above all, as are nurses, teachers, policemen, and soldiers, doctors are conscientiously driven by duty to the public to serve to the best of their ability. They are truly public servants.

Doctors working exclusively as single-handed practitioners or portfolio careers have tended to be the most satisfied with their lives. The former, despite providing a lifetime of service to a stable local community in which their own lives were embedded, are becoming obsolete; the latter, offering as it does a break from the daily pressure of clinical practice has become increasingly attractive to new entrants to general practice. The shift, whilst likely ensuring greater doctor retention at the front line, has come at the expense of the unique element that differentiated general practice from other medical specialties, the intimate bond that a doctor has with his or her patients. The loss of that relationship is likely to have a profound effect on how the British public view general practice.

Theoretically, GPs should be the happiest of men and women; yet many appear to be worn down and disillusioned. Ask any GP why this is, and they will reflexively respond that it is due to an unsustainable workload. GPs are good at solving problems, but this problem, despite 70 years of trying, has remained insoluble. Whether the posited developments detailed in this chapter provide a solution to this conundrum remains to be seen. British society should sincerely hope that there is a resolution to the issue of unsustainable workload. If not, we will inevitably lose the one asset that truly differentiated the NHS from the healthcare systems in the rest of the world, the family doctor.

The NHS was created in 1948 in response to the healthcare needs of British society of the time. It has continued to evolve sine then to meet those needs. The place of general practice in the future delivery of healthcare will depend on what society dictates. Whatever that may be, the role of the general practitioner will remain demanding and frustrating but ultimately there are few jobs in life that are more emotionally, intellectually, and financially rewarding!

Index

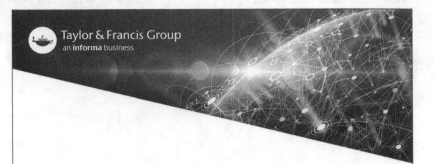

Printed in the United States
by Baker & Taylor Publisher Services

Printed in the United States
by Baker & Taylor Publisher Services